forms of living

Stefanos Geroulanos and Todd Meyers, *series editors*

Human Remains

Human Remains

Medicine, Death, and Desire in Nineteenth-Century Paris

Jonathan Strauss

FORDHAM UNIVERSITY PRESS

NEW YORK 2012

Fordham University Press has no responsibility for the persistence or accuracy of URLs for external or third-party Internet websites referred to in this publication and does not guarantee that any content on such websites is, or will remain, accurate or appropriate.

Fordham University Press also publishes its books in a variety of electronic formats. Some content that appears in print may not be available in electronic books.

Library of Congress Cataloging-in-Publication Data

Strauss, Jonathan.
   Human remains : medicine, death, and desire in nineteenth-century Paris / Jonathan Strauss.—1st ed.
       p.   cm.— (Forms of living)
   Includes bibliographical references and index.
   ISBN 978-0-8232-3379-3 (cloth : alk. paper)
   ISBN 978-0-8232-3380-9 (pbk. : alk. paper)
       1. Death—France—Paris—History—19th century.
2. Dead—Social aspects—History—19th century.   3. Public
health—France—Paris—History—19th century.   4. Medicine—
France—Paris—History—19th century.   5. Human body—Social
aspects—France—Paris—History—19th century.   6. Paris
(France)—Social conditions—19th century.   I. Title.
HQ1073.5.F82P377   2012
306.90944'3609034—dc23

                                                            2011026669

Printed in the United States of America
14   13   12   5   4   3   2   1
First edition

For Ludy

CONTENTS

All translations are mine unless otherwise indicated. I have tried to remain faithful to the meaning and different tones of documents written by authors from a wide range of disciplines and historical periods, while rendering them in an English that is as natural and readable as possible. In the text, the first time titles of works and institutions are mentioned, they will be followed by a translation in parentheses, unless their sense can easily be deduced from English cognates. All subsequent references will use the original French. The one exception to this is the section on Odilon Redon in chapter 6, where, to comply with the practices in art history and avoid very cumbersome constructions, I have used only the English versions of his titles.

ACKNOWLEDGMENTS

This book is the product of a long, ongoing conversation with many people in widely scattered settings. It has been a complex undertaking, covering a range of fields that were, in some cases, unfamiliar to me, and its evolution was at times unclear and ungainly. I would like to thank a handful of individuals who have taken a particularly active role in its creation and without whose aid this volume would not now exist. Jim Creech generously contributed his insight and intelligence to this project since its very inception and he provided an intellectual compass throughout its evolution. Marie-Claire Vallois was a pillar of support at difficult moments and a joyous accomplice in better ones. Marie-Hélène Huet's scholarship was a source of inspiration, while her careful readings and encouragement proved conceptually and morally invaluable.

I would also like to thank those who have read and responded to various versions of this text, in particular Geoffrey Bennington, Suzanne Guerlac, and Maurice Samuels, as well as an anonymous reader for Fordham. Colleagues at Miami have offered sustained and layered commentary, especially Tim Melley, Elisabeth Hodges, and Claire Goldstein. Others have intervened more punctually, but no less meaningfully. Bruno Chaouat has engaged various points of the argument and offered it hospitality at Cerisy-la-Salle. Marina van Zuylen gave advice and imaginative orientation, especially on sections relating to Odilon Redon. Martine De Groote helped me navigate the resources of the Bibliothèque Nationale de France along with its sometimes esoteric culture and history.

This book and its author owe a deep debt of gratitude to a host of interlocutors at conferences, colloquia, and talks, notably in the French sections of Emory, UCLA, Indiana University, and Cornell, where colleagues and friends helped me tease through various aspects of the argument. Two colloquia at

Cerisy-la-Salle stand out, as do several names: Dalia Judovitz, Elissa Marder, Patrick Bray, Maurice de Gandillac.

But more than anything or anyone, it is Jeanne Strauss De Groote who has made this book possible. She has brought to it a historian's acumen and a deep humanity.

Human Remains

Introduction: The Toxic Imagination

> The celebrated Méry used to say, as Fontenelle reports in his eulogy, that anatomists resemble the porters [*crocheteurs*] of Paris, who know all the streets, down to the smallest and most remote, but do not know what happens inside the houses. Still, it has occurred to me, if I might pursue this ingenious comparison, that in the present state of things, anatomists might try to find a way to penetrate into these houses and to discover a few of the secrets within them.
>
> —JEAN JOSEPH SUE[1]

On the night of April 7, 1786, a tumbrel-load of corpses left the Saints-Innocents cemetery in the heart of the French capital for catacombs outside the city's walls. With it, began the first in a long series of torch-lit processions that would trouble Parisians' sleep for nearly two years. The Saints-Innocents, which had accommodated the dead for nearly five centuries, was now choked with them. Its soil had grown so depleted that it could no longer decompose bodies. Its grounds were strewn with bones and heaved by the gases of putrefaction. Strange forces emanating from the graveyard were deteriorating nearby houses, and neighbors were falling sick. Newly discovered chemical agents, it was determined, had been leaching from the site, polluting the air with miasmas, tainting water sources, and poisoning the city as a whole. After half a millennium, the dead had become intolerable.

In order to be removed, however, the bodies had first to be disturbed and carried through the city, denuded of the earth that had previously covered and to some extent tempered the effects of their putrefaction. The cartloads of corpses moving through the nighttime streets of Paris must have created a strange and dramatic procession, surrounded as they were by an elaborate panoply of religious and hygienic prophylaxis.[2] A report read before the *Royal Society of Medicine* on March 3, 1789, gives some idea of the effect these macabre convoys had on contemporary imaginations:

> The great number of torches and the lines of fires burning on every side and casting a funereal light; their reflections on the surrounding objects; the sight of crosses, tombs, epitaphs; the silence of the night; the thick cloud of smoke that surrounded and covered the work site, and in the middle of which the workmen, whose operations one could dimly make out, seemed to move like shadows; the various ruins left from the demolition of the buildings; the soil heaved up by the exhumations, all of this gave to the setting an aspect at once imposing and lugubrious. The religious ceremonies added still more to the spectacle: the transport of the coffins, the pomp that, for the most distinguished sepulchers, accompanied these removals, the hearses and the catafalques; the long lines of funerary carts, laden with bones and winding past at the close of day toward the new site that had been prepared beyond the walls for the disposal of these sad remains.[3]

The smoky torches were intended not only to shed light but also to counteract the toxic effects of miasmas given off by the decomposing bodies, and taken as a whole the event represented a particularly elaborate staging of fears about the deceased, about a virulence that needed to be vigorously countered on spiritual as well as hygienic registers. It also marked a turning point in the relations between the living and the dead. For the deceased were not merely believed to be dangerous. They had become frightening in a new way, and that fear was expressed through concerns about urban space.

That those corpses would have to be moved at all represented a conceptual and social revolution, for Christians as a culture had shown themselves to be unusual in their willingness to abide their dead: unlike the Greeks and Romans, they had chosen to remain near their ancestors. During the early years of oppression, they had congregated in catacombs and even afterward, when they could emerge into the light of day without fear of immediate persecution, they still held their deceased close to the heart of their communities, burying them in and around churches and in the centers of cities.[4] In the eighteenth century, however, an unprecedented change took place in attitudes about the location of the dead, and for the first time in western history a broad movement took hold to expel them from the places of worship that they had previously inhabited, to drive them from the cities, and in general to break the centuries-old link that bound them to the communities they had left behind.[5]

The story of the Saints-Innocents is emblematic of this revolution. In 1737, the Parlement of Paris grew sufficiently concerned about the potential health risks of burials to commission a report on conditions in the city's cemeteries. Though alarming, the findings produced few results, and under popular pressure another inquiry was ordered some twenty-five years later, in 1763. On May 21, 1765, the Parlement finally took action, banning *intramuros* burials in all but exceptional cases and ordering the removal of existing parish cemeteries to outside the capital. The legislation, however, languished for several years and produced only a few isolated successes.[6] Over the four decades that followed, the same basic scenario would repeat itself periodically, with public outcries leading to investigations that led, in turn, to edicts that went largely unenforced. Still, the process reflected a general change in attitudes that had spread throughout Europe. In 1786, for example, the Hapsburg court promulgated laws about the transfer of cemeteries *extramuros*, which were largely similar to measures taken in Spain over the years 1785, 1786, and 1787.

And despite the hesitations and difficulties, slow but real progress was being made. The Saints-Innocents was closed and emptied. More significantly, plans were laid in 1801 to concentrate the Parisian dead in three extramural burying grounds, which would eventually be located at Montparnasse to the south, Montmartre in the north, and Mont Louis to the east. The process reached a double culmination in 1804, with the inauguration of Père Lachaise cemetery on May 21 and the Imperial Decree on Burials of 23 Prairial (June 12), year XII. The opening of the Montparnasse and Montmartre cemeteries in 1824 and 1825 left Paris almost entirely free of dead bodies, and burials for the city's inhabitants were confined to three modernized and highly regulated spaces.[7] Outside of the capital, however, progress still languished, and in 1843 a royal decree was required to eliminate exceptions to existing laws for smaller towns, thereby extending the laws' reach to cover all *communes* in France. Thereafter, no human remains were legally tolerated within thirty-five to forty meters of dwellings.[8] By law and, to a large extent, in practice, French urban spaces were now clear of the dead.

But it was not just a matter of moving the dead from cities and *communes*. They also had to be enclosed behind barriers, and the law of 23 prairial 1804 provided for this as well. The motivation for enclosure was originally twofold: on the one hand to protect the deceased from such molestations and indignities as animals or marauders, and, more importantly, on the other hand to inhibit the contamination of surrounding areas by the pestilential gases given off from dead bodies. As with removal, progress was often slow, due in large part to the tremendous expense that compliance entailed, but by the end of the nineteenth century, cemetery walls had become such a commonplace that they could serve by themselves as shorthand allusions to death.[9] This enclosure, especially of the newer burial sites around Paris, seems to have played a key role in one of the more startling and incongruous developments in the treatment of the dead during this period. In 1859, the city of Paris was officially expanded, and as a result, the dead who had been buried in the three *extra-muros* cemeteries created by Napoleonic decree in 1804 suddenly found themselves once more inside the city they had been forced to flee. The *conseil d'état* simply decided to make an exception, allowing them to remain within Paris in defiance of the previous law. The dead were near but separate, still virulent and frightening, as scientific publications continued to show, but sufficiently cordoned off as to represent a manageable threat.

All these changes resulted from contemporary developments in medicine. Scientific thought in general and medicine in particular had never previously enjoyed the credibility or influence that they acquired in the late eighteenth and early nineteenth centuries, when they entered into the very fabric of educated life as both a revolutionary system for explaining daily experience and objects of interest in their own right. An intelligent nonspecialist such as Louis-Sébastien Mercier could marvel at the progress of chemistry and adopt some of its most recent principles as a means to see deep into the invisible heart of the substances around him, to decipher the hidden agencies of his physical urban world. Under his transformed gaze, even the mud was different. No longer a mere inconvenience, it now distilled a venomous putrefaction that seeped throughout the city.[10] Caught up in the excitement of the moment, wealthy and inquisitive amateurs took to anatomizing as a hobby, purchasing human cadavers for home dissections and occasionally clogging latrines with the remnants of their entertainments. And in the aftermath of the 1789 revolution, an army of young bourgeois with more intelligence than capital filled the medical profession, making it a dominant social force.[11] Coupled with the funds unleashed by speculation and the newly created stock market, this force physically rebuilt Paris in the image of its ideals and fears. Principal among those fears were the beliefs that urban air was dangerous, that sewers and filth corrupted it, that corpses and feces were joined in a continuum of putrefaction, and that the latter was infectious, capable of penetrating into the stones themselves and then infiltrating living bodies. Because this putrefaction originated in dead matter and feces, human beings needed to be hermetically isolated from their own remains.

In the course of this social revolution, corpses became part of a more generalized category of the abject, and their treatment paralleled that of other noxious elements, such as human wastes and all substances subject to putrefaction. Everything that rotted entered into a broader, somewhat indistinct field of dangerous forces that worked insidiously against life and humanity. As these notions developed, death ceased to be simply one element among others and rose, instead, to become the master category, the name of the field itself. Rotting and evil smells were no longer seen as merely similar to death, but as material forms of it. As a state of being, as a material presence, death consequently had to be isolated from the dwelling places of the living, but this created another problem—the need to understand what death in itself *is*. The responses were troubling and often contradictory. At best, contemporary science seemed to indicate that death was, by its very nature, indeterminate and that it occupied an existential zone somewhere between the animate and the inanimate. This indeterminacy lent death a new horror by giving the impression that it clung inseparably to life, permeating the biological in much the same way that miasmas infected physical bodies. The abjection of the corpse instantiated, in this way, an ontological problem, which was the inability to distinguish between what should have been two absolutely different conditions of being. Moreover, as the dead destabilized distinctions between the organic and the inorganic, life and death, human and inhuman, being and nothingness, other categories interrelated with them also began to blur. The notions of the past, of history, of subjectivity, and of meaning itself threatened to move beyond the grasp of the human and into the realm of the dead. In that other zone, these notions might be determined, when not simply undermined, by obscure material forces inimical to human beings, indeed to life itself. The threat seemed so real, in fact, that the preeminent French philosopher of the nineteenth century, Auguste Comte, declared that the principal occupation of humankind should be "increasingly to unite all of living nature for a permanent struggle against the whole of the inorganic world" and he tried to rally what he called "the ongoing league of life against death."[12] The border between life and death was unclear, perhaps unknowable, and yet it had, at all costs, to be enforced. This is the crucial paradox at the heart of nineteenth-century attempts to recreate Paris according to medical principles.

Hygienists embraced urban planning to free Paris of noxious elements, but in so doing they also transformed the idea of what a city is. In their hands, it became a tool to establish biological distinctions between the living and the dead, even when those distinctions seemed elusive or impossible. The space inside the city's walls, according to this new paradigm, had to be not just physically but also conceptually clean. It should be an area in which the theoretical difference between life and death was explicit and enforced. As such, the city also became an ontological device, a way to create and apply basic distinctions and to permit the production of meaning based on the concepts of humanity and life. As the incarnation of biological ambiguity, the dead, on the other hand, were constitutionally antiurban, antisocial, and, indeed, antipolitical. Hygiene was not, consequently, just a matter of practical measures for safeguarding health, it was a key element in elaborate conceptual, political, and experiential structures that expressed themselves through urban space.

A Medicine of Desire

This book is about changing notions of death, but it is also about medicine in the aftermath of the Enlightenment and the French Revolution. The new conceptions of death that appeared during the first half of the nineteenth century were possible only through contemporary developments in the medical sciences. From the late eighteenth through the nineteenth centuries, medicine gained unprecedented credibility as a discipline. It redefined and asserted its legitimacy in respect to other institutions, notably the courts and the Church, while its theories and approaches gained a broader truth-value, extending their reach beyond the domain of health to issues of more fundamental social interest. In writings that influenced a generation of researchers on medical history, Michel Foucault argued that the rise of medicine could be best understood as an expression of power relations and that the discipline should be considered a form of bio-politics.[13] In the following chapters I will argue, however, that the rise of medicine was substantially propelled by a largely unacknowledged irrational element. How one is to make sense of that irrational element is therefore a central issue in studying the medicalization of death. Foucault faced a similar problem when he attempted to write the history of madness, especially its transformation into a medical category. His solution was to define the insane as excluded from discourse, to understand them as a silence and a blank.[14] The present study attempts instead to treat the nonsensical as fantasmatically present—a presence manifested in part through beliefs about the materiality of death—and to examine the influence of the irrational on the language of the rational. In this respect, I will follow Gaston Bachelard's descriptions of scientific thought more closely than I will Foucault's accounts of nineteenth-century medicine.[15]

Contemporaries themselves were sometimes aware of that irrational component and even attempted to devise technologies to represent and cure it. Such was the case of Etienne-Gaspard Robertson, who, at the end of the eighteenth century, created what he called a "ghost machine" in order to reproduce the fascination of the dead. Figures in literature and the arts, such as Balzac, Flaubert, and Odilon Redon, responded in their own ways to recent scientific theorizations, considering the materiality of death to be related, in important and revealing ways, to the materiality of their own aesthetic productions. This did not mean that scientific reasoning could somehow "explain" artistic production, as one is tempted to believe in reading texts such as Zola's *Roman Expérimental* (The Experimental Novel), but instead that artists had, through their own media and techniques, special access to the nonscientific elements of scientific discourse.

These irrational aspects of the interest in the dead were driven, I argue, by an inadmissible desire for the abject. Rather than an expression of power relations or bio-politics, that irrational component was thus a form of erotics. To understand that erotics, I will turn to two of the most powerful explanatory discourses of the twentieth century, looking first to psychoanalytic theories of anality and the fantasm and then, in an attempt to frame this same question in terms of meaning, considering fantasms of the dead in relation to language. By thus reading the history of the irrational in medical discourse as a textual event and by viewing the treatment of corpses in nineteenth-century Paris as a form of literature, it is possible to find a sense in the nonsensical components of nineteenth-century studies on material death. It will also be necessary, however, to acknowledge more generalized relations between the structure of language and the dead, as well as the role of the corpse in the production of any meaning.

I will, in short, examine the role of fantasmatic or mythical drives both in the definition of social space and in some of the dominant discourses that sought to shape that space. This is not, then, a history of any *real* nineteenth century, but rather an account of an *unreal* one, of a fantasy that exercised itself on the shape and meaning of the city as it was structured by medicine and hygiene. Indeed, it is not a history at all, since those mythical drives are by nature prehistorical. Nor is this a thematic study or the review and analysis of different appearances of a term in a circumscribed period and place. Instead, I will show how the corpse functioned as an *operator*, a broad, labile, and emotionally charged concept that focused cultural transformation in a way that was not otherwise possible.

The epigraph from Jean Joseph Sue, above, gives a compact and concrete example of these operations. Sue was one of the preeminent doctors of the early nineteenth century. He published two important studies on the limits between life and death. As an anatomist working on the same sorts of issues and with the same sorts of approaches as Xavier Bichat, he was focusing on questions central to what was then the most important field of medicine. He was doing so, moreover, in the heart of the most important community of medical researchers, Paris, at a moment crucial to the modernization of their discipline. And for him, the city itself could be understood as a figure for the subject of the anatomist—the two were cognate images of each other. Anatomy, in this respect, was a study of public space through indirect means. In calling for a change in the practice of anatomy, Sue framed the issue as the difference between two separate but related kinds of *savoir* or knowledge—on the one hand a descriptive knowledge and on the other a more intimate familiarity. This familiarity, which Sue proposes as the future orientation of anatomy (and therefore, by extension, of medicine as a whole) is represented as a penetration into living quarters, the ability to know "what happens inside of houses" and the "secrets of their interior"—a kind of knowledge that I will later attempt to clarify through psychoanalytic theories of the fantasm. Domestic secrets are thus the model for the future of scientific knowledge. But the work of the anatomist is a question of life and death performed—as Sue's own books attest—on the bodies of the dead. So the issues of material death are metaphorically inextricable from issues of the city and from family secrets.

That metaphorical aspect is crucial, since it is the key, in this particular text, to perceiving those connections—were one not to read this document in a literary way, that connection would disappear.[16] Sue is himself consciously performing a figural reading in this passage, since he explicitly refers to the "comparison" around which it is structured, but he is not entirely in control of that reading. Another metaphor, more disguised, appears in this short excerpt, and it too offers its own insights into the kind of reading that will be necessary to bring my "history" of medicine to a term. Méry, according to

Sue, dismissed anatomists as *"crocheteurs,"* who only know the outsides of buildings. The word *crocheteur* means porter, a person hired to carry burdens from one address to another. Such individuals would, of course, need to know the various streets of Paris in order to perform their tasks and would not normally be invited to linger inside. But the word had another, slightly older meaning: a lock picker. This second sense undermines the ostensible meaning of the passage, since lock pickers get into the very houses from which porters are supposedly excluded, but it does so by describing just the sort of intrusions into secret spaces that defines the future of anatomy later in the same passage: anatomists, like lock pickers, need to find the key to exploring an interiority that is hidden from them. The manifest sense of the passage is thus contradicted by another one, which, nonetheless, better expresses the stated desires of the author. In this uncontrolled metaphor, however, the author reveals a more transgressive aspect of medical science—the possibility that such knowledge could be illicit, illegal, and asocial in its longing to understand the city.

The quotation represents, in these respects, a figure for my approach to reading medical documents, an approach that sees them as a rich and complex literature that can be understood through aesthetic, psychoanalytic, and linguistic analysis. It is also an argument, I submit, for reading such documents as imaginative constructions of urban space, constructions that would be translated into material results under the impetus of hygienic reform.

Plan

As is probably already clear, the argument in this book is complex. By necessity, its form is, I believe, unprecedented. The fields covered are broad, and the various approaches adopted may not be intuitive for readers coming from different disciplinary backgrounds. For these reasons—and perhaps, too, for those who would rather scan the map of a book than pick its locks—the following, quick summary of its contents should prove useful.

As an entry into the larger issues of death, medicine, and irrationality, chapter 1, "Medicine and Authority," uses contemporary press accounts to reconstruct a spectacular case of necrophilia from the mid-nineteenth century. Sergeant François Bertrand's nocturnal visits to cemeteries left behind grisly tableaux that horrified the French public for over a year and eventually led to his court-martial in 1849. The details of his exploits immediately unleashed a series of analyses in the medical press, which agreed that his behavior touched the farthest limits of the pathological. What made Bertrand's crimes so disturbing was their object. More than the criminal himself, it was the dead who were in the dock, implicitly accused of inspiring an unfathomable attraction. The trial and its aftermath called on the expertise of qualified alienists to help explain this deviant behavior, but these witnesses quickly disputed the authority of the court to pronounce judgment on the case, asserting that it involved medical rather than legal issues. For Bertrand's contemporaries, understanding his behavior largely meant assigning jurisdiction over it. The dead, as expressed by his sexual desire, were on trial, but so were the right and power to make sense of them.

In order to establish the background to this struggle for authority, the chapter retraces the rivalry between the courts and doctors to the mid-eighteenth century. There were two principal points of dispute: on the one hand doctors argued that the medical profession should be self-governing (and largely, therefore, beyond the purview of the courts) and on the other they attempted to increase their influence on legal decisions, especially in their role as expert witnesses. By the middle of the nineteenth century, French doctors had met with mixed success. They had been able to retain some guild-like autonomies and a degree of self-governance. Certain significant cases had demonstrated both the dismissive attitudes of the courts toward these institutions and their own, probably unwitting, adoption of medical reasoning. On the other hand, to secure a position of influence and credibility within society, the medical profession also had to establish its independence from the Catholic Church, and it was even more successful in this respect than it was with the courts. The late eighteenth and early nineteenth centuries thus saw the rise in France of a new language for making sense of social and asocial behaviors, a language whose dynamics and importance were revealed in the disputes surrounding Bertrand. Indeed, society itself was a labile and contested term in these debates, an entity that was most fully instantiated, perhaps, in the very documents they produced.

Recent studies on the rise of the medical profession have tended to focus on the treatment of mental illness. Chapter 2, "The Medical Uses of Nonsense," picks up on this scholarship to argue that the very unintelligibility of the insane had a certain utility to the legitimacy of medical discourse: it represented a space outside of society that was nonetheless crucial to the definition of society. This was a fantasmatic realm, in the sense that madness was believed to force certain rational rules of organization—and dominant discourses—to yield before powerful irrational processes. In establishing their mastery over madness, doctors were using the very opacity of a nonsensical language to establish their own discursive credibility, and the legitimacy of medicine consequently depended on specific features of unreason. Some of these features were shared by death, which, while nothing in itself, nonetheless served as a space onto which crucial, extrasocial fantasies could be projected. Theories about death therefore played an equally—if not more—important role in giving content and shape to the unknowable and exercised an underappreciated force in the self-definition of nineteenth-century French society.

Previously, the social control of mortality had been administered by the court system and army and had been organized imaginarily by the Church. The judiciary used death as a punishment against individuals, while the military wielded it as a tool to combat other nations, and in both cases it served primarily as an instrument to protect sovereignty. It was the codes of war and the laws, bound at least in theory by a Christian morality, that had legitimized and regulated the imposition of death. But with the execution of the king and the rise of a secular ethics based on materialist principles, the fantasmatic, ethical, and practical hold on mortality needed to be rethought. In this sense, the revolution of 1789 had changed the meaning of death, and the control of it now had to be justified on new, nonreligious grounds.

Doctors were able to convince contemporaries first of the difficulty in interpreting the symptoms of illness and, second, of their own, unique ability to read the signs of death. In this way, they became the guardians of an ontological absolute with a crucial role in social organization. Some of the more practical consequences of this epistemological shift can be seen in the relations between the medical profession and the legal system. The courts, for example, delegated the determination of whether or not a person was dead to specially designated doctors; the transfer of human remains from the Saints-Innocents and other cemeteries was placed under medical supervision; and the guillotine itself, the emblem of a new social order based on a changed relation to mortality, was conceived and perfected by a medical corps.

As an unknown and unknowable, death acted as a source of power. Much in the same way that doctors proved able to speak the unspeakable language of madness, so were they able to delimit and potentially master the mysteries of mortality. Insofar as public authority was premised on the right to control death, and as medicine came to dominate death conceptually, doctors gained in authority. Even more important, crucial ontological distinctions—between being and nonbeing, between the present and the past—had become medical issues.

In taking control of death, however, medical research revealed certain problems with the absoluteness of that ontological distinction. The *Idéologues* and materialists of the Enlightenment had begun to speak of death as part of a physical continuum with life rather than absolutely distinct from it. These changes in the conceptualization of mortality opened the door to a new world of horrors and uncertainties while unleashing fears of an unmasterable continuity between the animate and inanimate. These anxieties were exacerbated by the belief that the conditions of modern life, especially the population densities of major cities, facilitated the mutual contamination between life and death. Chapter 3, "A Hostile Environment," examines ways in which urban space, and Paris in particular, was seen to embody death and describes some of the medical procedures that were used to combat that ambient toxicity, looking in particular at the metaphorical fluidity uniting its various manifestations. More important for this discussion, however, than particular practices, their utility, or their signification for the progress of hygiene as a means to combat disease are the theories of death underlying this notion of toxicity. Chapter 4, "Death Comes Alive," examines the most influential of these. Death, from the hygienic viewpoint, was a material presence: not a concept or abstract limit but a state. As such it necessarily obeyed physical laws, intervened in the environment, and enjoyed existence. Its essence, it seemed, could be located in putrescence, which was understood, in turn, as a form of fermentation. The principal figures in the study of material death in the early nineteenth century—and the leading figures in medicine in general—were the pathological anatomists, and they accordingly gave particular attention to the question of fermentation. From a close reading of key anatomical texts, an ambiguous image of death emerges, however. And this ambiguity opened a rich imaginative zone in which the living and the dead could share characteristics, a zone from which emerged the notion of an inanimate sentience hidden in the material world and vestigially present in human consciousness. This sentience was closely related to the sense of smell, through which human beings retain an experiential access to it. The sense of smell revealed, moreover, a capacity to reorganize the significance of mortality in its structural relation to the city, as is disclosed through a reading of Walter Benjamin's writings on nineteenth-century Paris.

So far, the images of material, or abject death, have been overwhelmingly negative, the source of anxieties and the object of elaborate prophylaxes. But certain intellectual, artistic, and social currents resisted this negativity. Chapter 5, "Pleasure in Revolt," looks at some of the ways in which the ambiguity of death could be interpreted as a positivity. Decomposing substances were observed to have fertilizing powers, and from this basic observation various imaginary systems of creativity were deduced. In the most basic sense, death was transformative, and as such it seemed to be the key for unlocking the dynamism inherent in matter itself. From this, one could extrapolate various sorts of conceptual and artistic potentials. Perhaps because they blended the notions of materiality and sentience, creating a link between thought and the physical world, human remains seemed to offer an image of aesthetic production, becoming a reference point and a model for the late eighteenth-century architects Etienne Boullée and Nicolas Ledoux. Feces, another human remnant conceptually linked to death through the forces of putrefaction, also instantiated this creative force. They seemed, for authors such as Pierre Leroux and Victor Hugo, to represent the possibility of social renewal and, indeed, the redemption of humanity itself. While these texts reveal the positivity of material death, another aspect of nineteenth-century Parisian society indicated the complexity of the affective components in abjection. Prostitution was treated, in nineteenth-century Paris, as a leading hygienic concern, the management of which had significant implications for society as a whole. In the debates that circled around them, prostitutes were consistently assimilated with waste disposal systems, especially the sewers. If prostitutes were abject like sewers, however, that suggests, conversely, that sewers were like prostitutes and therefore exercised some sort of erotic attraction. I draw that similarity out to argue that the hygienic response to the sex industry constituted a highly dissimulated expression of erotism in relation to human wastes, including the dead. Most important for the purposes of my discussion, the hygienic reactions to the bodies and persons of prostitutes allow me to read the medical theorization of material abjection on a new register, that of desire, and to see in the figure of the prostitute an initial, fantasmatic formulation of how that desire relates to individual identity. The history of the rise of medicine was shaped, then, not merely by Foucauldian discursive or bio-power, but also, and perhaps more profoundly, by a crucial, irrational element that can now be identified as a hidden erotics of the abject.

Chapter 6, "Monsters and Artists," looks at some of the more significant ways in which artists and novelists could use the aestheticization of material death and the abject desires associated it. The works in question built on a familiarity with contemporary science and medicine, but not merely in an attempt to thematize them. Instead, they drew on their own aesthetic materiality to examine cognate concerns about the relations between life and death. The painter and lithographer Odilon Redon used his conversance with anatomy, biology, and evolution to develop a pictorial universe in which death could be viewed from the viewpoint of the dead. Balzac took the issue further, by looking at the relations between putrefaction and the fictional status of literary characters. Flaubert drew on a metaphorics of dead bodies to imagine the complex relations between historical and novelistic narratives. In each of these cases, the medicalized knowledge of death offered a means for expressing and thinking through the materiality of artworks while offering insights into the imaginary and libidinal aspects of medical thought. As such, they represent a significant commentary on contemporary scientific theories.

In an attempt to formulate these aesthetic insights in more conceptual terms, chapter 7, "Abstracting Desire," turns to the psychoanalytic theories of anality and the fantasm. The corpse plays a crucial, if indirect role in these theories, which conceptualize the abject as a reduction of subjectivity into an object in the real. An instance of this can already be seen in the nineteenth-century literature on prostitution. But the positivity and desire that was observed in the interest elicited by abjection seems to be explained, in these theories, by the fact that fantasms relate, as a whole, to questions about beginnings. They form, in this respect, the structure for a mythical origin not merely of the individual but also of the city itself, especially insofar as it is imagined to be a space of reason and meaning. To trace the fantasmatic history of Paris, then, I consider key definitions of the city as a rational space. From these myths of enlightenment, there emerges an imaginary division between a viscous, sentient materiality of the dead and a pure, abstract sublimity of death. The modern city, in these myths, would be constructed on the basis of the latter in order to protect it against the former.

In my conclusion, "What Abjection Means," I apply a further twist to the myths of abjection at work in the relation between death and the medicalized city. In order to identify the role of meaning in the fantasmatic organization of desire, I reframe the previous description of the imaginary power of the corpse in terms of language and subjectivity. The abject dead represent, as noted earlier, the breakdown of subjectivity. But the subjectivity in question is, I now argue, the awareness of *other* subjectivities, represented in the very structures of language. The desire inherent in abjection may be the longing for a lost and mythical world of plenitude, in which consciousness spreads throughout material existence, unhindered by the constraints of the "I." But that lost plenitude—the mythical origin of the self and the city—can no longer be imagined without recalling that it entails the loss or killing of the other. This memory returns, ineradicably, as a remnant of that fantasmatic killing. It returns, in other words, as a corpse. The revulsion that cannot be dissociated from abject desire derives, then, from the attempt to expel the remnant blocking our appropriation of the material world. That obstruction is the dead other, who invariably resurfaces in the structures of desire themselves.

The fear of illness and abjection that motivates the medical history of nineteenth-century Paris is thus, on a deep and dissimulated level, the attempt to manage a recurrent and unspeakable erotic desire, which expresses itself obliquely, but richly, in medical documents, artistic production, and the very shape of the city. This book as a whole, then, recounts a mythical history of nineteenth-century Paris, in which the city is understood to be a fantasmatic formulation of the relation between life and death as manifested through scientific and aesthetic documents. It is a history of unreason speaking through the language of reason, a literature, if you will, of urban space—or urban space as literature.

ONE

Medicine and Authority

In 1849, a sergeant François Bertrand was brought before a military tribunal on charges of digging up human corpses and mutilating them. The ensuing trial captured the public imagination. Spectators thronged the court-martial, gasping in horror at the grisly testimony of expert witnesses and the accused himself. The popular press followed the case closely, while contemporary alienists, who treated the alleged crimes as a significant example of mental illness, analyzed their perpetrator in depth. Still, despite all the years that have passed and all the documentation devoted to the trial, a certain mystery still clings to it, for if evidence abounds for the tremendous interest that Bertrand's case excited, it is less clear *why* it should have been so fascinating. The medical reports that sought to understand the sergeant's behavior focused on the difference between destructive and erotic monomanias but made virtually no attempt to explain the significance of the peculiar object of his sexual longings, although it, more than anything else, set his crimes apart. The notion that the dead could be erotically exciting was in this sense a crucial but unexamined element of his case, and it is that desire—or rather its resonance on various imaginative registers throughout nineteenth-century Paris—that we will try to understand in the chapters that follow. Bertrand's case, and especially the reactions to it, indicate the importance of medical science in framing questions about necrophilic desire in that historical context—and indeed, as I will show, the relation between the living and the dead had become a medical concern by the time Bertrand appeared before the judges. But Bertrand's court-martial also reveals how unstable the value of medical insight was during this period, how it struggled both to assert itself in relation to other discourses, especially those of the courts and the Church, and, more generally, to establish its credibility as an explanatory system with a broad social reach. And if doctors gradually gained control over the knowledge of death during this period, that knowledge became a crucial element in their social legitimacy, so that while the meaning of death was embedded in medical theories, the value of those theories stemmed, in large part, from the mysterious nature of death. In this chapter, I will start by considering sergeant Bertrand's court-martial and the reactions to it as an emblematic moment in establishing the truth and social values of medicine—and, in that respect, as a first step toward appreciating the social value of death.

A Case of Necrophilia

Scarcely had I entered the cemetery when I began to dig up a young girl, who must have been between 15 and 17 years old. This body is the first on which I yielded to shameless excesses. I cannot define what I felt at that moment, all that one feels with a living woman is nothing in comparison. I kissed that dead woman on all the parts of her body, I pressed her against me as if to cut her in two; in a word, I lavished on her all the caresses that an impassioned lover might give to the object of his love. After having played with this inanimate body for a quarter hour, I set about mutilating it, tearing out its entrails as I did to all the other victims of my fury. I then put the body back into the pit and, having covered it once again with dirt, I returned to the barracks.[1]

Sometime around March 10, 1848, a young sergeant in the French army scaled the walls of a cemetery and had sex, for the first time in his life, with a corpse. The experience seems to have unleashed a long-suppressed need in him, and over the next year he pursued a second, hidden existence, breaking into graveyards at night, copulating with the dead, and then tearing them to

bits until he was shot in the act and brought to trial. Once the story of François Bertrand's crimes became known, the public reacted violently. Naming
him a "vampire" and "the dreadful monomaniac of Montparnasse cemetery,"[2] the press detailed his "horrible" and "odious profanations."[3] The
transcript of Bertrand's eventual court-martial is studded with parenthetical
notations of the crowd's shocked reactions to his testimony. For their part,
the doctors who wrote about his case were little more restrained in their
condemnations. Benédicte-Auguste Morel called his crimes "the most monstrous act that can be imagined,"[4] and Ambroise Tardieu, professor of criminal medicine at the Ecole de Médecine in Paris, qualified them as the "last
stage the perversion of the sexual instinct can reach."[5] Henri de Castelnau,
who had otherwise spoken with apparent sympathy of the twenty-five-year-
old officer's "light blue eyes" and his "gentle physiognomy," nonetheless
decried the "unheard of passion," the "horrible madness," and the "horrible
episode" of which Bertrand was at once the victim and the agent.[6] In time,
Bertrand himself seemed to have joined in his doctors' revulsion, for, in the
words of the man who treated him, he "feels only horror, and an unfeigned
horror, at the memory of the dreadful acts for which he is appearing before
the tribunal."[7] According to the sergeant himself, his crimes were incomprehensible even to him: "Even today" he stated at his trial, "I cannot grasp the
sensations that I felt in scattering about the shredded bits of corpses."[8]

> Q. When you opened the cadavers, did you not thrust your hands inside them?
>
> A. *Still unperturbed and in the most level tone of voice.* Yes, Colonel, I put my hands
> in to tear out the entrails and I often went as far as the upper regions, from which
> I ripped out the liver. (A shudder of horror among the spectators.)[9]

The case and its trial raise a wealth of incidental questions vastly more
important than the issue of Bertrand's guilt and help illuminate the complexity of a cultural moment in which the dead and their relation to the city were
in upheaval. The reactions of doctors and simple observers, both at the trial
and in the press, insist repeatedly on the uniqueness of the sergeant's crimes.
During his testimony in court, the doctor Charles-Jacob Marchal de Calvi
asserted that Bertrand's condition could not be compared to other forms of
monomania, that it was, somehow, *sui generis*, and this measured opinion was
echoed in all of the more excitable commentaries—even from doctors—that
spoke of the case in superlatives, finding in it the final degree of perversion
or the most monstrous acts that can be imagined.[10] But what made Bertrand

so different was the object of his desire, and so it was not so much the sergeant as the dead who were unique. Beneath all of his pathological criminality, they were the ones who lent their importance and horror to the case and who motivated the reactions of the public.

It is surprising that anyone should have found Bertrand's behavior more disturbing than, say, acts of violence against the living, but various sources attest to the extreme seriousness with which contemporaries viewed his crimes. Tardieu described his violations of the dead as the "last stage" of perversion. Other responses were still more extreme and physical. The watchmen at the Montparnasse cemetery, for example, protected the grounds with booby-trapped rifles that they aimed to strike an intruder in the chest.[11] The newspapers recorded the wounds that one of these "machines infernales" eventually inflicted on Bertrand: "three bullets penetrated deep into the upper and middle sections [of his body], and two ingots lodged in the flesh along with the pieces of clothing they tore off."[12] His injuries were serious enough to place his life in danger, and even months later, at his trial, he could only hobble to the stand on crutches.[13] The fact that he survived at all was attributed to his good luck, for as one of the newspapers concluded: "His passion must have been most violent, since on two occasions . . . his life was in peril."[14] In the eyes of the cemetery guards and of the newspapers that reported their tactics without condemning them, it was not unreasonable to kill someone for attempting to disturb a graveyard. The crime of mutilating the deceased was apparently more distressing than killing the criminal guilty of it. As absurd as it might sound, the dead could be more precious than the living.

The Authorities

For Bertrand's contemporaries, understanding his case largely meant assigning jurisdiction over it. The doctors involved vigorously asserted their authority, arguing that the sergeant should not be submitted to the military tribunal that did, in fact, eventually try him, but should instead be entrusted to medical analysis and supervision. "How," wrote Henri de Castelnau after the judgment was handed down, "before the positive affirmations of science, could a contrary opinion prevail without opposing debates between competent men, and how is it possible that a sick man was condemned as a criminal?"[15] In the midst of the trial itself, Dr. Marchal de Calvi, who took the stand as an expert witness, seized the opportunity to argue that since Bertrand was not in control of his actions he should be found innocent. Insofar as Bertrand's necrophilia was the expression of a monomania, which doctors alone were qualified to treat, he had not, Marchal reasoned, behaved as a free agent, and his actions did not, therefore, fall under the purview of the law. Marchal observed that in following this logic, the material consequences of being judged innocent would have been significantly worse for Bertrand. "He was not *free*," the doctor argued. "I know how serious this assertion is, how prejudicial to the accused, in the sense that if he is not found guilty he might be subject to administrative measures that could go as far as prolonged confinement, while, if he is found guilty, his punishment is in comparison very light."[16]

In contesting the tribunal's right to dispose of the young sergeant, Marchal was also asserting his authority over a vastly more significant object, for in making his argument, the doctor emphasized its broader implications for society in general. "In what I am saying," he testified, "in the judgment that I am offering, I have been at pains not to omit the interest of society, to which the individual's interest cannot be sacrificed but which dominates that partial interest in the same way that an indefinite number prevails over the unit. On reflection, it will be seen that the interest of society is protected by my interpretation, whereas it is not by the opposing interpretation, which consists in considering the accused as responsible, as guilty."[17] It is society itself that is at stake here, but Marchal's pragmatism leads him to espouse a surprisingly instrumental approach to the significance of the case: he does not contend that his view of Bertrand's behavior is more truthful, but rather that it is more effective. Furthermore, he argues, by choosing an approach to understanding Bertrand's acts, one is also determining their effects on society, such that the crime, its meaning, and its consequences depend on the conceptual paradigm used to make sense of the criminal. As a result, Marchal contends, the courts must recognize that in cases like this doctors understand and protect society better than the law and should therefore willingly surrender their authority. In Castelnau's frustrated outburst about the conviction, one can hear a certain incredulity that the "positive affirmations of science" had not even been heard and that truth-value, duly established according to the protocols of his discipline, could not guarantee his competency in determining public policy over social behavior. Marchal, on the other hand, abandons the notion of scientific positivism, at least for the sake of argument, in order to engage in the kind of dispute with the law that Castelnau had unsuccessfully hoped for, even if the results were no more encouraging. In Marchal's testimony, one hears a shift in the discursive approach, an attempt to establish a language of disagreement that will cross between the logics of two different disciplines. In this new language, the positivism of science becomes relativistic, tactical, and pragmatic.

The distinction between the two interpretive paradigms emerges primarily from their divergent approaches to the status of individuality. Marchal depicts the proposed transfer of jurisdiction from legal to medical authorities as a "domination" of (Bertrand's) relatively insignificant personal interest for the well-being of the collectivity. Since the difference between the monomaniac and the society that he harms is infinite, so too is the distance between the interests that the law, on the one hand, and the doctors, on the other, protect. What society needs, he argues, is an agency that can "dominate" the same individuality that Bertrand had asserted by pursuing his own perverted interests. Insofar as a person identifies with the social interest, as Marchal claims to do, he is infinitely more than himself. Conversely, the one who pleases himself rather than society distances himself infinitely, in that very pleasure, from the social. This distancing gesture is repeated in Bertrand's case: just as the sergeant occupies the "last stage of perversion," so is his own good infinitely separate from the collective good. It is his minuscule personal concern that the law safeguards, while the doctor protects the whole of society. And he protects it not from the individual himself, but from what he comes to incarnate—the pathology. It is not a person that Marchal inculpates; on the contrary, Bertrand is, to his mind, innocent. What *is* guilty—if the term has any meaning when applied to such an extra-judicial and extra-moral object—is the unfree and impersonal in him, that force that denies his individuality and agency. Even if he is unique, the medico-social issue, as Marchal describes it, is not Bertrand in particular but rather the transindividual condition that he embodies.[18] It is the illness that threatens society, not Bertrand. It lies beyond individuation, beyond the laws, and at the very edge of the human. This is what is dreadful in the soft-spoken young officer with his blue eyes and gentle demeanor: Bertrand's crimes occurred outside the social order. Indeed, to the extent that he indulged in them, he did not even instantiate that infinitesimally small but irreducibly necessary component of society, the individual. In his pathology, he was an illness that measured itself against the polity as a whole, that stood outside of the city and refused its structures, its laws, and its modes of producing meaning.

Bertrand's case is significant in setting these different authorities against each other at two especially important points of contact: madness and death. As I will show in the next chapter, these two areas hold a special significance for social order in that they both lie outside of rationalized experience, thereby relativizing the notion of reason and everything that depends on it. Now, certain other crimes, including any case of potentially monomaniacal homicide, touch on the issues of madness and death to some extent, but with Bertrand, the status of death changes entirely. First, it has been replaced by the dead, for instead of some abstract concept of nonbeing or transcendence, it is the physical remains of the deceased that are involved, or, as Bertrand's contemporary, Dr. Claude-François Michéa, put it, "of all these cases the most monstrous and disgusting is Bertrand's, for that madman sought out sensual pleasures not merely in death, he demanded them even from putre-faction."[19] Second, Bertrand's desires invert the value of the dead as decomposing physical remains. Corpses have shifted from objects of disgust to instruments of pleasure, from sources of aversion to powerful forces of attraction. The very lability of their affective value disturbs those subjectively internalized limits of sociability that are revulsion and desire. The edges of the social feel different for Bertrand, and that difference is overwhelming, voluptuous. That they could feel so different to anyone, even a madman, suggests that those affective borders are not natural laws and that society is built in defiance of a great and potentially horrifying disorder that reaches into the very individuality of its members. Medical science attempted to identify and master that disorder, and it did so as part of an attempt to establish its legitimacy in society. The medicalization of death needs, therefore, to be understood within that particular context, which I will sketch out in the following pages, focusing first on the relations between medicine and other dominant discourses, primarily the courts and the Church.

The Rise of Medical Science

From the late eighteenth through the nineteenth century, medicine gained unprecedented credibility as a discipline. It redefined and asserted its legitimacy in respect to other discourses, notably the law and the Church, while its theories and approaches gained a broader truth-value, extending their reach beyond the domain of health to other issues of social interest. Nothing better indicates the changed role of doctors in society than the way they revolution-ized their own economic and class status.[20] The sciences as a whole made great strides in this respect, as Nicole and Jean Dhombres have shown. Whereas in the years before the Revolution of 1789, d'Alembert could com-plain that "'the title and profession of scientist [*savant*]' were not considered to have much merit," the situation had changed radically by the end of the century.[21] With the Directory (1795–1799) and, even more so, the first Empire (1804–1815), scientists began to enjoy a level of wealth and recogni-tion that placed them among the most privileged members of society, while some of the most prominent among them entered the nobility under the title of "comte d'Empire."[22] With differences of detail and speed, the same gen-eral narrative held for members of the medical profession as well. By 1795, according to Jean-Charles Sournia, "they were in all of the major branches of government, honored, sometimes titled, and they played an active role in the government of *départements* and *communes*."[23] They fared even better under the Empire, as Sournia observed: "in all, Napoleon ennobled 51 doc-tors. Under the ancien régime, these practitioners never would have been able to obtain these positions, ranks, and titles. . . . The other doctors returned to their professions, but the idea was now established that they were significant figures and that they could even be men of distinction [*notables*]."[24] In the century that followed, doctors were able to consolidate and expand their hold on power, prestige, and wealth.[25] Their most elite representatives did proportionally better. George Weisz has analyzed the members of the Académie de Médecine in Paris at four different moments from 1821 to 1935 according to various indicators of social standing, including their addresses and the amount of money they bequeathed in their wills. The results for 1901 are astounding: "Among all the elites of the period," he wrote, "only the heads of business enterprises left significantly larger fortunes than did acade-micians."[26] What these accounts show is that medical professionals had fun-damentally changed their position in society, leaping forward as a body in credibility and power. Apparently, they were able to convince their contem-poraries that they were in possession of something unique and valuable for society as a whole. But to do so, they had first to demonstrate that there was something coherent about medical thinking and that it could not be subordi-nated to other, existing forms of authority.

Working in very broad strokes, we can say that the coherence of the medi-cal discipline was established theoretically through notions like that of the lesion and pragmatically through control over institutions, teaching, and practice. When Pierre-Jean-Georges Cabanis published *Du degré de certitude de la médecine* (On the Degree of Certainty in Medicine) in 1798, that consolidation was still mostly an ideal. "Yes," he wrote, "I dare predict that, along with the true spirit of observation, the philosophical spirit that must preside over it is going to arise again in medicine; science is going to take on a new appearance. Its scattered fragments will be joined to form a system as simple and fecund as the laws of nature."[27] If its detractors, according to Cabanis, argued that there was no certainty and no science in medicine, it was primarily because they could not find an underlying principle or set of principles that unified it as a field of knowledge. It was not even clear that one could speak of illnesses in general terms, since symptoms varied widely from patient to patient and the same individual might exhibit the same symptoms for different diseases.[28] Consequently, "semiotics, or the art of recognizing the different states of the animal economy by means of the signs that characterize them, is without doubt the most difficult, but also the most important part of medicine."[29] If the doctor's ability to see through the various symptoms to their underlying cause was the most important of his talents, its difficulty lay in the fact that, for Cabanis and others, it derived not so much from theoretical principles as from an imaginative and affective sympathy on the part of the practitioner. The apparent rules determining the production of symptoms are, the medical student quickly discovers, fluid and poorly respected by the patients themselves, so that often "it seems that the doctor's theoretical knowledge becomes worthless beside the sickbed and that all his practical knowledge resides in a sort of instinct perfected by habit. Ultimately, it is by identifying, as it were, with the suffering person, by joining in his pains, by the quick action of a sensitive imagination, that he sees the illness in a single glance [*coup-d'œil*], grasping all of its marks at once."[30] This idea of an almost mystical identification with the patient and its status as a practical and hermetic knowledge handed down through the corporate institutions of medicine will be important for the disputes between doctors and the courts, but as the basis for a scientific program, the sympathetic *coup d'œil* was a frail reed to lean on. Even Cabanis described this approach as an art rather than a philosophy or science. At the time of his writing, however, pathological anatomists had already been developing the idea that diseases could be attributed to localizable disturbances in the structure of organs and that these lesions were the determining cause of both sicknesses and their consequent symptoms.[31] The concept of the lesion would be disputed throughout its history, notably by F. J. V. Broussais and, more conclusively, by Claude Bernard in the 1860s, but it nonetheless provided a crucial service to the rise of medicine: it acted as an underlying theoretical principle derived from clinical observations and was thus able to join not only symptoms to diseases but also practical experience—in the clinic or at the bedside—to abstract concepts.[32] Even if it was eventually discarded, even if it was only one of several similar organizing principles such as monomania, the *coup d'œil*, or Bernard's *milieu intérieur*, the lesion provided a necessary conceptual unity to medicine, the science that Cabanis had raised as its goal.[33]

In organizational terms, medicine underwent a similar, if not cognate, centralization in the period following the Revolution.[34] As far back as the thirteenth century, the profession had been a self-regulated and more or less coherent discipline. As Jan Goldstein observes, until the late eighteenth century it was, "with respect to its organizational structure, no different from other town-based occupations" and functioned much like other guilds, with authorities from the profession itself monopolizing medical training and the conferral of the right to practice.[35] However organized it might have been, though, the medical profession in France was far from centralized under the ancien régime, and even up to the eve of the Revolution different localities had their own, exclusive corporate structures, which did not recognize the rights or credentials of practitioners from other jurisdictions. As a result, any doctor who moved to another city would most likely have to obtain certification from the competent authorities in his new place of work.[36] Teaching was even less controlled. Pierre Huard has listed some five different types of institutions that provided medical training, ranging from "*facultés* and colleges of medicine" through courses offered in hospitals or by the departments of war and the navy, to "private schools established by individuals or religious orders."[37] The first category alone was broadly decentralized, with France counting no less than twenty-two *facultés* and an equal number of colleges of medicine at the beginning of the eighteenth century. By 1793, this number had dropped considerably, but at sixteen it remained impressive: "Of these sixteen *facultés*," Huard observes, "five (Paris, Montpellier, Strasbourg, Reims, and Toulouse) retained an indisputable importance, and five still maintained a certain level of activity. . . . The six others were barely alive."[38] And this quick sketch does not even include the teaching of surgery, which was an entirely independent discipline, with its own guild structures and teaching institutions.

Like so much else, however, the Revolution swept away this fragmentation. First, for three wild years, from March 2, 1791, to December 4, 1794, anyone who wanted to could legally practice medicine.[39] Decrees abolished all "teaching bodies [*congrégations enseignantes*]" as well as colleges and *facultés*, so that under the Terror medicine was absolutely deregulated.[40] Very quickly, however, the pendulum began to swing almost as far in the opposite direction, moving toward a strong, centralized monopoly on the training, certification, and disciplining of doctors. Medicine and surgery were unified. Schools began to reopen. "Beginning in 1797, a national hierarchy was established for medical teaching, which had become a monopoly."[41] With the law of 15 ventôse year XI (March 10, 1803), which remained in force until 1892, the government declared that "no one may take up the profession of doctor, surgeon, or *officier de santé*" without a certification from one of only three schools of medicine, located in Paris, Montpellier and Strasbourg.[42] These schools then became *faculties* in 1808, when the Université Impériale was founded.[43] "Under the Empire," wrote Nicole and Jean Dhombres, "the medical profession was structured on the basis of the education one received and it was organized on a national level."[44] When the Académie Royale de Médecine was founded in 1820, under the Bourbon restoration, France acquired a single source of expertise for health-related policies and laid the foundations for an officially sanctioned medical elite.[45] The structures that had grown up locally under various patronages and institutional structures during the ancien régime had been replaced by an intensely centralized bureaucracy that would, despite minor variations and often heated internal struggles, endure throughout the nineteenth century.[46]

Law and Medicine

The consolidation of medicine as a coherent discipline with an authoritative voice in public policy was not only a matter of internal organization. Doctors had to establish their credibility in respect to other, more recognized social forces, notably the courts and the Church. Vernon Rosario has remarked that Bertrand's case "was the occasion for two battles: a heated professional dispute between physicians and lawyers, and a debate within the medical profession about the classification of mental diseases."[47] It is that first battle that is of interest here and for two reasons. First, it illustrates the increasing importance of medicine within broader theories of society as a whole, for discussions about the bearing of medical science on judicial issues tended to frame the matter in terms of social good. Second, it reveals how doctors and their advocates used certain medical principles not only scientifically or to solve problems within their own discipline, but also strategically to establish medicine's authority in relation to other discourses. In other words, medicine consolidated its credibility as a unique and singularly valuable discipline in part by promoting principles that were more effective legally than medically. This is not a new observation, but it is important to recall the polemical nature of medical truth in relation first to the courts and then to the Church before moving on to consider some of the irrational desires that were motivating that truth.

While there is virtually no mention of medical issues in the French civil or penal codes, concern about the relations between medicine and the courts mushroomed in the nineteenth century.[48] According to the catalogue of the Bibliothèque Nationale de France, the earliest book to contain a variant on the term *medico-legal* in its title appeared in 1634, and some form of the expression recurred in a total of seventeen others before 1800.[49] In the following century alone, however, it figured over seven hundred times. Already Félix Vicq d'Azyr's influential and encyclopedic *Médecine*, published from 1787 to 1830, had devoted two of its nine rubrics to "legal medicine" and "the jurisprudence of medicine and pharmacology."[50] In 1820, Louis XVIII founded the Académie de Médecine "to advise on questions of medicine and surgery, notably on questions of legal medicine."[51] With this impetus, the early nineteenth century gave birth to a series of periodicals devoted not only to medicine in general—which were themselves numerous—but more specifically to the relations between medicine and the law. In 1829, the doctors Esquirol and Mar founded the *Annales d'hygiène publique et de médecine légale* (Annals of Public Hygiene and Legal Medicine) on the principle that "the function of medicine is not only to study and cure disease; medicine has an intimate relationship with social organization, sometimes aiding the legislator in the drafting of laws, often enlightening the magistrate about their application."[52]

Relations between courts and doctors were not always so congenial, however, and disputes between the two parties arose primarily along two fronts. On the one hand, the doctors' struggle had a defensive aspect, with the medical profession seeking to maintain its autonomy by jealously guarding the right to regulate itself without inference from outside bodies. On the other hand, doctors began attempting incursions into the authority of the courts by insisting, with growing stridency, that medical opinions be taken into consideration in certain legal procedures, especially when they concerned madness and individual free will.[53] As has already been observed, the first of these two approaches can be traced back to the guild-like medical corporations of the thirteenth century, but by the middle of the eighteenth century the question of medical self-governance had again become a matter of spirited discussion. In 1762, for instance, the doctor and lawyer Jean Verdier dedicated a two-volume study to the organization and policing of the medical corps, which at that time was subject to the oversight of the *Juges de Police*. Arguing that without a highly specialized scientific training it would be impossible to understand, much less pass judgment on doctors' actions, he proposed that the medical profession should have its own police and judges. "It is therefore to be desired," he wrote, "that these crimes fall under the purview of a private tribunal of doctors, who alone would be competent to judge such matters."[54] He was, in other words, recommending a parallel legal system. While to a large extent, doctors got that system, at least through the end of the nineteenth century, the relations between the legal and medical disciplines remained fairly fluid and often contentious.

The crux of the issue was the notion of medical responsibility, or the degree to which doctors could be held accountable in courts of law for damages resulting from their professional practice. Under the ancien régime, magistrates were, for the most part, loathe to involve themselves in such technical controversies, about which they understood little, and as a result doctors largely escaped legal scrutiny for alleged incompetence or for injuries they might inflict in the course of their ministrations.[55] The situation remained essentially unchanged throughout the nineteenth century. The penal code had little to say about doctors beyond article 29 of the law of 19 ventôse year XI, which concerned a particular case of medical oversight, stipulating when a lower order *officier de santé* had to call on supervision from a fully accredited *docteur en médecine*.[56] The issue of medical responsibility was thus approached through the articles 319 and 320 of the penal code and articles 1382 and 1383 of the civil code.[57] These articles all concerned general issues of liability for damages or injury and made no specific mention of medical practitioners. This situation struck doctors and some lawyers as highly unsatisfactory, leading them to call for exceptions and "palliatives" similar to those accorded to members of the legal profession.[58] Things came to a head in two court cases dating from the early part of the century. "It has become classic," wrote Robert Gervais in 1986, "to consider that the principle of medical responsibility was established, for the first time, by the appellate court's judgment of June 18, 1835 in the Thouret-Noroy case," and he thus noted that "the first decision concerning medical responsibility, since the civil code, dates from 1835."[59] The trial probably was a turning point in the legal interpretation of medical responsibility, but Gervais is off in arguing that it is the first such case. Paul Brouardel, writing at the end of the nineteenth century, points to another judgment, handed down some five years earlier, that had revolved around the applicability of articles 1382 and 1383 to medical procedures. Now, for Brouardel, the final judgment in this instance marked a blow against the self-regulation of the medical profession, but some attention to the wording of the court's decision mitigates that conclusion and indicates the way in which leading doctors had, at this crucial juncture, laid the bases for a special status in relation to the law.

In 1823, a certain Dr. Hélie of Domfront was accused of criminal negligence in his treatment of a patient. The proceedings dragged on inconclusively until 1829, when a commission from the Académie de Médecine convened to examine the case. It found that the courts were not competent to judge medical malpractice and released a statement arguing that:

> the responsibility of doctors in the conscientious exercise of their profession cannot be justiciable by the law. . . . Concerning medical practice, therefore, as in matters of distributive justice, doctors cannot, any more than judges, be held legally accountable for the errors they may commit in the good faith exercise of their functions. In the former, as in the latter case, responsibility is an entirely moral question, a matter of conscience: no judicial procedures can legally be opened unless it be in cases of improper solicitation, deceit, fraud, or prevarication. So concludes an accurate understanding of private interests.[60]

In its final judgment, the court in Domfront quoted this passage, concluded simply that it was a "way of thinking that the tribunal cannot share," and found Dr. Hélie guilty.[61] Despite its credentials as the preeminent medico-legal institution in France, the only legal power that the Académie de Médecine enjoyed, even in a minor local court, was its ability to argue and, perhaps, persuade. Despite its pretensions to autonomy, the Académie—and those it represented—were simply subjects before the law. While the discrepancy between the Académie's lofty claims and the court's brisk dismissal of them suggests the medical profession had no leverage whatsoever in the judicial system, the actual arguments for Hélie's guilt indicate that scientific thought had made its way more insidiously into legal practice. The final judgment found that because he neglected to exhaust the "various means that the [medical] art indicated to him and to consult with colleagues; and having neglected to do so and having, instead, acted without prudence and with an incredible haste, [Dr. Hélie] is guilty of a serious fault, which renders him responsible for damages resulting from the Foucault child's mutilation."[62] In short, the court accepted the criteria for treatment established by the medical profession itself and limited its own intervention in the case to determining if the doctor's actions had been consistent with the principles that his "art indicated to him."

The doctors defined the rules for conscientious treatment; the courts decided if they had been observed. But in order to reach that decision, the magistrates would have to acquaint themselves with a language and specialization that were not their own. They would have to become, if not doctors themselves, at least students of its science. Now this in itself does not create a special status for medicine in relation to the law. Shoddy carpentry, poor engineering, or ill-conceived architecture could, for instance, all bring grievous consequences, and the magistrates presiding over such cases would need to familiarize themselves with the principles of the relevant disciplines. Indeed, courts systematically call on outside expertise without finding the need to set up alternative judicial systems. But doctors argued, and argued with a great deal of success, that they were different. The outlines of their reasoning can be seen in a commentary on the 1835 Thouret-Noroy case, in which Charles Dalboussière, a lawyer before the Cour Royale de Paris, took up the doctors' cause. "A doctor is brought up on charges of ineptitude!" he wrote. "But who will be his judge? . . . One would thus turn the judicial setting into a debating chamber for the various medical doctrines that succeed each other in society and that often divide it in the midst of some controversy provoked and sustained by ardent proselytes and heated convictions."[63] The principles of architecture, carpentry, and engineering may not all be entirely simple, but they are not in endless flux, and that distinguishes them from medical science. For medicine, as an experimental discipline, was so fluid and so open to different theories that even doctors themselves disagreed about almost everything but the most standard practices. If doctors, who were experts, could not decide what was or was not a plausible technique, approach, or determination in respect to a particular patient, how could a magistrate? And, in fact, throughout the nineteenth century, the courts continued to venture only reluctantly into these technical debates, so that in practice doctors were sanctioned only in the most grievous and clear-cut instances of malpractice.[64] Medicine was thus protected in practice if not in theory by its own experimental and clinical methods, by its uncertainties and fluidity as a discipline—in short, by the very absence of the scientific grounding that seemed so crucial to its acceptability as an authoritative discourse.

Concerns about the governance, oversight, and discipline of the medical corps continued throughout the nineteenth century, without doctors' ever being able to establish the sort of judicial autonomy that the Académie de Médecine's special commission had proposed in the Hélie case. Still, in practice doctors enjoyed an almost complete immunity against charges of professional incompetence or negligence. In other ways as well, medicine defined itself as a uniquely privileged discipline in relation to the law. In 1894, the Conseil Général du Gard declared that in its present state forensic medicine constituted "a genuine peril to the nation" and offered the following suggestions: "1) that there be created in France a medico-legal institute for the purpose of training specialists; 2) that in the future the status of forensic doctor be conferred only on medical doctors who have completed an internship (whose duration is to be determined) in the medico-legal institute."[65] Far from resolving themselves after more than a century of debate and sparring, the conflicts between the legal and medical professions had become a social crisis. The proposed solution entailed creating a hybrid institution to produce a subcategory of doctors specifically trained to assure communication between legal and medical practice. In effect, the Conseil's recommendation acknowledged both the distinctive nature of medicine within the legal sphere (there are, for instance, no institutes for forensic music or carpentry) and the perilous consequences of mishandling the relation between the two disciplines.

Another crucial element in the extra-judicial autonomy of doctors was the so-called *medical secret*, a long-standing principle that was reaffirmed in 1810 by article 378 of the penal code.[66] According to Paul Brouardel's *La responsabilité médicale* (Medical Responsibility), legislators recognized the "social interest" of discretion in certain professions and acknowledged that in order to be treated effectively, patients needed to communicate openly with their physicians, which meant free from the fear that information supplied during consultations could subsequently be used against them in other contexts.[67] Although Brouardel's study dates from 1898, the question of patient-doctor confidentiality was being hotly debated at the time of Bertrand's court-martial. In 1845, a major congress of French doctors had convened in an amphitheatre of the Ecole de Médecine to discuss it and other related topics.[68] At the trial itself, the issue reappears quickly but significantly in what seems to be a testy exchange between Dr. Marchal de Calvi, on the witness stand, and the presiding magistrate:

> *Le président*: Since the accused and his counsel themselves both ask that you read this document, I enjoin you, doctor, not merely to read the document but also to inform the court of all the facts that have been brought to your attention by the accused in the various conversations you have had with him, unless they are protected by doctor-patient confidentiality [*confidences faites sous les réserves de votre caractère de médecin*].
>
> *Dr. Marchal de Calvi*: I am perfectly aware of the full extent and the full burden of my duties.[69]

The tone of Marchal's response, stressing emphatically that he understands "*perfectly* the *full* extent and the *full* burden" of his responsibilities, hints that he is irritated by something in what the magistrate has just said. His insistence on his totalizing mastery of the codes regulating his own profession suggests, in turn, that what he resents is the judge's arrogating the right to impose those responsibilities on him: they are not the magistrate's to apply or remove, since they have been developed by the medical profession itself in the autonomous exercise of its self-regulation. Not to grasp that principle is to misunderstand that the "medical secret" was a privilege that the doctors won for themselves through the legitimacy of their own disciplinary approach to knowledge. By forcing its acceptance as a legal principle, the medical profession was able to create for itself a zone of silence separate from the judicial system, a realm in which aberrant and socially intolerable behavior could be discussed freely, in which the ill and their illnesses could speak and be understood.[70] These were the protocols for deciphering the sick. Or such, at least, was the argument.

Now, it might seem that legally recognizing the "medical secret" to be in the interest of society, as Brouardel recommends, would mean ascribing as much importance to individual concerns as to respect for the laws. In practice, however, accepting the social utility of such secrets meant considering individual health as not really an individual but rather a collective issue. This attitude was the product of concerns about contagion and communicability and the observation that diseases passed among individuals, linking them through bonds that often had no respect for legal categories of responsibility and innocence.[71] It was crucial to make the patient speak, not for his or her own sake, but for the sake of hearing, recognizing, and battling potential illnesses, which, if untreated, could go on to infect others and threaten the community.[72] In a routine check-up one still has the strange sense that the doctor is interested in something very close to and yet somehow other than the patient. Virtually every adult has learned that when a physician on duty enters the room and asks, "How are you?" the question is different from normal conversation. The expected response does not involve, say, descriptions of recent artistic accomplishments or gripes about siblings' unreasonable demands. Usually, the patient has sufficiently assimilated medical protocols to respond instead with details about the functioning of his or her organism and betrays, in that way, a familiarity with the medical alienation of individuals from their own body. In responding, the patient enacts a certain cleavage between at least two discourses and two subjects, one of which is properly medical and somehow impersonal.

Three years before the publication of Brouardel's *Responsibilité médicale*, Marcel Proust remarked with some wonder on this transformation of the patient and emphasized the extra-judicial quality of this new kind of individual. In his novel *Jean Santeuil*, his narrator observed:

> The doctor who treats a young man will not allow him to leave if he is still sick, whatever interest the law might have in arresting him or the military authorities in drafting him. But once, out of love for professional truth—which is for him the most important thing—he has forbidden the young man to leave, he will side, energetically and cordially, with the young man's claims and will have nothing but hostility toward civil justice and the military authorities, whose interests do not take that truth into consideration.[73]

The "medical secret" protected its subject from interference by another sort of person, who normally fell under the purview of the law. As Marchal argued during Bertrand's court-martial, there was an infinite distance between these two subjects; only the medical one, he contended, truly represented the interests of society. And as Proust remarked, this medical subject was the product of a special, discursive relation to a notion of truth. In these discussions there thus emerged a certain image of the general good and the vague but powerful notion of a subjectivity defined by it—a good and a subjectivity that could only be understood through medicine.

To recognize such an incompatibility between the behavior of illnesses and the normal judicial needs for disclosure of information is, moreover, to acknowledge incompatibilities among the various connections that draw people together into a social group. And once such divergences are accepted, the silences, such as the "medical secret," that separate different discourses of collectivity, notably the law and medicine, become symbols of the inconsistencies fissuring the conceptualization of society itself, figures for the impossibility of imagining it as a whole. This impossibility was, of course, a self-imposed one—in the most basic practical terms, information could be shared, jurists and doctors could, conceivably, know the same details about patients—but it was a necessity nonetheless, since in order for the legal and medical disciplines to function, such sharing of knowledge had to be prohibited. As a consequence, the social order as a whole might be theoretically or abstractly intelligible, but for its participants, it would always be full of impenetrable but indispensable mysteries. There could be no panoptic position from which actual society could be known to any of its members, and individuals would be held together through the circulation of information available only to others.

This was the social order at the moment of Bertrand's trial. A tissue of disputes. Not somewhere outside of them, but the disputes themselves, which tirelessly invoke a common good. One cannot describe that order as a whole without losing the feeling of its texture, the panic of its blind spots, and the anxieties that brought it to life for contemporaries. Within this context, doctors were able to create a distinctive place for their discipline in relation to the law. They were able to make that relation an issue of social utility, thus expanding their own concerns into concerns about society, its definition, and its good. Within these disputes, doctors were able to preserve a unique legal autonomy by instrumentalizing the incomprehensibility of their discipline, its conceptual fluidity—what I will term, in the next chapter, its nonsense. As a result, medicine was able to reshape some of the most basic social categories, such as subjectivity.

Medicine and the Church

To secure a position of credibility and influence within society, the medical profession had to establish its independence not only against the legal system, but also in relation to the Catholic Church.[74] Often, the two disputes echoed each other, as when the priest and doctor Pierre Debreyne drew on military metaphors to describe the clergy's need to "reconquer the high ground of intellectual and scientific influence," words that recall Philippe Pinel and Henri Legrand du Saulle's statements about the relations between jurisprudence and medicine.[75] Under the ancien régime, the Church exercised considerable control over doctors. French medical schools were normally attached to universities, whose chancellors, with only two exceptions, were representatives of the Pope.[76] In the course of their practice, moreover, doctors and surgeons were legally constrained to obey certain directives of the Church. A key example of this emerged in the delicate and emotionally charged moments when an individual's life hung in the balance. In 1712, Louis XIV had made law a prescription, dating back to the fourth Lateran council, that medical practitioners invite any patient to confess whom they felt to be in imminent danger of death.[77] Just before the Revolution, the clergy of Tours attempted to refine this law. For the *cahiers de doléances* drawn up in preparation for the 1789 meeting of the Estates-General, they submitted a request that "doctors and surgeons should be forbidden to examine a patient on the third day of his illness unless he has obtained a certificate of confession."[78] Jean-Charles Sournia has remarked that such a stipulation was undoubtedly motivated by a pragmatic concern: any patient who had already been sick for three days was presumably in danger of death. But for Sournia, the real significance of the priests' request lay elsewhere. "In reality," he observed, "the demand went further, for it granted the Church control over sickness and doctors."[79] The Revolution upended all of this.[80] The universities were placed under the authority of the state rather than the Church, even if ecclesiastical figures such as the abbé Frayssinous would subsequently be called on to head some of them.[81] Legally, doctors no longer had to bow to the demands of the clergy, as reforms swept away laws such as Louis XIV's 1712 declaration and the civil and penal codes fell silent on the relations between medicine and religion.

But theoretical debates still shook those relations. The secularization of the state under the Revolution and the early successes of militantly atheist scientists rapidly gave way in face of a reinvigorated Church. Chateaubriand's 1802 *Génie du christianisme* (The Genius of Christianity) played a crucial role in this revival, for it argued broadly and convincingly that the sciences were inadequate for resolving social and philosophical issues.[82] It was not until the early 1820s that the intellectual disputes about the relative merits of faith and scientific thought came to an uneasy stasis, which would last through the mid-century.[83] The baron Augustin-Louis Cauchy summarized the situation in his 1844 *Considérations sur les ordres religieux adressées aux amis des sciences* (Considerations on the Religious Orders Addressed to Friends of the Sciences), writing that "the very titles of Catholic and geometer . . . impose on me duties that I cannot shirk. As a Catholic, I cannot remain indifferent to the interests of religion; as a geometer, I cannot remain indifferent to the interests of science."[84] The two vocations had their own demands and their own sorts of truth, and the key to their reconciliation in the same individual, or the same society, would be achieved through an acceptance of that difference. Many scientists, including numerous doctors, were able to reconcile the two parties in their own lives, as were the institutions of medicine and the Church overall.[85] Despite atheistic and materialist trends stemming from the Enlightenment on the one hand and attacks on the sciences inspired by Chateaubriand and similar voices on the other, throughout the first half of the century, Church dogma and medical theory were largely able to define separate and compatible spheres of validity. Indeed, some clerics recognized the value of the new movements in the sciences and attempted to appropriate a measure of their authority. Father Pierre Debreyne, for instance, proposed that priests verse themselves in the new discoveries of the sciences so that they could compete on a more even footing with medical practitioners. The clergyman, he wrote, "must create for himself a new type of influence, an influence based on enlightenment and science."[86]

In practical ways, however, doctors were already asserting their independence from ecclesiastical oversight, and the priests represented a very different sort of adversary from the courts. At least in the first half of the century, physicians, churchmen, and some nuns enjoyed a similar, intimate contact with the ill. Doctors were present at their charges' final moments, in many cases hindering or displacing the priest's attempts to administer one of the Church's most emotionally powerful sacraments, while the old control that the Church had exercised over doctors in this regard had disappeared with the ancien régime. The clergy was concerned that in other ways as well medical practitioners might interfere with the application of God's laws on earth. Out of a reluctance to create useless psychological pain, for instance, doctors had a tendency to hide from their terminally ill patients the gravity of their condition, which meant that the latter were inclined to defer extreme unction until it was potentially too late.[87] There was also a distrust of physicians in cases of possible suicide, a suspicion that out of sympathy for bereaved families they were only too willing to offer false causes of death so as to facilitate unlawful burials in consecrated grounds.[88] But it was often not the priests themselves who were the principal source of friction. The hospitals were, for the most part, still staffed by nuns, even after their secularization in Paris. Frequently obstructionist, seemingly omnipresent, these women had, in many cases, enough medical training to make them skilled adversaries.[89] As Jan Goldstein has written in reference to the particularly exasperating experiences of Dr. Antoine-Marie Chambeyron, "in calling nineteenth-century carceral institutions 'panoptic,' Michel Foucault was referring only to the constant visibility of the inmates to the experts. Inattentive to the continuing lively presence of religious personnel in most of these institutions, Foucault failed to point out that the public space of hospitals and asylums was regularly the site of another penetrating gaze: that directed toward medical men by angry and suspicious nuns."[90] The physicians finally resorted to more vigorous methods and began to remove this religious personnel from medical facilities. In 1878 the Sœurs de Saint-Vincent-de-Paul were expelled from the Laennec hospital, and the trend continued until 1908, when the Sœurs Augustines were finally driven out of the Hôtel-Dieu of Paris.[91]

If the doctors encroached on practices and relationships, such as those with the dying, that the clergy might have preferred to control, the latter attempted, in turn, to appropriate some of the privileges of the medical profession. The scientific primers intended for the use of clergymen by such authors as Tillie and Debreyne are one rather innocuous manifestation of this tendency.[92] The illegal practice of medicine by uncertified priests was a more insidious problem, and it was not until the latter half of the nineteenth century that the Ecole de Médecine was able to bring it under some sort of control.[93] But, as if in response, advocates of the Church tried a new and potentially devastating approach. Reaching back to the provisions for freedom of instruction enshrined in the charter of 1830 and the constitution of 1848, they argued that the Ecole de Médecine's monopoly on the training and certification of physicians violated the country's most basic laws.

Almost immediately, an acrimonious debate on the subject erupted in the pages of the *Union médicale*. The doctor Edouard Carrière argued that medical instruction had to be subjected to a single "authority" derived systematically from a priori principles and contended that "physiology itself teaches the limitation of freedom."[94] The editor in chief, Amédée Latour, on the other hand, advocated open competition among various medical schools, all of which would be under the supervision and control of a single, independent body.[95] Needless to say, this would have undone all of the attempts, dating back to Verdier, to consolidate medical authority and autonomy within a single, self-regulating discourse and would have facilitated a return to the decentralization of the ancien régime. The particulars of this debate warrant some scrutiny, since they indicate how medical knowledge could be instrumentalized to other ends. The arguments on behalf of medicine are surprisingly slack intellectually and seem almost transparently motivated by other concerns than scientific rigor or social justice. A certain materialist determinism drives Carrière's justifications for centralizing authority in a single, elitist institution, and his reasoning, which is often stretched or specious, could easily be applied to other, less benign forms of social control. According to him, the same interpretive activity that distinguishes sign from symptom also produces discoveries in science, for the latter are not merely observations or even analyses, but rather inductions dependent on the autonomous activity of the mind. He terms this activity "authority," and views it as the great underlying principle of advancement both in the sciences and in society as a whole. "Progress is not merely compatible with authority," he writes; "it is by authority that progress is produced and that it advances with that firm and steady step that is as solemn and imposing as true science."[96] But Carrière seems unfazed by the idea that the solemnity of scientific authority might sometimes prevail over its tendency to move forward:

> It is, however, most unfortunate, some will say, that Galileo should have been imprisoned in a dungeon for having discovered a great truth. It is terrible that in the name of this authority genius should succumb at the moment when it should illuminate, and when power and the public should lend themselves to the propagation of that light. I will first make this observation. An institution with a tradition of great thinkers, that is invested in the protection and the conservation of society, is such an institution to yield to the first appeal, to the demands of a single man? It cannot relinquish its great responsibility before an individuality that is but an insignificant atom in matters concerning the interests of a whole world. Catholicism could sense the rise of Protestantism when it took measures against scientists [*savans*]. Galileo's innovation was not dangerous; others are. In such a case, is it not better to act with prudence than to permit a series of struggles and insurrections?[97]

Curiously and somewhat perversely, Carrière uses the example of the Catholic Church's repression of Galileo's discoveries to argue for the medical profession's right to repress the unauthorized teaching of medicine by the Church. Feigning, literally, to be more Catholic than the Pope, he agrees that the clergy were right to gag scientific discovery because they had an obligation to protect society. Carrière presents himself as preaching prudence rather than anarchy on the one hand and, on the other, the need to recognize an infinite incommensurability between the social order and individual interest. His argument nonetheless sets truth against authority, forcing one to conclude that progress is driven not by the former, but through the autonomous workings of authority itself. Rather than the expression of a new and more enlightened way of making sense, authority is fetishized as a self-justifying force in its own right. There are other unsettling aspects to Carrière's reasoning. Later, when Latour defies him to identify the single, a priori principle or law from which medical knowledge derives and by which it deserves the title of science, Carrière limits his responses to *ad hominem* attacks. All in all, one is left wondering whether Latour was not justified in his contentions that the opposing party had confused social and natural laws, that they had attributed an ontological necessity to structures that were, in fact, the results of social power dynamics.[98] The victory, at least for the moment, went to Latour and his colleagues. On March 15, 1850, the *loi Falloux* was passed, "which gave members of religious orders the right to open schools without any professional qualification and introduced strongly clerical councils to regulate the universities."[99]

Given polemicists like Carrière, the fact that doctors ultimately succeeded in protecting their privileges—in relation to medical training at least—is not without its mysterious aspects, and it is difficult to avoid a vague unease at how they reached their ends. If the Church, as part of a broader renaissance of Christian identity marked by monuments such as Chateaubriand's *Génie du christianisme*, had enjoyed a broad dominion over the nascent medical profession in the first half of the nineteenth century, its hold loosened rapidly over the course of the following years.[100] In the second half of the century, the courts began vigorously to prosecute clergy for the illegal practice of medicine.[101] Pasteur's breakthroughs in germ theory and immunization gave a dramatic and widely publicized credibility to medicine in service of the social good and seemed decisively to confound previous arguments from the Church about the very possibility of progress.[102] Then, in the last three decades, the Third Republic moved to secularize government institutions, a process that undid most of the *loi Falloux*'s practical effects and culminated in the 1904 separation of churches and the state. After a century of struggles, the doctors' pursuit of credibility and distinctiveness within established power structures had born fruit. One of the most prominent signs of this success was the dramatic change in their social status, and this, in turn, served to reinforce their apparent legitimacy and to consolidate their gains against the clergy. In Pierre Guillaume's words, "in this context, the relations between the practitioner and the priest cannot remain the same. The Church must abandon its affirmation of the latter's superiority over the former."[103] If the revolution of 1789 had swept the bourgeoisie into power, the Enlightenment, for its part, had offered doctors access to that newly enfranchised class and given them a conceptual capital that they could parlay into an unprecedented legitimacy within the highest ranks of the established social order. True, the Church kept a close eye on its new rivals, and priests, who still enjoyed moral influence over their parishioners, could exercise a tremendous control over their patronage of individual physicians.[104] Nonetheless, over the course of the century, the position of the medical profession had been fundamentally transformed in relation to the Church. At key moments in that transformation, however, the medical profession made an almost cynical use of dubious reasoning to promote its credibility and authority and to instrumentalize medical science as a social force. And if, in the first decades of the century, doctors had generally been willing to accept the notion that science and religion governed separate aspects of society and different classes of truth, by the end of the century medical practitioners had vastly expanded their domain, often to the detriment of the Church.[105]

The Truth-Value of Medicine

Documents from the nineteenth century claimed that the authority of medicine had a wider scope than access to hidden knowledge about the body, no matter how important that particular knowledge might have appeared.[106] We have already seen doctors contend that the nature of their discipline conferred certain privileges on them, such as an indispensable role within the courts and an inherent right to self-legislation, especially in relation to teaching and the certification of competence. Their arguments pushed farther, however, for these claims to a special status were motivated by an underlying conviction that medical thought as such was not only unique, coherent, and powerful, but that it also enjoyed a general conceptual superiority over other disciplines.

One finds evidence of a determination to use the protocols of medical science to resolve problems in other fields as early as 1799, when François-Emmanuel Fodéré described legal medicine as "the application of physico-medical principles to the administration of justice."[107] The way he phrased the sentence indicates that he was not speaking of merely introducing medically produced knowledge into court cases—in the form, say, of expert testimony—but rather of subordinating legal processes to medical ones. Two years later, Nicolas-Pierre Gilbert took Fodéré's approach to extremes by contending that "these benefits of forensic medicine know no limits. There is not an action, not a movement made by Man in his social state that cannot make use of it. It is of all times and all places: it is the first, the holiest of magistracies, for it has always and only for object the happiness of mankind, the peace and safety of citizens."[108] It is difficult to imagine how one could distinguish between legal medicine and other forms of jurisprudence on the basis of Gilbert's description, but evidently he believed that medical thought promised a systemic redefinition of human experience in its totality. His very inability to identify clearly or distinctively what it was about medicine that made it universally useful indicates, however, some of the irrational fascination that the new discipline exercised over late eighteenth-century imaginations. Medicine's conceptual power seems to have extended beyond its proponent's ability to conceptualize it—to have derived, in other words, from an unidentifiable, unmastered elsewhere.

In his 1798 *Du degré de certitude de la médecine*, Cabanis made similar claims, framing them in terms of education and morality. Medicine alone, he wrote, "can make known to us the laws of the living mechanism . . . [and] it lays bare to us the physical man, of whom the moral man is himself but a part."[109] He attempted, moreover, to locate the origin of medicine's social utility, arguing that "it finds in the eternal laws of nature the foundations for man's rights and duties. In a word, it illuminates the study of understanding and outlines the art by which we guide and perfect it."[110] With privileged access to the workings of the human body and the hidden laws of nature, doctors were, according to Cabanis, best positioned to understand and reveal the fundamental structures of human behavior and society. They were, in this sense, the true legislators and the rightful architects of a new freedom. Medicine was, in this respect, a unique form of thinking that reached into the very foundations of society itself. Fodéré, Gilbert, and Cabanis may simply come across as over-excited promoters of their chosen discipline, but their positions on the truth-value of medicine were part of a larger discussion about the utility of the sciences in general. Nicole and Jean Dhombres have shown how this notion of utility set two significantly different schools of thought against each other. On the one hand, Rousseau and his followers, such as Robespierre and other members of the Convention, understood scientific advances to be useful because they helped resolve practical problems and prepared youths for a profession.[111] On the other hand, the encyclopedists, such as d'Alembert, Lacépède, Monge, and Carnot, argued that the true utility of the sciences was of a more theoretical and moral nature. Like Cabanis, they tended to emphasize its social value.[112] For figures such as these, as Dhombres and Dhombres have put it, "science became a school of civics."[113] They have traced the vicissitudes of this second, more theoretical approach to the value of science over the years following the Revolution and up through the second decade of the nineteenth century, noting that while it continued to attract partisans, the latter tended, for the most part, to be isolated figures and their ideas cut off from institutional support.[114]

What Dhombres and Dhombres have termed the "encyclopedist" approach did not, however, entirely disappear and it continued to influence discussions about the value of medicine. It is a somewhat subtle point, and one has to listen carefully, at certain key moments, to the discussions about medical issues to detect its ongoing presence, but this belief in the general applicability of medical principles to social questions was a crucial aspect of their broader importance during the nineteenth century and after. This can be seen in the 1849 debate between Edouard Carrière and Amédée Latour that I discussed earlier. Carrière defended the notion that medicine, like the sciences in general, enjoyed an inherent authority that derived from its status as a conceptual system. "Authority," he wrote, "is not and must not be an empty word. It entails submission not to the whims of an individual will, but to an order of ideas or principles of which a man or a collective is the representation." From there, he went on to assert that medicine was not merely "a science of observation of facts, a science of analysis," but also, "a science of induction" with its own "a prioris."[115] It was, in short, the form of medical thought, its method, that gave it weight and credibility. And this method was, as Carrière understood it, identical to the order that structured both human individuals and associations. The principles of medical semiotics did not simply, therefore, express the basic laws of the physical world, they could also serve as instruments to understand those other forms of representation—those sign systems—that were, for him, men and their communities.

Carrière immediately put these theories to practical use. Basing his reasoning on an analogy between biological and social processes, he argued that "physiology itself teaches the limitation of freedom" and attempted to prove that the restriction of medical teaching to institutions authorized by the

Ecole de Médecine was dictated by the very laws of nature, as revealed by medicine itself.[116] Although in this case Carrière's descriptions of methodological authority were marshaled to protect the self-governance of the medical corps, they could just as easily have been applied to other social structures and have served as a basic paradigm for all sorts of legislation. Latour, on the other hand, disputed his colleague's assertion that medical practice was, in fact, built on the sort of underlying law that could confer upon it the title of science. "If this word signifies general principles, primary and principal facts, general rules, all of which express the same thing," he wrote, "I no longer recognize medicine's right to call itself a science; it is in vain that I seek, in this supposed science, a single law that, like attraction in astronomy or affinity in chemistry, would allow one to explain, to discover the causes of, or to predict phenomena."[117] Although, for him, the term *medical science* was an oxymoron, he did not contest the basic principles underlying Carrière's reasoning, *viz.* that it is the intellectual formalities of a discipline that establish its authority—and indeed he used those principles as the basis for his own rebuttal. In arguing that other forms of medical training, notably at ecclesiastical institutions, should be legally accredited, however, he obliquely introduced other criteria to justify authority, writing:

> the instructor must not only be free from the obligation to cut his science and his doctrines to the official pattern of teaching, but the student must also be free to look for science not in the places where it resembles official science, but in the places where it is best. . . . . [State teaching] must be subordinated, for the same reasons and to the same extent as all teaching, to a separate, independent, and impartial surveillance, which, in a word, holds all teaching in its scales and gives preference only to the best and most useful. The deregulation of teaching thus culminates in the separation of the teaching corps from the corps of students, and this is an essential characteristic.[118]

Latour demanded that authority be justified not by dogma but by quality. Quality, in turn, must be established on the basis of autonomous criteria that were left unclear, and this very vagueness concealed the crucial problem in these polemics. Latour never rejected Carrière's contention that authority could be derived from the formal characteristics of a discourse or discipline, but he never explicitly embraced that idea either. He stated categorically that the process of judgment must be independent and impartial and derived the "essential characteristic" of medical training from this structural particularity. It was thus the formal aspects of the procedure of judgment that allowed one to make determinations of value, but for Latour, they were not enough in themselves. And the sole criterion for giving preference that he explicitly offered—aside from the unexplained term *better*—was utility. Utility was, as I will show in the next chapter, a value cited throughout these debates, and often from the most unexpected quarters. Ecclesiastics such as Debreyne and Ferrand used it to argue against the monomania theory, while doctors, such as Marchal de Calvi, advanced it to defend the contrary. The guiding principles not only for certifying the general social validity of medical thought, but also for establishing systems of deontology and ethics thus became formal, discursive characteristics and utility. Truth was not treated in these debates as the fundamental criterion for establishing the worth of medical thought, and the principle of goodness—with all of its ethical implications—was largely reduced to the notion of usefulness.

But the notion that medicine gained its value from a unique and privileged relation to truth gained a significant currency. This change can be gauged in the credibility that was attributed to medical thought in other domains of social life, in the role that doctors began almost naturally to assume in moments of public crisis, and by the reverence with which some of their most brilliant contemporaries in other disciplines viewed these scientists' peculiar approach to knowledge. These different strands came together in what was probably the most important cultural event in France at the end of the nineteenth century. The Dreyfus affair started as a court-martial for treason and then developed into a national cause célèbre about anti-Semitism. Solicited by the editors of the newspaper *Le temps*, the director of the Institut Pasteur in Paris, Emile Duclaux, lent his signature to a petition demanding a review of Dreyfus's original condemnation. He added as justification: "I tell myself that in principle a judgment handed down in such a troubled period, after such a press campaign, and without any subsequent corroboration, such a judgment might be irregular, or false, or guilty. It does not satisfy my desire for justice and truth."[119] He speaks in the first person, but it is a very special subject position he adopts, one certified by his medical training and a century-long history of doctors' repeatedly positioning themselves as the mouthpiece for a higher and impersonal common good. Speaking as a scientist, Duclaux is not himself, but rather a concern for social order based in a characteristically disciplinary way of speaking. That, at least, is how Marcel Proust understood the authority of scientists when he described their contributions to the Dreyfus controversy. "It is always with a joyful and virile emotion," he wrote in *Jean Santeuil*, "that one hears singular and audacious words come from the mouth of men of science, who, as a pure point of professional honor, come to tell the truth, a truth they care about simply because it is the truth that they have learned to cherish in their art."[120]

Doctors' authority depended on a specific relation to the truth, one that was peculiar to the late eighteenth and nineteenth centuries and that involved, as I will show, a highly original notion of sign systems, which they dubbed semiotics. This authority was premised on a new subjective relation between the figure of the scientist and the language he or she spoke, a language that, in turn, generated other, novel forms of nonsubjective personality, such as the madman, the illness, and the patient. Given the public bickering—indeed, cynicism—about power and truth on the part of medical practitioners and their opponents, it is difficult to imagine how anyone, especially as clear-sighted an observer as Proust, could subscribe to the belief that scientific reasoning was a disinterested pursuit of knowledge. His reaction indicates some of the mysteriousness of doctors' rise in social credibility and their ability to seize a leading role in shaping social issues— not only as legislators, members of a favored social class, or expert witnesses, but more importantly as purveyors of a unique form of truth. The issue is not whether Proust was right or wrong, whether he believed what he wrote or not, or whether nineteenth-century French society was indeed shaped by medical theories. What is important is that Proust could have expressed such a vision so clearly and felt that it would represent a recognizable and significant position. In the next chapter, I will examine in more depth that mystery at the source of medical legitimacy, the ways in which doctors were able to instrumentalize to their own ends irrational fears, desires, and fascinations, especially concerning madness and death.

The Medical Uses of Nonsense

In 1816, Philippe Pinel, the great revolutionizer of psychiatry, warned that his discipline "opens such a vast field to research that I am still very reluctant to offer an outline of it. One cannot hide the fact that its fundamental bases are little known and that the reciprocal limits between the domain of juris-prudence and that of medicine are still far from having been established."[1] The science of madness became one of the crucial areas for defining the reciprocal competencies, rights, and authorities of medicine and the law. Since the tense negotiations between the two disciplines over the meaning and status of the insane have been abundantly and often brilliantly examined, I will only briefly retrace some of those findings. My interest in discussing these debates is to consider the role of irrationality as a legitimizing force within them—to discern, in other words, the ways in which the very incom-prehensibility of the mad created a mysterious and extra-social language that the rising medical profession could adapt to its own purposes.

In the previous chapter I indicated how the unintelligibility, indeed the internal incoherence, of medical discourse created a privileged space for doctors in respect to their civil and criminal liability, providing them with an exceptional degree of autonomy from judicial oversight. In this chapter, I develop a similar argument in respect to the unintelligibility of madness before turning to examine another, less frequently discussed element in the legitimation of medicine—doctors' increasing mastery of death. Here again, it was the foreignness of death, its extra-social status, and its role as an imaginary construct that gave it force. In the late eighteenth and early nineteenth centuries, the medical profession learned to harness that irrational force to establish its own credibility and usefulness.[2]

Madness Between Medicine, the Law, and the Church

At the same time that doctors attempted, with mixed success, to secure their self-governance outside the legal system, they were also trying to impose their own discipline on the workings of the courts, principally by insisting that medical interpretations be taken into consideration for certain kinds of legal procedures, such as admittance into insane asylums, establishing *tutelle* (that is, the legal guardianship of an incompetent), and especially in cases involving mental debility and its effects on the principle of individual responsibility. What was new at the end of the eighteenth century was not, however, the notion of medico-legal expertise as such, but rather the increasing clarification, standardization, and consolidation of its status within the legal system. As Robert Castel has argued, this change was propelled, in large part, by the medicalization of madness, for the control of the insane passed from the police to the medical profession in the period from Louis XIV to 1800.[3] Jan Goldstein has shown that in the final years of the ancien régime "the foundations of psychiatry were inconspicuously being laid," and that the social importance of this new discipline was quickly acknowledged by the creation of special institutions.[4] In the late seventeenth century, Louis XIV had established a *hôpital général* in each city, but these were not intended to provide care for the sick; instead they were designed to isolate all sorts of marginal or undesirable individuals from the general population.[5] The mad made up a small but significant portion of their inmates, and by the latter part of the eighteenth century, their status within these institutions began to shift, as it was determined to be at least theoretically possible to cure them.[6] Under the care of specialized doctors, the insane could, in principle at least, be reintegrated into society. Their status within the group of social undesirables accordingly changed, and the institutions originally designed to isolate them started to become instruments to effect their cure.[7] As Castel has suggested, the medical understandings of mental illness under the ancien régime were not necessarily incompatible with the system for isolating the mad developed under Louis XIV, but they were also not particularly important to that system. "It is when the keystone to the edifice is decapitated," he writes, "that its constituent elements will become incompatible. The medical aspect will then acquire an entirely different meaning: where once it was subordinate, it will become dominant, for it will constitute the axis of the new equilibrium."[8]

Castel has described how the Napoleonic regime brought the control of the mad into its vast—and overwhelmingly successful—project to centralize and standardize the bureaucratic administration of France. On March 25, 1813, an imperial decree mandated that all prefects undertake a census to determine the number of mad people under their jurisdiction and to evaluate their condition. The tenor of this new order, the force of its organizational and financial concerns, still resonates in an explanatory document circulated by the Ministry of the Interior later that year: "This state of things creates organizational problems in book-keeping, uncertainties about the sums that must be allocated in budgets, and continuous obstacles both to the administration of public establishments and to their occupancy by the insane, who need, nonetheless, to be sequestered from society."[9] Castel, in a particularly brilliant and perverse turn, isolates this question of sequestration as the crucial moment in the rise of psychiatric medicine, which he views, in a Foucaultdian light, as the product of rivalries for power among different disciplines and discourses. While it was clear that the government could not allow the mentally ill to disrupt the public order by their violent eccentricities, and while some of the mad could be restrained only by internment in special institutions, the idea that a third party could be designated the legal guardian of a mentally incompetent individual and, in that role, order their consignment to a hospital for a potentially indefinite period raised considerable alarm. With this mechanism of *tutelle*, the more affluent classes in particular feared a return to the ancien régime's *lettres de cachet*, which had allowed families to reassert control over their more unruly members through preemptory and indefinite imprisonment.[10] The institutions themselves, moreover, raised apparently intractable administrative problems, since they did not fit easily into existing bureaucratic paradigms. But when the concept of "therapeutic isolation" was introduced into these discussions, their aspect changed completely, according to Castel.

The idea that isolation could promote the mental health of the deranged, that it was not merely in the interest of families and the public but also, and perhaps foremost, a benefit to the mad themselves, even if they could not yet appreciate it, abruptly transformed the imprisonment of the insane into their treatment. Their prisons became asylums. While the compatibility between medical and judicial approaches to the mentally ill had been a happy but insignificant accident under the ancien régime, in the Napoleonic order it became crucial. As Castel puts it:

> the medical notion of a "special establishment" allows administrators to escape from the aporia of the hybrid "mixed establishment" and from the insoluble problems of management and financing that it creates: to what budget line should it be attached, to what ministerial department should it be assigned, etc.? But through this technical solution to a managerial problem, the political solution to a question of principle is discovered.[11]

In other words, this administrative godsend was also a profound conceptual breakthrough, which allowed for the reconciliation of public and private interests. One can see how this was so from the Marquis de Barthélemy's arguments in support of the 1813 *Législation sur les aliénés et les enfants assistés* (Legislation on the Insane and on Child Assistance). He had stated that:

> this legislation must see to it that the ills of a suffering and unfortunate man be mitigated and that his cure, if it is possible, be obtained, while at the same time taking steps to remove from a person dangerous to others or himself the means by which he might do harm. To attain this double goal, the legislation must prescribe the isolation of the insane, for this isolation, even as it protects the public from their eccentricities and excesses, offers what is, in the eyes of science, the most powerful means of cure. Happy coincidence that, in the application of rigorous measures, reconciles advantage to the sick with the public good![12]

The potentially contradictory "double goal" of the legislation had been resolved through the introduction of a specifically medical concept, which enabled lawmakers—and the public—to see the "happy coincidence" that had until then escaped them, to appreciate the previously hidden compatibility between the interests of the insane and those of society, and to exit the apparent impasse of the *tutelle*. There is one observation in particular that should be added to Castel's readings of these debates, and that is the crucial role of a specifically medical discourse in their resolution. As a discipline with its own protocols for making sense, medical science intervened in the administration of the mad with a sort of providential force, and by allowing behaviors and situations to be understood in new ways it freed the government to act on these problems in manners that would previously have been impossible or impractical. Pinel, in this sense, had not merely liberated the mad. He had also freed the government.

This conceptual breakthrough for medicine did not, of course, end the disputes between the legal and medical professions concerning madness. An 1826 doctoral thesis on "medical jurisprudence as it relates to the insane" for the Faculté de Médecine in Paris sought to reassure jurists that they did not have to "fear that justice will be invaded by medicine in those matters that concern it."[13] The author, Jean-Léon Bonfils, then offered a vigorous interpretation of the articles 489 and 504 on mental alienation in the civil code. These sections of the code established certain procedures for determining mental illness but nowhere made specific mention of a medical exam. Bonfils took it upon himself to demonstrate that only such an exam could fulfill the demands of the law and that the law therefore implicitly required it. His argument was essentially that judges were not competent to make evaluations of mental alienation and that only trained doctors could possibly satisfy the conditions of the statutes. "It is an appointed judge, assisted by a clerk and accompanied by a royal prosecutor, . . . who must certify the existence or non-existence of an illness, its nature, and its degree," Bonfils observed and then objected:

> Unless the judge, who is there to verify and testify before the tribunal to the truth of the depositions made by the witnesses, touch, for example, upon the monomaniac's soft spot, he will find against the declarations of the witnesses. . . . How then is the judge, who is not a doctor and is not familiar with the actions of various impressions upon the mind of a feeble man, let alone a sick one, and cannot therefore take them into account, how is he going to respond to article 489?[14]

The doctor knows how to touch the weak point, to put his finger on the special place that triggers the actions of the hidden illness, knows, alone, how to make it speak. For the greatest of monomania's deceptions is its intermittent nature, its ability to remain latent for prolonged periods and then to emerge suddenly in its full, florid violence as a response to certain stimuli. "From one moment to the next," Bonfils writes, "the monomania, which previously did no harm to the reasoned exercise of the citizen's rights, can either change its subject or transform into mania or dementia, placing the insane person in such a position that he no longer freely controls his actions or can undergo a judicial hearing, but is instead silenced and even imprisoned. Here again are circumstances in which a judge, no matter how much instruction he has received, can certainly not conduct an examination without the aid of a doctor."[15] The language of madness that the medical professional was able to understand and translate did not, it would seem, function on a level that could be transmitted through "instruction" alone. It played, somehow, on other registers not available to the judge, and it is this peculiar relation to madness that separates the medical practitioner from the jurist. Only the doctor, whose training goes beyond theoretical principles to the actual frequentation and treatment of the mad, possessed this almost mystical sensitivity to the nature of their illness, only the doctor shared this special bond with the monomaniac's irrationality. Part of the doctor's authority thus derived from a skill that could not be taught, from a message that was spoken in a language he could learn only from the mad themselves as aided by his own disciplinary pre-disposition. This irrational and unspeakable element formed a crucial part in Bonfils's ideas about the specificity of medical practice, about its form of knowledge and its status as discourse. The mad, it would seem, lent the power of their otherness to the legitimacy of medicine.

But the secret meanings of the insane formed only part of a larger language that was accessible to scientists and doctors alone, a language that gave rise to its own rules and codifications, its own systems of decryption. And it is not an anachronism to speak of semiology in reference to these studies, for the word *séméiologique* was pervasively used in them.[16] Indeed, it originated in the eighteenth century as a medical term for the science of the body's signs. The rise of this semiology helped define medical discourse as a distinctive code endowed with unique abilities to understand certain otherwise incomprehensible aspects of human nature.[17] Like many doctors, Pierre Debreyne used the difference between two different kinds of indicators to demonstrate the uniqueness and importance of medical discourse—its very existence, in fact—explaining that the symptom was a physical anomaly inseparable from a pathological condition, while the sign was that same symptom as interpreted and explained by competent authorities. The former was a physical condition, the latter "the fruit of an intellectual combination or operation, that is to say of a judgment." And for this reason, while anyone might notice that a patient was, say, coughing up blood or having trouble breathing, "these phenomena, for the ordinary man, remain in the state of symptoms; the doctor alone knows how to convert them into signs."[18] In this sense, when alienists such as Bonfils contended that they spoke a special language, they were basing their arguments on a rigorous notion of sign systems and the ongoing self-definition of medicine as a unique and dynamic form of discourse. Cabanis had already described some of the difficulties of medical *séméiotique* in his 1798 volume *Du degré de certitude de la médecine*, arguing that the ability to see through various symptoms to their underlying cause came in a single *coup d'œil*, whose almost spiritual power derived from the physician's sympathy with the sufferer.[19] He had gone on to draw broader conclusions about the transmissibility of medical knowledge, writing: "The knowledge that one acquires in schools or in books can neither impart nor cultivate the wisdom of the senses. The rules of poetry do not make a great poet, nor those of music a great musician. Talent is rare and cannot be passed down. The true knowledge of our art is not a more or less complete set of impressions gathered at the bedside of the sick."[20] Doctors knew, from practice, how to touch and provoke, how to make nature speak and respond. Our very term semiotics is based in this distinctive medical intercourse with an unintelligible other, this codification of a mystery that could not be taught.

In conclusion to his long argument about the incompetence of judges to identify madness, Bonfils quoted one of the leading proponents of the monomania thesis, Etienne-Jean Georget: "In Paris, no director of a mental institution should accept a sick person without a certificate from his attending physician attesting his mental alienation."[21] Georget's presence is not surprising, for as psychiatry became the leading edge for a more generalized border dispute between medicine and the courts, within psychiatry itself the main force of the conflict was further localized onto a single point—the diagnosis of monomania.[22] Georget was not only one of the most visible figures in the monomania debate, he was also one of the most controversial and became a convenient target for opponents. Elias Regnault, for instance, also cited him, but in order to dismiss the entire concept of monomania. "A new word has made its way into criminal law," he wrote in 1828. "MONOMANIA has, for several years, been constantly invoked in the court of assizes. The lawyer has seized hold of this medico-legal entity as the final hope in a lost cause; the doctor thinks he has found a new glory to exploit; and the juror has encountered only a new series of uncertainties and troubles in a task that is already so difficult."[23] Regnault was, in large part, simply reiterating arguments that had been made earlier, even among some in the medical establishment itself. In 1826, for example, the doctor Urbain Coste had already dismissed the reasoning employed by authors like Bonfils. "In good faith," Coste wrote, "there is not a single man of sound judgment who is not as competent as Mr. Pinel or Mr. Esquirol in these matters and who has not the advantage over them of being a stranger to any scientific prejudices. Unfortunately, doctors have taken the polite gesture of the tribunals seriously, and in examining the questions submitted to them have all too often replaced the natural light of reason with the ambitious ignorance of their parochial interests."[24]

Despite the ongoing controversy about the sheer existence of monomania and the competence of judges, or other nonspecialists, to identify the symptoms of insanity, the importance of medical opinion in the control of madness was nonetheless officially recognized in a law passed on June 30, 1838. The legislation marked a turning point in the legal status of psychiatry and, more generally, medical science. As Castel has observed, this was "the first great legislative measure to recognize a *right to assistance and to care* for a category of indigents and sick people. It [was] the first to set in place an entire aid mechanism, which included the invention of a new space—the asylum—the creation of an initial corps of government doctors, the establishment of a 'specialized knowledge,' etc."[25] With this move, madness became not only an "affair of state," as Castel puts it, but so did medical opinion.[26]

The legislation might have redefined psychiatry's legal status, but something of the pragmatic, perhaps disillusioned approach that Marchal de Calvi had brought to bear in his arguments about the value of medical testimony at Bertrand's court-martial continued to inflect theoretical and nosological discussions among doctors. It surfaced in an exchange about monomania between the doctors Alexandre-Jacques-François Brierre de Boismont and Bénédicte-August Morel, both of whom had written articles on the sergeant's case. Although Brierre seems to have sided personally with his colleague's skepticism about the existence of monomania, he felt it inexpedient to express such hesitations in public, especially when they might be taken up by members of the judicial system to cast doubt on the legal competence of medical science. "My opinions on monomania are, then, basically similar to those of Monsieur Morel," Brierre wrote. "Only I believe the moment has not yet come for arguing this [antimonomania] thesis. The true ideas that Esquirol's doctrine leads us to propound are far from being accepted in society, and I fear that their numerous opponents would seize on this dissension among doctors in order to stage a new protest." Brierre went on to add that Morel "does not share our fears about the benefit that the jurisconsults could reap from this disunion" among medical theorists.[27] In short, the relations between doctors and the courts about the status of madness were intense, often conflictual, and sometimes surprisingly cynical. They were also grounded in the notion of an almost occult knowledge of the human organism.

As with the jurists, the question of madness played a central role in the relations between the Church and the medical profession, and here again, the debate centered on the notion of free will and individual responsibility. Although the priest Pierre Debreyne, for instance, accepted the general notion of monomania, he was deeply troubled by certain subcategories of the condition advanced by alienists. "We repeat," he wrote, "that we cannot accept the theory or principle of monomania with irresistible inclination and without delirium in the act, because it seems to us dangerous, in the sense that it suspends the effects of free will, destroys the morality of human actions, and tends to encourage the impunity of crimes; for if the inclination is *irresistible* and without delirium in the act, what becomes of free will?"[28] Although in this passage he speaks only of crimes, on the next page he will expand his concerns to the realm of the more properly religious in arguing that "this doctrine of forensic doctors (monomania without delirium) obviously tends to destroy free will or the *moral liberty* of human actions."[29] Similar to Carrière, Debreyne does not assert that his opinion about monomania is more *true* than that of the alienists; he contends, instead, that it is less *dangerous*. The criterion for its acceptance is not epistemological but practical, and its danger is that, if accepted, it could destroy the notion of free will and, with it, the category of subjective responsibility. For both the clergy and the jurists, this new medical diagnosis threatened the very subject that underlay their access to and control of individuals.

A Specifically Irrational Legitimacy

As doctors pressed their claim that the value of their intellectual approach reached far beyond the scope of their discipline itself to broader social issues, the irrationality of madness began to play an increasingly crucial role in establishing the specificity and impact of medical discourse. Robert Castel has written that psychiatry was the first medical specialization, the field in which modern medicine initially defined itself as a determinate and authoritative body of knowledge.[30] We have already seen that process of accreditation at work in the relation between the legal and medical professions and in the way that psychiatry lent doctors an unprecedented authority in respect to the court system. A core element of their argument was, as I have shown, the unique relationship that they supposedly enjoyed with insanity, the special access to the mad that they claimed to enjoy. Bonfils maintained, for instance, that his colleagues possessed an understanding of monomaniacs that could not simply be learned through theoretical principles, but that must be acquired by a careful frequentation of the mentally ill. From this perspective, the protocols of scientific thought shaped the behavior of doctors, so that something about medical practice, about the demeanor even of the practitioner, created a special familiarity and understanding between him and the insane. The paradoxical result was that the proponents of a rationalized science presented themselves as the only members of society capable of understanding unreason and grounded their legitimacy as a social force in that very understanding, in that fundamentally unspeakable relation to insanity. This can be seen again in 1864, when the doctor Henri Legrand du Saulle rejoiced, somewhat prematurely, that the legal credibility of medical testimony had finally been established and that "in a criminal trial where a question of morbid psychology is debated, the juridical consequences must be the necessary consequence of the diagnosis that is made."[31] To hear him tell it, the real center of power in courts had moved from the judges' bank to the witness stand, for it was, in his view, expert testimony that determined the findings of the magistrates and bore, in this sense, the ultimate responsibility for assigning guilt. The decisions of the justices were, in this regard, a mere extension of the doctors' opinions. He went on to claim that:

> there is no longer any disagreement about the need for doctors' participation and the usefulness of their assistance: interpreters of a language unknown to the magistrates, they translate in the course of a trial impressions of the loftiest order. We have a right to be proud of the role that has been entrusted to us, and we must try always to fulfill it; but nothing is more difficult than to hold a conquered soil intact [*conserver intact un sol conquis*]. . . . We have wanted to protect the failings of a damaged brain from the harsh rigors of the law, and our deposition has been classified among the sentimental eccentricities of the defense. We have wanted too, in face of an utterly shipwrecked free will, to save the head of someone who suffers from an incurable disease, and our influence has often led to nothing more than a senseless [*inintelligent*] verdict.[32]

Some of the metaphorics is familiar, such as the evocation of a battlefield to describe the rivalry between medical and legal discourses. The idea of a "*sol conquis*" led Legrand, however, along different semantic resonances towards the "sentimental eccentricities" of which the doctors stood accused. Their knowledge lay somehow outside: closer than others to the zones of sentiment, affect, and irrationality, they spoke from beyond the limits of reason, from the *carte du tendre* and the realms of the mad themselves. A strange reproach against the language of science: it is too irrational, too sentimental. It calls from those spaces that sergeant Bertrand had by his own account sought out—the fringes of society, of the intelligible, of the human. For in Enlightenment theorizations of the state, the mad were the region outside: as Diderot and Rousseau had argued, the bonds of the social order are the laws of reason, and those who refuse them are, by definition, irrational and inhuman.[33] Indeed, madness and social exclusion were almost one and the same thing for them, a form of inhuman animality. The verdicts handed down by justices under the sway of medical arguments had too often, according to Legrand, been "senseless." The threat of an encroaching subrational nonsense haunts his conception of expert testimony, but his defense against this danger was to better understand the relation between doctors and their patients. The medical practitioner did not himself speak in the language of the mad, but instead translated it. Somehow, through medical intervention, the utterances of the inhuman could paradoxically be made human, sense could be found in the nonsensical gibbering of the insane, reason in the irrational. Never, perhaps, had the task of the translator been greater or more crucial: the doctor reincorporated the very principle of the nonsocial into the social. But the translation did not render the patient into a typical legal subject; he or she was socialized only within the protocols of medical interpretation. To treat the sufferer as a normal citizen would amount to punishing the innocent or to liberating the dangerous, and consequently when courts treated the mad according to their usual criteria, it was the verdict—and justice—that became senseless. What the law by itself could not recognize or accommodate, then, was how mental illness transformed the very nature of the responsible individual subjectivity on which modern jurisprudence and Enlightenment social order were grounded.

For the space inhabited by the mad lay also, in various and complicated ways, beyond the reach of justice. In his 1826 medical dissertation, Bonfils wrote of them that "for all time and among all civilized peoples, these unfortunates have been considered to be outside the law [*hors la loi*] in respect to social duties, to the culpability of their actions, and to the punishments which for other men ordinarily follow on their crimes."[34] Unintelligible, unmappable, the actions of the insane fell under no sure jurisdiction because, in some way, they passed unrecognized, invisible, and inaudible to the courts. A chorus of voices corroborated this conception. Even though he argued against the monomania thesis, Elias Regnault acknowledged the possibility, at least, of a madness that would be visible only to a doctor, a case where only such a specialist could "declare the existence of that sickness and recognize it, when it is still hidden to the world."[35] Some seven years before Legrand du Saulle described doctors as "interpreters of a language unknown to the magistrates," and noted how, in that capacity, they themselves had been misunderstood and their testimony in court "classified among the sentimental eccentricities of the defense," the neurologist Jean-Martin Charcot had argued, like so many of his colleagues, that medical expertise was necessary to translate the spontaneous symptoms of nature into a system of intelligible signs.[36] Only doctors could appreciate the transformation that madness forced on the notion of legal subjectivity and they could appreciate it only because of their special relation to the language of unreason. But in their ability to see what others could not, to speak an idiom that for their contemporaries was noise when even audible, in penetrating a realm beyond the law, doctors themselves ran the risk of incomprehension, of being judged to have passed *outside* into the meaningless realm of eccentricity and sentiment. Their brief, in this case, was therefore to argue the value of that eccentric space, to defend the significance of affect, and thereby to enlarge the notion of the social by including in it a vast expanse unmastered by the legal system. By arguing that one could be mad and human, they created an extra-legal, purely medical person.

On the one hand, even Latour acknowledged that there was something useful about medical thinking, whether or not the latter was a science. On the other, psychiatry was one of the principal fields through which doctors established the credibility and unique value of their discipline. And since, as I have argued, the legitimacy of psychiatric medicine was grounded in the unintelligibility of the mad, medicine's usefulness appears to have derived from its relation not to truth but to untruth, despite the contrary impressions of later commentators like Proust. Doctors' social credentials thus depended paradoxically on the illegitimacy of the unsocial. The extraordinary force that propelled them from relative obscurity into their modern position of relative dominance came not from within the social order, not from the protocols of reason or the power of legal argument alone, but more importantly from some strange outside, some meaningless elsewhere. Whereas the utterances and behavior of the mad could be translated into juridically comprehensible statements, the laws governing their language remained different and even unspeakable. The precarious and often incongruous arguments about the utility of medicine were thus subordinated to another logic—or rather illogic —of the irrational, which revealed its significance not to the clarity of organized thought but to other, more obscure sorts of processes, which were caught up in the fabric of experience and ethics. These other laws revealed themselves only in practices like the frequentation of the mad. But if medicine was useful to society because it made the mad intelligible in their unintelligibility, the mad were useful to medicine because they conferred on doctors a special, extra-judicial authority. And if the eccentricity of the mad made doctors eccentric, it was because their status beyond the laws moved their caregivers and interpreters beyond the law as well. On the disputed terrains, the borders, and the *sol conquis* between medicine and the law, the space of insanity was off the charts, a rich and uncivilized continent to be colonized.

By affirming two contradictory propositions, doctors were able to resolve a fundamental dichotomy that the Enlightenment had opened up in the relation between the social order and its others. Medicine offered the promise that those others were not, in fact, so different as they had seemed, that their alterity could be grasped and controlled. Its usefulness derived not only from an increasing success in curing ailments or from more detailed and compelling descriptions of the animal body, but also, and most importantly, from the ability to *translate* an irrational language into a socially recognizable and meaningful idiom. That translation assured that madness did not represent an alternate worldview but was rather an epiphenomenon of reason, a deviant and defective version of the same natural laws that were becoming intelligible to science. The doctor's trained ear was thus an organ that guaranteed against a Manichaean world in which alternate primal realities vie against each other and promised, in its place, a rational natural order, troubled only by incidental lapses and flaws. At the same time, however, doctors argued conversely that the others of society—the mad and their companions among the former denizens of the ancien régime's hospitals—were indeed so different that they could be incorporated into the community only if the community transformed itself and effectively became other to what it had been. A new, extra-legal subjectivity would be required, along with an entire discipline to accommodate it. Medicine derived its authority from its privileged relation to this unknown, this asocial being that dwelt outside the city, this thinking that was inimical, indeed hostile to humanity. Insofar as madness represented a zone ruled by irrational sentiments and affect, a zone where subjective projections and fantasies passed for truths, it was the realm of the purely imaginary.

Death Becomes a Medical Condition

Madness was not the only manifestation of uncivil alterity. Despite psychiatry's importance to the rise of medicine, another domain of scientific inquiry was probably even more crucial to its history, for during the Enlightenment and its aftermath, doctors played a key role in revolutionizing the understanding and mastery of a deeper and more universal mystery of human existence—death.[37] As a social category, mortality had previously fallen largely under the purview of the Church, which ministered to it through pastoral care, and the government, which administered it either as punishment or in war. Except in the case of legitimate self-defense, the individual appropriation of the power to kill was generally criminal and as such fell outside the social order. During the eighteenth century, however, the power over death increasingly lost its one-sided meaning as the ability to kill and acquired a converse value as the capacity to stave off mortality. It would be difficult to exaggerate the breadth and significance of this transformation but difficult, also, to perceive it, since it has become so much a part of our own relation to the human condition. One can detect, however, echoes of the almost incredulous excitement these changes inspired in the pages of Louis-Sébastien Mercier's *Tableau de Paris* (Picture of Paris), published just before the revolution of 1789. "The beautiful and new experiments performed on the decomposition and recomposition of air," he wrote, "offer us useful aids unknown to all of antiquity."[38] The formulation is strange and striking, perhaps difficult to appreciate at first, but what Mercier is saying is that antiquity has just ended and that its end is marked, effected in fact, by just these kinds of experiments. They are beautiful and new; already, that the two words should go together marks a separation from the aesthetics and ideology of the past, not so much an echo of the quarrel between the ancients and the moderns as that turning point in the idea of novelty that will eventually develop into an anxious longing in Baudelaire's poetry. The studies themselves concern decomposition and recomposition. I will discuss shortly the value of the first term in relation to contemporary theories of death; the second is perhaps even more remarkable. Putrefaction, the work of death, has its own, singsong obverse: in the very notion of such "recomposition," the work of decay is reversed, the air purified, life restored. A strange hope haunts the very word. Mercier continues:

> and to the extent that the government is inclined to encourage these curious dis-coveries (which hold the promise of others), the great cities will have one less scourge to bear. It is impossible that indolence and insensitivity should close the government's eyes to the miracles of chemistry. This science, freed from its old formulae, seems at last to bring before benighted humanity the true remedies that it had previously misunderstood. . . . The work of the chemists has reduced the number of accidents occasioned by emptying latrines, wells, and cesspools [*fosses d'aisance, puits & puisards*]. We now know what for so long we did not, *viz.* what mephitic air is, and in what manner we can combat its dangerous and deadly influ-ences. The benefits of chemistry are each day more numerous and offer methods that are in the essential interest of humanity.
>
> More than ever before the government consults these useful physicians.[39]

He is writing about emptying latrines, and yet, in these unexpected corners of Paris, a miracle is taking place. Finally, the science of chemistry has come into its own, full with the promise of endless advantages to the fundamental concerns of humanity. But among the accidents that plague the city, the only one that Mercier identifies even indirectly is death—this is the exemplary concern of urban space. At last one can combat "dangerous and deadly influ-ences." One can fight death. One can, to some extent, even win. As Mercier's contemporary Antoine-Alexis Cadet-De-Vaux put it: "Such are the means, at once so efficacious and so simple, to annihilate mephitism and to command, in some manner, over life and death."[40]

By the early nineteenth century, however, the focus of scientific studies on death had shifted from chemistry to physiology, almost entirely under the impetus of Xavier Bichat's *Recherches physiologiques sur la vie et la mort* (Physio-logical Studies on Life and Death), first published in 1799 and then reissued throughout the following century.[41] It is difficult to exaggerate the impor-tance of Bichat for modern medicine, for he was probably the key figure responsible for the rise of the Paris school and for the central role that clinical pathology assumed there.[42] Life, for him and his followers, could only be understood through its context and effects, or as Bichat himself put it: "Such indeed is the mode of existence for living bodies, that everything around them aims to destroy them. Inorganic bodies constantly act upon them; they themselves exercise upon each other a continuous action; they would soon succumb did they not contain a permanent principle of reaction. This princi-ple is that of life; unknown in its nature, it can only be appreciated by its phenomena."[43] This notion of reactivity was fundamental to Bichat's conception of animation, and he summarized his approach in what was to become the slogan of the vitalist movement for the next half century: *"Life is the set of functions that resist death."*[44] Life, for him, was negative, a force whose underlying principle resided in the continuous struggle against the more primordial actions of a surrounding inorganic world.[45] Although the vitalist movement began to fade by the middle of the nineteenth century, the power of Bichat's theoretical paradigm endured much longer, moving through various metamorphoses in Magendie and the latter's student Claude Bernard.[46] Freud adapted Bichat's basic proposition in 1920 when he speculated that *eros*, or sexual desire, acts as the counterforce to *thanatos*, the regressive urge toward a more fundamental, inanimate state.[47] The core of Bichat's innovation was to isolate life and death as objects of study and to recast them in terms of physiological conditions. For him, the two forces could be conceptualized as such only through a specialized knowledge of the body. As objects of study they had, in other words, become part of medicine.

Auguste Comte, somewhat forgotten now but one of the most important French philosophers of the nineteenth century and a disciple of Bichat's vitalist theory, sketched out some of the implications of his revolution:

> the sheer notion of life presupposes existences that are not endowed with it . . .
> Ultimately, living beings can only exist in inert media, which furnish them with
> both a support and a source of direct or indirect nourishment . . . If everything
> were alive, no natural law would be possible. For variability, always inherent in
> vital spontaneity, finds itself truly limited only by the preponderance of the inert
> medium.[48]

Inorganic matter—the stuff of death—was thus the great legislator of the natural world, the unbending and regular force that lent system to the impulses of life and laid down the bases of its laws.[49] For Comte, the principal occupation of humankind should, however, be to resist this legislation, "increasingly to unite all of living nature for a permanent struggle against the whole of the inorganic world," and to "direct all of living nature against dead nature, in order to exploit the terrestrial domain" in what he called "the ongoing league of life against death."[50] This was the basic ontological imperative of humanity for him. Death is everywhere, and it must be the primary concern of the living, not by preparing for some potential afterlife, but through the ongoing resistance to a relentlessly destructive force. Our very being hinged, for Comte, on our relation of dependence and allergy to inanimate matter; this relation bound us together with all that lives and confronted us—as the strongest and the most able—with the moral imperative to defend all weaker living beings. This resistance was the most basic form of the progress that Comte, in the epigraph to his *Système de politique positive*, called the goal of humanity, its inherent ethical responsibility to all manifestations of life, down even to plants (which might help explain the strange dedicatory poem entitled "The Thoughts of a Flower" that opens *Système*). The result of over half a century of research and debate in the field of physiology, Comte's monumental, perhaps deliriously optimistic system indicates the defining role that medicine had acquired as a field, for to fight death, as he proposed, one must know it, and those who knew death were the doctors, since they alone could speak its newly discovered language.

But endlessly and inherently fugitive, life as such escaped definition. As Bichat wrote, its principle, "whose nature is unknown . . . can only be appreciated through its phenomena." Or Félix Gannal, in 1868: "it is by its effects, and more as a result than a principle, that one observes life."[51] This elusiveness was complicated by the fact that life's opposite was just as indeterminate in its essence, a problem that led Eugène Bouchut to observe in 1849: "One day, perhaps, we will go farther if we succeed in discovering the secret of the material conditions of life, and then, instead of purely and simply observing that act, to which so many different phenomena are attached, we will point to life and say: here is what death is."[52] One knew only the remains of the vital force itself, the inanimate signs of its fleeting passage. Every physiological study was thus like a murder scene, for it attempted to reconstruct a missing existence through the circumstances of its absence. It is probably no accident that the detective novel emerged as a literary genre during this same period, since it resolved, in narrative form, a new but fundamental intellectual problem—the identification of a life through the particulars of its disappearance.[53] Such a connection between abstract philosophy and popular entertainment might seem improbable, but there were practical consequences to the conceptual indeterminacy of life, and these problems seem to have created the kind of generalized anxiety among the nineteenth-century French that would have stimulated popular literary production and consumption. A segment of the public had become aware that vital signs could sometimes be so illegible or so deeply hidden in the complexities of inorganic matter that they might fool even the most practiced eye, as in certain cataleptic states that could easily be mistaken for death.[54] The idea of such confusion led to a pervasive fear of premature burial, and as a consequence a specialized literature arose, intended to help physicians identify death.[55] Both Gannal and Bouchut authored monographs on the subject, while in the United States, Edgar Allan Poe—more appreciated by intellectuals in France than in his home country—devoted a short story to the dreadful futility of such efforts.[56] One could interpret these developments to mean that any interest in the more abstract issues of life and death stemmed from concerns about their practical consequences—there could, for instance, be serious inconveniences in being mistaken for a corpse. Or, conversely, one could see these practical concerns as displacements of a more fundamental anxiety about a particular conceptual indeterminacy. The sheer fact that the public grew fretful about premature burial during this period suggests that it did, in some way, perceive a change or destabilization in the category of death. To worry about being buried alive was, in this respect, to ask in a nervous, popularized form: what is death? And the response—like the question itself—could no longer come from lawyers, priests, or other representatives of the traditional social order. It was now expected from doctors. They were the ones who were called on to verify the end of life. And their new role was recognized officially in the person of the "doctor of the dead [*médecin des morts*]," the physician who was authorized by the government to determine if an individual had deceased.[57]

The Medico-Legal Status of the Dead

Further evidence of this epistemological shift in the principle of life emerged in the relations between the medical profession and the legal system. The fact that in 1785 the Lieutenant General of Police placed the exhumation of the Saints-Innocents cemetery in Paris under the control of the Société Royale de Médecine mostly reflects the hygienic concerns raised by the unearthing and transfer of noxious substances; it also shows, however, that the dead already fell under that category and that their disposal and treatment were thus beginning to be officially recognized as medical issues.[58] In contrast, moreover, to ongoing disputes about the qualifications necessary to identify madness, nineteenth-century courts accepted the need for medical expertise in certifying that someone was in fact dead. "As soon as a death is declared," wrote Paul Brouardel, "the verifying doctor, whom the public calls somewhat ironically 'the doctor of the dead,' presents himself at the home of the deceased in order to perform the examinations required by law. Aside from the officers sent to verify, and as a measure of quality control, the Prefect of the Seine nominates a certain number of doctors as inspectors, who must examine at least one corpse in three. This service is very well organized in Paris and it offers all possible guarantees; in all the large cities, in Lyons and in Bordeaux, there is an analogous service."[59]

Despite the Hypocratic oath's injunction to cause no harm, the doctors' participation in helping the courts identify death and the police quarantine it was probably less important than their role in causing it, for nowhere did they intervene more decisively in its jurisprudence than with the administration of capital punishment. The historian Robert Favre has argued that the instrumentalization of death played a crucial role in Enlightenment theories of law and social order, which largely heeded Montesquieu's warning in the *Esprit des lois* (The Spirit of the Laws) that "one must be careful not to inspire in men too much contempt for death: otherwise they will escape the legislator."[60] The newly ascendant medical profession played a central role in this social use of death. It was a doctor, Joseph Ignace Guillotin, who first proposed to the Constituent Assembly, on December 1, 1789—less than five months after the fall of the Bastille—that the "method of punishment shall be the same for all persons on whom the law shall pronounce a sentence of death, whatever the crime of which they are guilty. The criminal shall be decapitated. Decapitation is to be effected by a simple mechanism."[61]

It was also a doctor, Pierre-Jean-Georges Cabanis, whom the Assembly entrusted with overseeing the design and testing of the machine. Although the basic equipment already existed and had been used in other countries, two aspects of its implementation made it, as a punishment, unique to the French Revolution, which, in Cabanis's words, "seems to have taken the guillotine as its standard."[62] First, its adoption was determined by a national legislative body that considered it to be a central element in the ideology of their nascent state. As Cabanis would put it some six years later: "The death of a man, ordered for the public interest, is without doubt the greatest act of social force."[63] The adoption or rejection of the machine to effect that act of social power had, furthermore, to be argued on the basis of its relation to the goals and nature of a republic that was itself still very much in the formative stages. The state, consequently, would not merely be a criterion to determine the fate of the machine; the machine, for its part, would also become a criterion by which to shape the nature of the state. For Hegel, who addressed the issue at length in the *Phenomenology of Spirit*, the guillotine was more than the mere emblem of the French Revolution: it was the very embodiment of its fundamental ideological principles, the instantiation of a social structure which generally, everywhere and for everyone, sought to annihilate individual particularity and experience through an identification with the absolute concept of freedom.[64]

Second, the legislature handed over the pragmatic aspects of that instantiation to doctors. After effecting some modifications suggested by a surgeon, the *administration des hôpitaux* (hospital administration), with the participation of Cabanis, subjected the guillotine to a series of tests. In recommending its use, Guillotin had promised that his machine would deliver a painless death, a pure cessation of being, and that its blade would, in this sense, section the new republic from the ancien régime of theatrical torture executions. To make that determination, however, it was not enough simply to observe the functioning of the mechanism or its physical effects on animal bodies, for the victims could not report on their experiences. Because the latter had to be deduced, it was necessary to interpret what one saw by translating symptoms into signs. For that, a highly specialized knowledge was needed, one grounded in a reliable theoretical and semiotic system that was capable of making the silences of the animate world speak. And so, when Cabanis wanted to ascertain whether the subject did or did not feel pain, he approached the problem by trying to identify the physical position of the *moi*—or "I"—within the body. "We are speaking here of sensations relative to the individual's 'I': these are the only ones that concern us," he wrote, adding a few pages later:

> Microscopic discoveries have taught us that life is everywhere; that, as a result, there is everywhere pleasure and pain; and in the very organization of our fibers there can exist innumerable causes of individual lives, whose correspondence and harmony with the whole system, by means of nerves, constitutes the "I." . . . [T]he "I" exists only in the general life: and the sensitivity of the fibers, when they are isolated, no more corresponds to it than does the sensitivity of the animals that can develop in various parts of the body.[65]

The guillotine engages the individual as a whole—that is the "I" that is in question here. Its death is understood to provide access to the subject as subject, for the latter exists only in the elusive principle of life itself, diffused throughout the bodily system as a whole rather than concentrated in any of the particular organs or cells that populate it. In a newly and at least theoretically democratic society—indeed in a suddenly and convulsively democratic one—the individual votes and dies as such. What is more, the person on whom the social order, in its greatest act of authority, imposes death can be identified only through medical theorizations such as Cabanis's. The guillo-tine was, in this regard, as much a clinical as a judicial instrument, indeed perhaps more so. Its conceptualization and functioning reveal not only that death had become a medical category, but also that any subjectivity grounded in death had consequently become one too.[66]

With their training in physiology, doctors had learned to read the silent language of corpses in a way that no one else could. They alone were able to determine reliably whether people were alive or not and how they died. If pure death replaced torture executions and assumed the status of maximum punishment under French law during this period, it was, at least in part, because physiologists had acquired the theoretical understanding necessary to identify and deliver such a condition. The guillotine, by suppressing the art of the executioner and the spontaneous individuality of the executed, rep-resented an attempt to isolate death as a mechanical intervention within two systems: on the one hand the judicial process, in which it was held to function as a uniform standard for all capital offenses, and on the other the organic life of the criminal, which it was supposed to end with an almost conceptual precision. As such, and with a unique symbolic significance within the social order, the guillotine expressed human law as an extension of those larger laws of nature to which scientists alone had access.[67]

A somewhat paradoxical relation consequently emerged between medicine and the law in respect to mortality, for on the one hand doctors' vocation and training opposed them to death, while on the other they were becoming the sole members of society who could understand and interpret it, and as such were emerging as its administrators. Cabanis wrote, "I vote with all of my heart for abolishing punishment by the guillotine . . .," but not from any concern over the pain it might cause or from an opposition to capital punishment itself. Instead, he felt that its appearance should be made more spectacular and terrifying. "As long as capital punishment is preserved," he wrote, "it will be necessary at least to make its apparatus imposing . . . That apparatus itself must make the punishment more rare and difficult."[68] Despite all the Enlightenment efforts to free mankind from a senseless fear of mortal-ity, Cabanis found himself arguing that one fights best against death not by minimizing its importance but, on the contrary, by making it even more terri-ble.[69] Still, not all of Cabanis's colleagues would have agreed with him, and even if, as Robert Favre has written, the "legal terror" of death, "inscribed in physiological and cosmological nature, inseparable from the conflicts stemming from social life, is the unshakable rock" of human life and the source, in some perverse way, of its stability and order, doctors continued to militate against this legislative force of nature in their very attempt to over-come death.[70] The complicated ethical position of medical practitioners in relation to capital punishment was probably best encapsulated by Edouard Carrière in one of his 1849 articles on the principle of authority in medicine. "Like you," he wrote, "I want to put an end to burnings at the stake and do away with guillotines, but I think that authority must be respected and must make itself respected."[71] His "yes, but" approach to abolishing public beheadings and burnings sums up the ambiguous and uncomfortable moral position of his profession at the middle of the nineteenth century, and it is telling that his reservations about combating mortality and minimizing pain—which must surely count among the fundamental principles of medi-cine—emerge from a concern about authority. Death was the enemy, but the medical profession had gained a unique social legitimacy through *intelligence* with it. Suppressing the guillotine and other forms of execution apparently would have represented a loss of status and power not only for the govern-ment, but also for doctors, who had become necessary to the conceptualiza-tion and administration of capital punishment.

Authority over the Dead

Despite its interest in death as both crime and penalty, the legal system seems to have shown only a modest concern for corpses, offering them little in the way of specific protections. Although article 360 of the 1810 penal code established punishments for various crimes committed in cemeteries, includ-ing those that occurred as part of an *attentat aux mœurs* (indecent act), when sergeant Bertrand was finally apprehended, there was no law that directly addressed the issue of corpse rape, and he was consequently arraigned on the relatively minor charge of "violating a tomb or sepulcher."[72] Indeed, one of the expert witnesses at the court-martial brought attention to this anomaly, protesting the disproportion between what the soldier had done and the legal categories for recognizing and punishing it.[73] From the expert's point of view, it seems, Bertrand's actions exceeded the imagination of the law, so that their full horror could be appreciated only by a different sort of discourse. The penal code and courts were concerned with the corpse only insofar as it rep-resented an extension of the person it had once embodied. On the other hand, the alienists who commented on the case concentrated on the person of the criminal and spoke of his victims only as features of his pathology. In approaching the issue from this perspective, they indirectly attributed a certain, unspoken agency to the deceased as deceased. The problem, from the alienists' perspective, was therefore not so much what Bertrand did to the dead as what the dead did to him. The horror of his case resulted, for them, from his subjectivity and its unusual relation to cadavers. By the alienists' reasoning, the latter had clearly infiltrated Bertrand's sense of self-identity in a way that could not be countenanced by society, even if it was not clear why that particular relation was so objectionable. Bertrand's court-martial indicated that while the dead were still active in society and could affect fundamental legal categories such as subjectivity, they nonetheless escaped, in some crucial way, the grasp of the law. And yet, for their own part, the alienists did little better in trying to understand the psychological significance of the dead, for they made no attempt to explore the fantasmatic specificity of human remains, the way in which they embodied an extreme pathological agency—not only for Bertrand, but also for the public that found his crimes at once so exceptionally horrifying and fascinating. In the discussions surrounding Bertrand's case, the dead were recognized, at least indirectly, as a significant legal and medical problem, but there was as yet no legal or medical apparatus available for dealing with them.

The Church had long enjoyed a near monopoly on the dead, who fell almost entirely under its care spiritually and physically. The rising importance of medicine, however, challenged the clergy on both these points. In respect to spiritual issues, one can trace the conflict back to the eighteenth century, when the *idéologues* had attempted to resolve or reject the Cartesian notion of a dichotomy between the body and soul.[74] While many of the members in the group, including Buffon, Condillac, and Helvétius, had difficulty in excluding an immaterial principle entirely from their conception of life, their more radical colleagues, such as the Baron d'Holbach and Cabanis, argued for an entirely materialist explanation of consciousness and other mental functions. The activities of the mind could be explained completely, according to these thinkers, by the constitution and behavior of the body. This meant that philosophy, anthropology, and ethics should all be dependent on medical science, or, as Destutt de Tracy wrote: "What is called *idéologie* is not, cannot be, and should not be but a part and derivation of physiology; one cannot ever be an *idéologue* without first being a physiologist."[75] These men and other like-minded contemporaries—such as the German neuroanatomist S. T. Soemmering, the Englishman Robert Whytt, and

the group around Bordeu, Barthez, and Fouquet at the School of Montpellier—had a tremendous influence on subsequent generations of thinkers,
leaving their impress on some of the most important scientists, philosophers,
and even artists of the nineteenth century.[76] For a significant number of intellectuals and other educated individuals, in short, physiology was not merely
a study of the body it was also a fundamental intellectual paradigm. And
although Maine de Biran would spend his last years as a devout Catholic, the
principles advanced by the *idéologues* as a whole contested one of the basic
tenets of Christian belief: the existence of an eternal soul. The priest Pierre
Debreyne would thus have reason to complain, in 1845, that physicians were
"too often unbelievers or of very little religious faith," for as members of a
profession almost entirely shaped by intellectual tendencies such as *idéologie*,
they were virtually by definition antipathetic to Church doctrine.[77]

By redefining mortality as a purely organic process, philosophical movements such as *idéologie* mounted a direct and pervasive challenge to the
Church's positions on the transcendental value of death. Simultaneously,
under the influence of new findings in medicine and physiology, the meaning and appearance of corpses began to change. No longer a mere *memento
mori*, they had now evolved into agents of death, who were believed to cause
life-threatening illnesses through the effects of miasmas and putrefaction.
This emphasis on the dangerous physiology of decay led doctors to advocate
changes in public policy that had, in turn, direct practical consequences for
the clergy. Over the course of the eighteenth century, hygienists, for example, exerted increasingly successful pressure on the government to force the
removal of corpses from churches and adjacent spaces into cemeteries
located safely outside the city. As the police and government yielded to the
hygienists' proposition that even when buried the dead represented a public
health concern, ecclesiastics responded with steady and vocal resistance.
Their arguments, however, generally accepted the premise that cadavers
were insalubrious and as such legitimate medical concerns, thus yielding the
most significant element in the new epistemology of death. At the same
time, they tended to emphasize the pragmatic or monetary difficulties that
changes in policy would entail, rather than their implications for dogma or
the spiritual identity of the Church. In a handwritten response to a series of
edicts from 1763 and 1765 that proscribed the burying of corpses inside the
capital, the parish priests, or *curés*, of Paris accepted the idea that corpses
gave off dangerous gases, but they argued that the new laws would create
delays that would only increase exposure to those gases. And although the

authors observed that "the removal [of sepulchers] . . . must soon accustom Christians to think that the dead are no longer anything or that they no longer need anything," they spent more time enumerating the inconveniences that the mandated innovations would cause for parishioners and priests, especially those who had to conduct funerals and accompany the dead to their grave.[78] The document focused in particular on the devastating economic consequences the edicts would supposedly inflict on *fabriques*— the groups of clerics and lay people that oversaw parish administration and enjoyed exclusive rights to providing funerary materials and services, such as decorations and the transportation of dead bodies.[79]

Despite a general acceptance of hygienic arguments and the difficulties allegedly created by the new laws, the Church and its satellite organizations were able to maintain their monopoly over funerary services throughout the nineteenth century. The decree of 23 prairial, year XII (1804) set out the basic conditions regulating funerals, and they remained in force for exactly one hundred years, ending only with the 1904 law establishing the separation of churches and state. Under the supervision of the clergy and local government, the *fabriques* drew up detailed schedules for the different levels of pomp and their prices, and exceptions to these practices seem to have been virtually impossible.[80] The final pages of Balzac's novel *Ferragus* offer a mordant description of the bureaucratic travails awaiting any individual who might want to depart from established funerary procedures, and ultimately, the novel claims, such variations could be effected only by moving outside legal channels and calling on powerful criminal intervention. It is not surprising that the Church would have expended so much energy on protecting its privileges. Funerals represented an important source of income for parishes, and indeed in many cases they were almost the only source of income, as other revenues, such as money from pew rentals, steadily declined over the latter half of the nineteenth century. In the 1860s, Xavier Riobé lamented the deteriorating financial situation of the clergy while optimistically noting that "wherever care has been taken to offer the public the means to celebrate their funerals with brilliance, significant results have been immediately obtained, and the *fabriques* have gathered in unhoped-for fruits."[81] Although Monseigneur Charles Freppel argued that the "decency of funerals disappears when the idea of the immortality of the soul is absent, and it is religion alone which can guarantee the respect due to the dead," the Church was clearly also driven by more venal reasons to defend its privileged relation to the dead.[82] When the republicans came to power in 1876, they swept through a series of anticlerical laws, and the Church's hold on funerary practices was so hotly debated that even the generally anti-clerical republican newspaper *Le Temps* expressed reservations about the tenor discussions had taken in the Senate, writing, "it seems that the calm and serenity that ought to surround death must not be confused with politics."[83] Despite the clergy's readiness to defend their financial interests in the funerary business, arguments like Freppel's continued to portray the Church as simultaneously rising above such pragmatic concerns, and this apparent disinterest—along with a general reluctance to treat the deceased as simply another political or commercial issue—kept legislators from withdrawing the Church's monopoly. Across nearly three decades of republican resistance it was consequently able to preserve its rights over the dead, losing them only with the law of 1904. It had, by that time, taken over one hundred and fifty years to loosen the Church's legal hold on the departed, and although the final break resulted from a global severing of church and state that did not directly involve doctors, the law itself was made possible by a more general rationalist ideology that they, as a body, had espoused and legitimized. More important, over the course of a century and a half, the Church had been forced to yield a crucial conceptual point by accepting the notion that, even when buried, dead bodies were toxic substances best understood by the medical profession. Even at the time, this was recognized as a profound intellectual and cultural shift. In their handwritten document, for instance, the *curés* of Paris already attested to the significance of this transformation: if the dead become simply a medical concern, the *curés* claimed, if their condition is accepted to be a physiological one, then death too will change. It will disappear. It will be nothing. Through their apparently pragmatic concerns, doctors—hygienists, in fact—were altering one of the most basic structures of human existence.

The Ethical Status of the Dead, or the Limits of Medicine

A 1974 medical thesis on necrophilia bears witness to the durability—and conceptual limits—of the new, medical approaches to death. The author, Pierre Desrosières, used François Bertrand's case as one of his principal reference points, and his analysis seems to be unique in actually considering the role of the dead in the sergeant's pathology. As I have argued, previous medical discussions of Bertrand's necrophilia all focused on issues of taxonomy or erotic drive without ever asking why their so-called monomaniac would have been fascinated by corpses in particular. And while contemporary doctors generally agreed that Bertrand's crimes represented a uniquely egregious form of mental deviation, none of them sought to explain just why they were so awful or tried to connect the singularity of the perpetrator's madness to the objects of his desire. That necrophilia would be the last degree of sexual perversion was treated as a given, leaving one to wonder how the defining characteristic of Bertrand's behavior could pass so thoroughly unexamined during a period when both madness and death were being redefined by doctors and scientists. Desrosière's analysis attempted to rectify this failure. "The necrophiliac looks to defy the Law of Death and the interdictions that attach to it," he wrote.

> By becoming a "criminal," he wants to operate the passage from life to death on his own. He thus attempts to enact a fundamental myth by staging it in a way that he tries to control. Through this "laboratory experiment" that he performs, he seeks an understanding of the functioning of death, and therefore a certain mastery over its reversibility. In delving into the body of a cadaver, the necrophiliac follows the subverted path of an autopsy.
>
> The originality of this procedure lies in its imminently solitary nature, which allows one to understand how it differs radically from the approach to death in archaic societies, where, it is true, staging plays a fundamental role, but one whose function is perfectly understood by all.
>
> In his actions, the criminal pervert occupies the place of a veritable demiurge. This undertaking, which situates him outside of the human and its rules, allows him, in a certain manner, to perform a short circuit that avoids death, even as he inflicts and autopsies it.
>
> This profound refusal of death's reality is to be placed in the same class as the refusal of the reality of castration, which offers the spectacle of the separation of the sexes. The pervert could thus formulate his justification by paraphrasing E. MANNONI [sic]: "I am quite aware that death exists, but nonetheless I at once dominate and defy it."[84]

Even in such a short passage, Desrosières's description of necrophilia plays across a wide range of different metaphorical systems that include the social, religious, mythic, and medical. It is the latter that is of most interest here and it functions in a very curious way. To explain the criminal's understanding of death, Desrosières describes him as attempting to ape the activities of doctors through strange variations on laboratory experiments and autopsies. Now, it is important to bear in mind that it is Desrosières and not Bertrand who is speaking in these lines. He is imagining Bertrand imagining what doctors do, and in this sense, the fantasies in this passage are more directly the doctor's than the patient's. The image of the doctor that emerges here is, moreover, essentially the same one I have already exposed in Enlightenment authors: a scientist who struggles heroically and potentially successfully against death, who can understand its functioning, master and perhaps even reverse it. So although it is projected onto a long-dead lunatic, this text documents an idea about the relation between death and medicine that remained largely unchanged from the late eighteenth to the early twenty-first centuries. Indeed, the paraphrase of Octave Mannoni that summarizes the necrophiliac's relation to mortality could be applied more appropriately to Cabanis and Desrosières than to Bertrand, and perhaps, in the best sense, to the medical profession as a whole: I know that death exists, but still . . .[85]

In depicting doctors in early-nineteenth-century terms, Desrosières observes something like a rivalry between them and the necrophiliacs they are expected to treat. Not only are the goals of the doctor and the pervert essentially identical—that is, to understand and control death—but on some basic level the means are the same as well, since each, in his own way, performs autopsies and laboratory experiments. The criminal, according to Desrosières, wants to be a physician but fails, unable to grasp the full import of the discourse he mimics. In Desrosières's view, it would thus seem that Bertrand does not suffer from a pathological relation to death; he suffers from a pathological relation to medicine. But the "short-circuit" that he mentions appears, in this respect, to be his own, since he cannot, or at least will not, imagine an understanding of death significantly other than the doctor's. Bertrand is not, in this way, fundamentally different from medical practitioners, he is only worse. There are good doctors and bad doctors, but there is no other approach to death in the world that Desrosières conjures up here. In fact, by shifting the focus of the necrophiliac's interest from death to medicine, he actively forecloses the very possibility of another, nonmedical discourse for thinking these questions and reduces Bertrand's ostensibly unique language to a sort of pidgin-doctor. Desrosières speaks and hears a medical language even in the most unexpected places and in so doing he refuses the sergeant a certain, fundamental difference. Bertrand, according to Desrosières's analysis, wants to be a physician, but insofar as it is Desrosières who is offering up this fantasy, it is more certainly his own desire that is expressed in this passage. And that desire would seem to be that the madman not be fundamentally different, that he have nothing new or valid to say about death.

The sergeant himself was, however, more circumspect about the meaning of his own behavior. At his court-martial, he described his actions as unspeakable and unintelligible even to him, saying: "I cannot say what was going on in me. . . . Even today, I cannot grasp the sensations that I felt in scattering about the shredded bits of corpses."[86] If one can rely on the document supposedly written by Bertrand that Ambroise Tardieu included in his *Etude médico-légale sur les attentats aux mœurs* (Medico-Legal Study on Crimes of Indecency), the necrophiliac was familiar with the case histories written about him and had his own opinions about their value. In a letter to Marchal de Calvi, reproduced by Tardieu, Bertrand catalogued a series of factual errors that had crept into the final medical and legal reports that had been filed about him.[87] He then made a more general observation about their psychological diagnosis:

> As to erotic monomania, I maintain that it never preceded destructive monomania. . . . Yes! Destructive monomania was always stronger in me than erotic monomania, incontestably so; and I believe I would never have placed myself in danger in order to rape a cadaver if I could not have destroyed it afterwards. Therefore [*donc*], destruction prevailed over the erotic, no matter what they say, and no one is able to prove the contrary; I know better than anyone, it seems to me, what was going on inside me.[88]

Whatever Bertrand was seeking so passionately at the bottom of the common grave, it was not really, he insisted, about sex. The uncharacteristic animation of this passage will surprise any reader who has grown accustomed to the necrophiliac's normal prose style. While he described even his most sensational crimes with a detached, even numbed, objectivity (the transcript of the court-martial noted that he spoke "*unperturbed and in the most level tone of voice*," a tone that carried over to his writing) he comes across here as almost vivacious. For the only time linguistically or otherwise in these texts, he explicitly ejaculates, punctuating his argument with an exclamatory "Yes!" With that affirmation, his outburst signals itself as the crux of his written testimony, the point that engages him emotionally in its subject, where he commits himself as a person—reasoning and feeling—to his own story. The style here is, moreover, polemical. Its author tries to set out an organized argument, breaking with his habitual parataxis and beginning a subordinate clause by the more nuanced conjunction *donc*. Like more socially accredited madmen of his period such as the Gérard de Nerval of the opening chapters of *Aurélia*, the sergeant contests the diagnosis of the medical authorities who have handled his case by opening an argument with them.[89] He appeals to personal experience as a higher authority than science. The lunatic or deviant has a right to speak, indeed has an *authority* to speak, according to him, because his subjective position gives him knowledge to which no one else has access except through his mediation. By the simple act of arguing, Bertrand asserts the value of his behavior and his person, contending that his testimony, and more significantly his opinion about that testimony, are as important as the pronouncements made by certified practitioners of medical discourse.

This is also the only passage by Bertrand himself to betray any belief in the importance of interpersonal relationships. Indeed, it is the one time in the Tardieu text that Bertrand even acknowledges an interlocutor: "Rest assured," he writes to Marchal, "that everything I have told you is the exact truth. It would be a poor way to recognize what you have had the goodness to do for me, who am a stranger to you, were I to lead you into error."[90] There is no practical reason why this *déterreur de cadavres* (unearther of cadavers) should want another person to understand him, since he seems to have been able to satisfy his sexual needs with corpses and he knows himself better than others can. Why should he want the understanding of another individual? What is lacking about himself—for here it is his self that is at issue—that must be sought out not by digging in the earth but in persuading? His call to the doctor reveals the importance of the role played by another in his self-awareness, for although the sergeant already knows more about himself than anyone else does, he wants to share that insight. Indeed, he treats the information as a gift that he wishes Marchal to accept. Another, in the person of the doctor, thus assumes significance to Bertrand's very self-identity, and by deploying a nuanced variety of rhetorical modes, he indicates both that his activities have meaning and that he wants to establish that meaning within a shared discourse. And when he articulates this desire to be understood, turning at last to confront that other with the vocative, "M. le Docteur," he turns also to a language of ethics. His relation to Marchal concerns goodness and truth, the doctor's *bonté* and the *vérité* that the *déterreur* feels he owes him. And the one to whom he calls is that other of extreme alienation who grounds the ethical relation: the stranger, the person to whom nothing is owed and to whom we therefore give out of goodness.[91] In his very foreignness, the stranger reveals our own identity as one possibility among others, letting us see ourselves through different eyes, making us strangers to ourselves, and opening the possibility of learning. The place of social alienation, of strangeness and estrangement, that Bertrand once inhabited as a necrophiliac he now adopts as an interpersonal position. Truth changes, in this rhetorical turn, from a medical and legal category to an ethical one, and the *déterreur* thus shifts the terms in which his necrophilia is to be understood. The story about his mutilation of corpses, he indirectly argues, can be thought of as an issue of goodness.

Desrosières refused to consider Bertrand's relation to death as fundamentally different from his own or as involving interpersonal relations. He insisted, instead, on the isolation, almost narcissism, of the necrophiliac's relation to corpses, despite the fact that almost all the accounts of his crimes emphasize their spectacular nature, how Bertrand littered cemetery grounds with body parts and festooned trees with human entrails. It is true that in his first desecrations he had been careful to hide the traces of his passage, painstakingly reinterring the bodies he had mutilated, but later his mutilations took on a public aspect, as if they were intentionally offered up for view—even though the attention attracted by these displays would only make them more difficult to perpetrate in the future.[92] By leaving behind these horrors, Bertrand thus privileged the communication of his crimes over the pleasure he derived from committing them. They represented, in this sense, the staging of a relation to death, a material language that expressed the mystery of his desire. Rather than narcissistic, Bertrand's acts appear to have had an important interpersonal—indeed, social—component. And once he was in custody, although his actions and his relation to death remained largely unintelligible, they nonetheless acquired an ethical value within a conversation across two discourses, one belonging to a man of science, the other to a madman. In this sense, another value predominated over comprehension, since something significant was occurring in the very *attempt* to understand a behavior, even if, in the end, that behavior was never understood. A certain mystery was shared between doctor and patient, and the ethical functioning of this mystery represented something of a triumph on the part of the madman, for it was the intransigent incomprehensibility of his actions—incomprehensible, as he said, even to himself—that organized the relations between the two interlocutors, drawing the incongruous pair together in the mutual endeavor to understand a series of crimes.

Marchal himself may not have agreed that his attempt to understand Bertrand's pathology was by nature interminable, but the uniqueness of the necrophiliac's aberration forced him, nonetheless, to treat corpses as a relation between two people rather than as an organic condition. Bertrand, as he himself observed, held crucial information about an alternate view of the dead, and his notion of truth was different from those that were being brought to bear on his case: for him, it was not the disclosure of a hidden meaning, nor was it the tactical instrument wielded by pragmatists such as Brierre de Boismont, Latour, Ferrand, or Debreyne, or the medico-centric fantasy of Desrosières. For Bertrand, it was grounded instead in the recognition of a mystery and the belief in an interpersonal goodness. Nonsense as such could, he demonstrated, operate within social and ethical relations in a positive, indeed constructive way. Bertrand, the *déterreur de cadavres*, deterrorized death by de-ontologizing an ontological category, transforming the terrible sublimity of nonbeing into a deontological encounter between two living people, brought together not by a shared knowledge but by the mystery that separated them. This mystery was the compatibility of their desires: Betrand's for the dead, Marchal's to comprehend him. The physical desire for the dead was matched against the intellectual desire to understand that desire.

A certain aesthetic quality predominated, moreover, in Bertrand's descriptions of his actions. He spoke primarily about sensations, feelings, physical longings and behaviors—in general, about a material and affective world. If such distinctions are valuable—and they certainly were held to be valid at the time—Bertrand was living in the world not of science but of art—an art that had a public, that exerted a powerful emotional response from its spectators (as evidenced by the transcripts of the court-martial), but that refused explanation, even by its practitioner. The dead were, in his case, a gift—not only in the sense of a gratuitous act of care that one person offers to another, but also in the sense of a unique and unexplainable talent, the genius that individualizes the artist to his or her audience.[93]

The Force of an Illusion

Michel Foucault argued that medical knowledge underwent an epistemological revolution at the turn of the nineteenth century. "With Bichat," he wrote, "knowledge of life finds its origin in the destruction of life; it is at death that sickness and life speak their truth."[94] Previously, he contended, doctors had studied life by observing the living, but with the publication of Bichat's *Anatomie générale* a new conceptual instrument fell into their hands. By isolating death as a specific moment in organic processes, Bichat allowed them to separate life clearly from its other and to define it in terms of that absolute opposition. At the same time, his clinical use of cadavers granted access to hidden physiological connections that could never be observed in a living body. "Morning to night for twenty years you could have stood by sickbeds taking notes on the ailments of the heart, lungs, and gastric viscera," he wrote, "and all would have been a confusion of symptoms that, since they were attached to nothing, would offer you only a series of incoherent phenomena. Open a few corpses: right away you will see the obscurity vanish that observation alone could not dissipate."[95] The dead offered something more than could be derived from mere observation: their bodies held, somehow, the interpretive key that transformed an endless proliferation of symptoms into meaningful signs.[96] The Rosetta stone to the physiological processes of life, they provided the place on which was written the code that brought those phenomena into a coherent language.

To trace the movement of death across the animal organism, it was not enough, however, just to open a few dead bodies, for although autopsies exposed otherwise hidden organs to view, the secret line between life and death was not, Bichat remarked, accessible to direct observation. To determine its intervention in the body, one needed instead to view the inner workings of the dying, the ways in which their organs reacted to death and, as one or the other failed, how they acted internally on one another. And so Bichat vivisected dogs, forcing single organs to fail and then following the ramifications across the still living flesh of the animal. Foucault spoke of death, in this epistemological moment, as an "impassable limit" and "a dividing line without thickness that indicates nosological time in the same way that the scalpel indicates organic space."[97] Its "atemporality" removed it, according to him, from the confusion of physiological processes and created an analytical distance from them.[98] But the vivisections tell a different story from the autopsies that Foucault cites; it is through the former, not the latter, that death was identified, and it was identified not as a timeless condition, but as a progressive force locked in combat against the resistance of life. In itself, death was perhaps an unknown force, but set against the living body, it found expression: a mobile writing that flashed up and then disappeared as the organs successively failed, an active, if fleeting presence in the flesh. Death itself, death in the body, mingled with the living, taking on a quasi-life of its own that continued independently after the organism as a whole finally succumbed.

Scientists and philosophers continued to debate the ontological and epistemological statuses of death throughout the nineteenth century. Certainly, death manifested itself as a force hostile to life, but unlike other invisible attractions, such as gravity, one could not define it through a set of constant, physical laws. In itself, it remained a mystery—or perhaps nothing at all. That lacuna troubled many in the medical community. The biologist F.-R. Buisson, for instance, contested Bichat's proposition that life was the set of forces that resisted death on the grounds that it amounted to a tautology. "A false idea," he wrote, "since to die signifies in every language to cease to live, and so the supposed definition is reduced to the following vicious circle: life is the totality of functions that resist the absence of life."[99] For Hegel, writing some five years after Buisson, the apparent nothingness of death could be understood as the vital force of the negative that allowed individual and historical progress.[100] The key to understanding life for Bichat, a tautology for Buisson, the force of the negative for Hegel, death was, in all cases, an unknown or a negative. On the biological level, it expressed itself only through its effects on the living. On the conceptual level, it existed only through projections and fantasies, through a discourse that made sense of those signs without ever being able to perceive their referent as such. And yet, despite its purely speculative nature, death had been determined to function physiologically as an absolute. This dual status as pure construction and determinative absolute helps explain the importance that the concept of mortality played in the rise of medicine. Nothing perceptible in itself, death was moving, like madness, conceptually beyond the reach of established nonmedical discourses. Like madness, too, it had implications for the very structures of subjectivity on which depended the notions of individual responsibility, suffrage, and citizenship—the city, in a word. But unlike madness, death had a conceptual, even philosophical purity. In much the same way that doctors were able to speak the unspeakable language of the insane, they were also able at least to delimit the unknowability of death and instrumentalize it to both diagnostic and punitive ends. Rather than merely the skilled observers of natural phenomena, doctors had become the masters of a fantasmatic absolute.

THREE

A Hostile Environment

Doctors and medical theorists were able to capitalize on death's status as a defining limit to increase their social legitimacy in the early nineteenth century. They also played, very skillfully, on fears about death as a physical state. Some of these developments can be traced to the encyclopedists, who described death as a physical condition that could be managed and perhaps even cured—not an absolutely but rather a relatively different state, part of a potentially reversible continuum of degeneration and physical decline that included the other physiological processes of life.[1] An entry on the subject argued that "in reality, there is perhaps less distance between old age and youth than between decrepitude and *death*, for here one must not consider life as an absolute thing. . . . *Death* is not armed with a sharp instrument, nothing violent accompanies it, and one stops living by imperceptible nuances."[2] The first words here are the most important: "*dans le réel*." This is not death as a concept, a metaphysical state, a spiritual vocation, or the pure abstraction of nonbeing, but as something *in* the real. A new generation of thinkers was refusing to imagine death as a transcendental category and argued instead that it was a physical process located in the animal body. These conceptual shifts offered the promise of an increased mastery over suffering and mortality—for they treated death more as a manageable illness than an immutable destiny—but they also opened the door to a new world of horrors and uncertainties, to fears of an uncontrollable continuity between life and death. These anxieties were in turn sustained by a belief that the conditions of modern life, especially the population densities and physical peculiarities of major cities, facilitated mutual communication and contamination between the animate and inanimate. As I will argue, this new concern would later find expression in vast projects to transform urban space, but it also made itself felt in more subtle and intimate forms, like the late nineteenth-century esthetics of symbolism and decadence. In his novel *Bruges-la-morte*, Georges Rodenbach, for instance, conceived of death as something that could become conceptually and affectively embedded in physical entities like a lock of hair or a town, while Joris Karl Huysmans, intrigued by recent discoveries in chemistry, imagined, with caustic humor and considerably less poetry, the possibility of preserving the fragrant essence of loved ones in the ptomaine residues exuded from their decomposing corpses.[3] This esthetic of death—this conception of death *as* a sensuous object of aesthesis—could also betray itself in the slightest of stylistic choices, as when, late in the century, Octave Mirbeau wrote of doors that opened out "on to Death [*sur de la mort*]."[4] The use of the partitive *de la* indicates that he, like the encyclopedists, imagined death not as an abstract and indivisible absolute, but as something that could be apprehended and meted out in indeterminate but distinct quantities, as if there could be more or less of death or a bit of it—as if it functioned, in short, like a physical substance. And Mirbeau's partitive is all the more telling for being an almost imperceptible detail: rather than the object of a conscious argument, this materialized perception of nonbeing had entered into the fabric of language itself, integrating itself into the texture of a literary movement.

In this chapter and the next, I will look at the medical theorization of this materialized death and the efforts to combat it through public health policies. I will first describe the role of hygiene in early nineteenth-century Paris and the way that it located vectors of disease in environmental conditions, especially the quality of air. The scientists behind these studies attempted to identify noxious agents and concentrated on urban spaces, which they considered to be particularly dangerous because of the density of their populations. They found that cities housed pathogens, that these pathogens were products of human biological processes, and that they formed a continuum of toxicity that had to be separated from inhabitants. In the next chapter, I will demonstrate how this notion of environmental toxins became identified with death itself, as if the latter could itself be physically present and even, perhaps, sentient. The point of what follows is not, however, to recount the emergence of hygiene as a discipline, since that history has already been brilliantly and abundantly detailed by other authors, but to understand the rise of public health as part of an intellectual and imaginative labor that sought, sometimes consciously and more often unconsciously, to understand the role of death in relation to society, especially as it manifested itself in the city.

Hygiene

Powered by recent theoretical developments in the physical sciences, especially in chemistry and the study of gases, the late eighteenth century marked a turning point in the attempt to clean, control, and rationalize urban space. While the squalid conditions in cities had long been linked to illness, the involvement of the police in urban health changed fundamentally in the last quarter of the eighteenth century.[5] Jacques-Hippolyte Ronesse remarked on the difference in 1782, noting that "for several years the object of the greatest solicitude for the Police Administration has been the cleaning of the streets; an object of the highest importance, since it . . . concerns the health of the citizens."[6] Almost simultaneously, Louis-Sébastien Mercier denounced many of the same problems that caught the attention of Ronesse: the filth that accumulated in Paris, the pollution of such animal necessities as food and wine, and the dangers that this generalized negligence represented for the well-being of the city's inhabitants.[7] Mercier explained the changed attitudes toward these problems as the direct and sustained result of recent developments in the sciences. "The old method used by cesspool cleaners," he wrote, "has just been abolished by the government, and they are obliged to adopt a new method, proven by experience and approved by the Academy of Sciences."[8] He then went on to observe that:

> the government consults these useful physicians more than ever. Because of them,
> it has proscribed the old habit of using only copper vessels to transport into Paris
> the milk that is consumed there . . . for the least decomposition of that metal is
> deadly and the cause of ravages hidden in the animal economy; and it has been

necessary not only to instruct the people on this, but also to protect them from it by means of authority.

It is on the recommendation of the same chemists that the police has prohibited wine merchants from using counters and tables made of lead.[9]

The capital, as Mercier saw it, was being transformed around him, recreated according to principles that had never before existed. Guided by experimental method and the self-governing Academy of Sciences, it was now physicians and chemists who determined the organization and laws of the city that was emerging, literally, from the detritus of old Paris. And this transformation, if not total or instantaneous in its material application, nonetheless took hold rapidly and durably as a general reconceptualization of urban space. The power of this theoretical restructuring was remarkable, even in the eyes of contemporaries. By 1822, the surgeon and alienist Claude Lachaise would write that "one may only conclude that nowhere does the police exercise such an active vigilance" as in respect to "causes of insalubrity."[10] But the police, he remarked, could not operate without the constant supervision of specialized scientists, since "there exist a thousand abuses that escape the eye of authority, or over which it could not extend its action, and whose deadly effects can often be recognized only by a doctor."[11] The dangers of filth were a secret process, perceptible only to specially trained scientists, and the logic of the new and more salubrious city was thus increasingly withdrawn from its inhabitants, locked away in the mysterious coils of physical nature and the body itself—"hidden," as Mercier put it, "in the animal economy."

In theory and in practice, nineteenth-century Paris embodied the rise of a new subcategory of medical science. The word *hygiaine* may have entered the French language in 1575, but the discipline itself did not begin to exert a significant influence on social behaviors until the late eighteenth century, when the importance of safeguarding public health through state intervention began to acquire widespread currency, making its way first into scientific publications and legislative debates and then into urban planning.[12] Understood as a government responsibility, public hygiene was related to the notion of a *police médicale*, in the more archaic sense of a civic policy for enforcing order and safety. As the nineteenth century progressed, the term became increasingly confused with *médecine légale*, an expression that previously had been used only to describe the application of medical expertise to judicial matters.[13] Public hygiene thus became another arena in which doctors worked through their complicated relations to the courts, the police, and the legislative system, but also one of the areas in which they exercised the most pervasive and enduring influence on daily life, for the physical shape of Paris and other nineteenth-century cities was revolutionized in large part as a result of contemporary hygienic theories.

Historians have traced the origins of this revolution to the mid-eighteenth century, especially in central Europe.[14] Somewhat later, as part of a general return to Hippocratic principles, certain schools of thought began to emphasize the way that environmental conditions could affect the health not merely of individuals, but of whole populations, leading to the fields of meteoropathology, which studied the effects of weather on the progress of illnesses, and medical geography.[15] The body politic was increasingly viewed as a physical body, with needs that exceeded those of its constituent members and that could only be addressed by dedicated medical specialists. Those needs, however, covered a broad and often unmanageable field that varied over time. During the Revolution, debates on the subject in the Assemblée Nationale Constituante mentioned the oversight of mines, cemeteries, slaughterhouses, and dyers, along with the wholesomeness of foodstuffs and the salubriousness of lodgings.[16] Subsequent proposals added concerns about epidemics, drugs, and state-run institutions such as prisons and hospitals.[17] In 1793, it was recommended that special commissions be entrusted with supervising the quality of air and comestibles and with visiting all public spaces to assure their conformity to sanitary policy.[18] When the Conseil de Salubrité de la Ville de Paris (Committee on Salubriousness of the City of Paris) was created in 1802, its responsibilities comprised these established concerns, but to them were soon added first aid, especially for victims of drowning and asphyxiation. Fourcroy's reforms of 1803, which created three schools of medicine in France, gave an unprecedented level of official recognition to the new discipline by endowing each with a chair in hygiene.[19] Louis René Villermé's work on the relations between illness and social conditions and his emphasis on statistical methods laid the groundwork, starting in 1810, for more holistic and unified approaches to the notion of public health.[20] It was not, however, until 1825 that the Conseil de Salubrité turned its full attention to what would become an obsession of urban planning and a system for bodily connecting all individual members of the city into a single biological organism: the sewers.[21]

The *annus mirabilis* was undoubtedly 1829, which saw the founding of the first journal in France dedicated to hygiene, the influential *Annales d'hygiène et de médecine légale*. The publication provided a powerful forum for the new discipline, and its very title argued for the central role of public health in the relations—and rivalries—between law and medicine. Even the term *annals* was charged, for it brought the notion of a historical breadth to the undertaking: time itself would now be counted not merely in years, but also in the progress of this science, which needed to be debated, publicized, and recorded. The unsigned prospectus in the journal's first issue offers some idea of the utopian scope that the editors envisioned for their undertaking. "Medicine has not only for its object the study and healing of illnesses," they held, "it has intimate connections with the organization of society. Sometimes it aids the legislator in the creation of new laws, often it enlightens the magistrate in their application, and always it watches with the government over the protection of public health."[22] Doctors' work was no longer confined to the needs of isolated patients. They had, it would seem, become guardians of the social order itself. On the one hand they observed whole populations, studying their behaviors and their needs, and on the other they enlightened, explained, and instructed their peers in other fields, telling the government how to treat the vast body that had been assigned to its care. And the doctors, according to the hygienists, had a unique and *intimate* relation to the social organization. I will return in chapters 5 and 7 to the question of that intimacy by looking at the fantasmatic and erotic elements underlying the efficacy of medical science in shaping society, but for the moment I will concentrate on the excitement that hygienic developments aroused among their practitioners. That excitement, and the reasoning propelling it, must have been contagious, for the pretensions of these specialists were not only weirdly grandiose, they were also, to a surprising extent, realized in the Paris of the nineteenth century.

Some of that reasoning was laid out by Hyppolite-Louis Royer-Collard in the inaugural lecture for the course he gave over the academic year 1845–1846 at the Faculté de Médecine in Paris. At the Faculté, Royer-Collard occupied the foremost among the three chairs in hygiene in France, and in that capacity he was probably the most distinguished representative of a field that was enjoying an unprecedented legitimacy in public policy. "Hygiene," he wrote, "is the direction, the conduct, the government of health."[23] His metaphorics immediately established an analogy between political and physiological principles, and although the former seem to explain the latter and, therefore, to underlie them, that order of precedence was soon reversed, for in subsequently attempting to define hygiene, Royer-Collard described it as "that part of medicine that teaches us how to regulate [*régler*] the life of man."[24] The discipline was thus a system for subordinating human life in general to medical principles and as such it represented an organization of the human condition across cultural boundaries. This is what Royer-Collard seems to have meant by the "government" of hygiene: a more fundamental, more universal human order. And this order itself derived from an ability to interpret and comprehend the functioning of the physical world, since, as he put it,

> medicine, considered as a whole, has two goals. It seeks to discover 1) the laws that govern organic phenomena, whether in health or in sickness and 2) the means by which to maintain or restore order in the functioning of the living economy.
>
> So you see, two things: *laws* and *means*. As a result two things in medicine as well: a *science* and an *art*.[25]

Medicine is a science because it is organized according to codes that define the very structures of the material world. But it is also an art in the sense that it is caught up in the specificities of the material world, in the individual cases that need to be interpreted and managed, but that sometimes demand the uncodifiable human sensitivity and the practical experience of the accomplished physician. This, it would seem, is part of the privileged and intimate knowledge that doctors alone possess, the untheorizable aspect of medical insight that reached back to Cabanis's belief that a practiced and sympathetic *coup d'œil* could alone reveal the nature of an illness. For such a trained medical observer, when the physical world speaks to and through human intelligence, it not only reveals the laws determining who we already are, it also legislates who we ought to be in the future. And it does this, first of all, by dictating how we should think. "So we are now led by necessity . . .," Royer-Collard continued, "to identify also an *intellectual and moral hygiene*, specific in its essence to the human species and destined to intervene constantly in man's properly physical and corporal hygiene."[26] Hygiene was, in this sense, the active and persistent intervention of thought in the material world, initially as limited to the human body, but subsequently extended to its physical environment as well—it was, consequently, the medical practice of subordinating matter to thought. And since human beings live together, their environment comprised, above all, the network of relations, both physical and immaterial, that create social space. As Royer-Collard wrote, "every meeting or collection of individuals forms a body, a sort of living unity, which has its own hygiene just like every other individual. This is what by common accord we call *public hygiene*."[27]

For the mid-century hygienist, this collective body had come to manifest itself most significantly in the city, and the latter must, therefore, be configured so as to better subordinate animal needs to reason. The first order of business in this undertaking was order itself, especially the physical and conceptual separation of things that must not be confused, such as the salubrious from the insalubrious, the living from the dead, and the dead from death. Without this medical intervention, the city, from Royer-Collard's point of view, could not attain to its rationalized form, could not become the political entity that it was *supposed* to be, and consequently would remain both unnatural and inhuman. In his description of the applicability of hygienic principles to urban space, he therefore recast the structures of social order in terms of health, reducing the administrative apparatus itself to an instrument for implementing scientifically dictated policy.

> In respect to the order of government, the topics for discussion and research that present themselves to us are almost infinite: the general policing of cities, which is to say the care for cleanliness, lighting, oversight of markets and food stalls, the sale of comestibles, the falsification and doctoring of food and drink, inhumations; the construction of streets, squares, dwellings, sewers, and canals; public establishments, prisons, hospitals, hospices, asylums, madhouses, charitable works, poorhouses, prostitution; institutions of public education, schools for deaf-mutes and the blind, etc.: all of this lies within the scope of public hygiene.[28]

The realm of medical intervention reached, in Royer-Collard's imagination, throughout the city and down to the meanest aspects of urban life. But the very wealth of social relations and their material expressions seemed to overwhelm him, as if he had lost hold, for a moment, of the organizational principles that were supposed to structure his contact with the city. His description degenerates into a congeries of telling details that create, if only briefly, the image of a space in which funerals jostle against doctored foods and road workers. But it was through the very incongruity of these elements that Royer-Collard was able to illustrate the notion of a boundless world caught up within the walls of Paris. This was the physical, but also the moral and intellectual space that must be mastered by an endlessly vigilant medical program.[29] And the enemy that at every moment awaited the hygienist in the infinite meanders of this potential confusion was death. This, it would seem, was the utility and justification for his entire, unsleeping system of human organization: it was an application of the great Enlightenment promise to banish mortality from human existence.

The initial successes of this program were striking. "Before the Revolution," Royer-Collard recalled, "the number of deaths was one in thirty. Today it is one in forty five. The probable length of life in Paris is twenty-six years, and the average lifespan about thirty-four. Certainly, a host of causes have helped produce such a result, but no one can doubt that these causes themselves are intimately connected to that universal renewal that has brought the light and benefits of civilization down into the very depths of society."[30] But the death that the hygienist struggled against was not the death of sublimation, which could be mastered in such concepts as the infinite or nothingness—or death itself; it was, instead, an uncontrolled death, which sprang up, unexpected and unwanted, from the material conditions of the city, a death that insinuated itself into the fabric of life, spreading unforeseeably and disease-like through the habitations of the living. Death as punishment, as organizing principle, was still being administered in the city. The guillotine still functioned. In Germany, Hegel had recently defined death as a philosophical principle, one that would underlie the notions of subjectivity and history for the next two centuries. What was being driven out was, instead, wild death, material death.

The excitement propelling the rise of hygiene derived, at least in part, from its extensive social significance and its crucial position at the juncture of medicine, law, and public policy. In that capacity, it also conferred on doctors a special, untransferable role in understanding and controlling the social order, for their "artistic" intimacy with the body operated like a secret and indispensable language. And they were surprisingly effective in imposing that language on the cities that were being rebuilt over the course of the nineteenth century. Paris, as I will argue, was transformed largely in conformity with their recommendations. This acceptance of medical privilege was motivated, in turn, by a fear of death and the concomitant promise, hidden in the arguments about scientific progress, that it could be beaten or at least tamed.[31] But if death had become the great threat lurking within the density of urban populations, it was a special kind of death, at once impersonal and material, a death caught up in the body and its environment, and as such, strangely labile, subject to the vicissitudes of the physical world and an apparently uncontrollable series of metamorphoses. In the hands of the artist-hygienists who attempted to understand and master it, this death expressed itself through a proliferation of metaphors.

Miasmas

With the rise of medicine as an explicative system and hygiene as a means for implementing it, urban space became a tool for transforming scientific theories into practice. Over the course of some hundred years, Paris in particular responded to contemporary medical discoveries in a way that would have been unthinkable earlier, knocking down buildings, tunneling out elaborate sewer systems, and transferring the contents of entire cemeteries beyond the city walls. The theories motivating this transformation are nowhere more clearly exposed than in discussions about the quality of Parisian air, which arose out of a complex history of experimentation and speculation. Now, animals are bound to their surroundings not only by their nutritive needs, but also through their senses, and of these the one that Enlightenment thinkers associated most intimately with materiality itself was smell. Because of this peculiarity, our ability to detect odors was thought to expose human beings more acutely than their other faculties to the dangers of the physical world. Although eighteenth-century discoveries in chemistry would transform it into an article of faith for the scientific community and for the free-thinkers they influenced, this theory of smells stemmed from a much earlier tradition. In the seventeenth century, Thomas Sydenham, for instance, had approvingly cited Hippocrates's attribution of epidemics to the qualities and disturbances in local air and had written of the illnesses produced by "occult and inexplicable changes in the bowels of the earth" that affect the atmosphere.[32] Already one finds in this description the notion, which will return much later among hygienists like Royer-Collard, that a force is hidden in matter itself, a force not merely unexplained, but inexplicable. Though almost imperceptible, air was, according to Syndenham, a material substance that harbored deadly and unintelligible dangers in a particularly insidious way.

His approach was pursued by other scientists, such as Stephen Hales, who at first attributed the noxiousness of air to variations in its elasticity, or the compressibility that allowed it to penetrate into porous bodies and thereby act on them. Hales's 1727 volume, *Vegetable Staticks*, argued that plants imbibed and retained air, thereby suggesting that organic bodies somehow combined with its substance. He also maintained that air could lose its life-sustaining qualities to become "spent," and on this basis he proposed, in 1741, new systems for ventilating crowded spaces, like jails and hospitals.

Even more important than his discoveries themselves was, however, his experimental method, which allowed him to trap specific gases, even though he was not aware that air itself was a compound. On the basis of these methods, Joseph Black of Scotland was able, in 1754, to isolate carbon dioxide, which he called "fixed air," and combine it with a solid, thereby demonstrating the chemical, and not merely mechanical properties of air. He was also intrigued by the observations that certain gases would not support a flame and that animals, when held in the enclosed space of a bell jar, would eventually die from their own exhalations. A series of experiments by Daniel Rutherford, one of Black's students, showed that the presence of carbon dioxide alone could not explain these facts, which the two men accordingly attributed to concentrations of "phlogiston" (now known as nitrogen), which they deduced had been produced by respiration and burning. Once air was saturated with this element, they reasoned, it would no longer support combustion. In the 1760s Joseph Priestley discovered that gases could dissolve in liquids and went on to isolate several distinct components, including oxygen, which, since it encouraged combustion, he thought to be dephlogisticated air. In the following decade, Antoine Laurent Lavoisier, who had been quantifying chemical reactions by meticulously weighing his materials and instruments before and after inducing those reactions, abandoned the phlogiston theory, determined that combustion was necessary to life, and gave the name *oxygen* to Priestley's dephlogisticated air.[33]

With breathtaking rapidity and sweep, a series of minute observations had forced the material world to reveal an unprecedented wealth of secrets, even from its most invisible hiding places. As this evidence appeared, it quickly became the source of speculation in various other fields. These findings also affected people's perceptions of everyday life, as demonstrated by the attempts, beginning with Hales's ventilators, to apply new scientific discoveries to practical concerns. Black's observation, for instance, that gases could insinuate themselves into solids came as a stunning, and deeply disturbing, revelation for some, since it suggested that odors affected not merely the senses, but could enter into the composition of the body itself. Certain smells were no longer merely unpleasant, but came to be viewed as dangers in themselves. Some of the separation between individuals and their environment dissolved as well, for people now had to imagine themselves immersed in a chemically active solution capable of penetrating into the smallest, most hidden recesses of their person and bonding with them. Little by little, they would, unless precautions were taken, become like the air around them.

Miasmas, or the vaporous products of decomposition, played a central, nervously observed role in these beliefs. Identified variously with different gases, such as phlogiston and "fixed air," these substances were thought to be released in the process of decomposition and to enter into the atmosphere, where they threatened to break down the chemical structure of bodies by infecting them with the same putrefaction that had given rise to the gases in the first place. But putrefaction was a very broad concept applicable to any sort of decomposition affecting organic matter, and it included the whole gamut of rotting, including those processes necessary to sustain the health and life of an organism. While the digestion of foods reduced them into their constituent nutritive elements and as such was indispensible to the health of the body, it did so only by decomposing them, thus exposing the stomach and intestines to the dangers of a potentially unrestricted decay: the putrefaction that began in the ingested food could, theoretically, spread to those organs in contact with it. The intestines were thus a locus of intense ambivalence, according to this scheme. Their products, on the other hand, since they concentrated putrescence while no longer contributing anything to bodily sustenance, could only be viewed as pernicious, and fecal matter was thus understood as a particularly potent source of disease.[34] In 1783, Louis-Sébastien Mercier accordingly lamented the fate of "vuidangeurs," who were constantly subjected to "pestilential miasmas" in the course of work that condemned them "to descend daily into cesspools [*fosses*], there to breathe an impure air, exposing all of their senses to the fetid and poisonous vapors that waste, consume, and dry them and that give to their face the livid and premature pallor of the grave."[35]

Inspired by often dramatic experiments, such as Rutherford's and Priestley's, but divided among various theories such as "phlogisticated air," "inflammable air," and "fixed air," scientists of the period sought to determine the chemical principles underlying this olfactory contagiousness, and as late as the last quarter of the eighteenth century, Félix Vicq d'Azyr and Jacques de Horne were still attempting to describe in some definitive way the noxious effects of putrid gases on living organisms. According to the former, those consequences could be attributed to several causes, the principal of which was an "odorous vapor" that "acts in a slow . . . manner on the animal fluids, which it clearly alters."[36] For Horne, the poisons generated by decomposition could impregnate and accumulate in the materials with which they came into contact and subsequently lie dormant until disturbed by the living, whom they could then infect.[37] The air we breathe, our physical surroundings, our very bodies and their excreta, all carried within them, according to these chemists, the constant threat of organic dissolution, the slow rotting of our persons into their constituent parts and our gradual, but inexorable reconfiguration into new compounds.

Death spread through odors, accumulating in the materials that imbibed them and then moving, sometimes through slow infusion and at others with the speed of lightening, into other material substances, including organic bodies. An open tomb was no longer merely a reminder of the end that awaits us all, but a noxious agent in itself. The recent science on this question became so generalized, in fact, that it acquired an almost mythological status. In 1737, the French parliament had responded to complaints from inhabitants in the center of Paris by commissioning two doctors and an apothecary to study the dangers of the Saints-Innocents cemetery. Based on the team's credentials, it is apparent that the issue was already perceived to be a medical one, but while their report noted the presence of fetid odors, the investigators insisted more on the discomfort those smells caused than on any possible toxicity.[38] By 1745, however, when the *abbé* Charles Gabriel Porée distributed a tract militating for hygienic reforms in the handling and storage of corpses, the situation had fundamentally changed, and part of this difference can undoubtedly be attributed to the publication of Hales's proposals for ventilating enclosed spaces in the intervening years. Porée now argued that the smells of death were not merely unpleasant but outright dangerous. "The germs of an infinite number of diseases are sealed up in our churches and in our cemeteries," he wrote. "These cemeteries and these churches are adjacent to our houses. Around and inside them, there is formed an atmosphere of corruption, destruction, and death."[39] His arguments were mostly a combination of anecdote and conjecture. Drawing on the most recent scientific theories, he based his reasoning on minute descriptions of the invisible properties of air and the effects of decomposition on them:

> Provided one be no stranger to physics, one cannot be unaware that the air is continuously filled with the corpuscles that emanate from bodies. If more solid materials, if minerals, if metals hidden in the earth at considerable depth constantly exhale particles that fly about in the air, how many such must come from bodies composed of fluid parts? On the basis of this principle, judge for yourself the abundance of liquids that ooze out of corpses heaped up one upon the other, especially in freshly reopened graves [*fosses*] where the bodies have only half rotted.

Then vapors and exhalations flow in torrents, with which the surrounding air finds itself completely impregnated.

But it is not necessary to disturb them: through the layer of earth that hides them they sweat night and day. . . . Now examine the nature of these corpuscles: how many vitriolic, sulfurous, saline, and arsenical parts are mixed into these excretions that the air we breathe carries right into our entrails.[40]

After such a document, corpses could no longer be the same. Suddenly they had begun to breathe, exhaling odors not merely unpleasant but deadly. Day and night, they sweated pestilential fluids that impregnated the surrounding earth with a complex array of active substances that then spread into the air above, where they crept insidiously into the bodies of the living. Cemeteries were still public spaces where children played, cattle grazed, and merchants conducted business, but above them the vapors of the buried were now seen to form "those fogs of an unbearable odor, fogs pernicious to any who find themselves in such noxious surroundings."[41] Chemistry had revealed a toxic continuity between the living and the dead. The science would evolve over the coming decades, and Porée's belief that air was an inert substance filled with corpuscles would yield to theories of gases and miasmas, but his tract had formalized a conceptual approach that would revolutionize the way the dead were viewed, leading eventually to their expulsion from churches and cities and entirely altering both urban space and the relations between the living and the deceased.

That transformation was long and arduous, however. An abundant literature followed in Porée's wake, arguing relentlessly that the dead poison the air and that they must therefore be removed from inhabited spaces.[42] One study by Scipione Piattoli, translated into French in 1778 with a long preface by Vicq d'Azyr, took as its starting point a dramatic series of deaths that had occurred several years earlier in a parish church at Montpellier. A tomb had been opened to receive a new corpse, but when a workman descended into it he lost consciousness. Of the four individuals who attempted to retrieve his body, three ended up dying on the spot of asphyxiation. The fourth, who was seized by convulsions, remained pale and disfigured for the rest of his life and was thereafter known throughout the city as the "resurrected."[43] With slight variations, this kind of scene was so frequently repeated in the popular and scientific literature of the time that it became something of a set piece. Another version published in 1786, for instance, described a disaster that befell parishioners in the Burgundian town of Saulieu: when workmen opened a tomb in their church, the "malefic exhalation" that was emitted killed the curate, the vicar, forty children and two hundred other by-standers.[44] The vague threats that Porée had cited some thirty years earlier had by now crystallized into detailed scenarios that seemed to derive much of their force from sheer extravagance and repetition. The four deaths of the 1778 report had swelled into a massacre eight years later. This apparently fantasmatic impulse was dutifully recorded and carefully analyzed by students of the physical sciences, whose explanations evolved over time. While Porée had ascribed the dangers of cemeteries to the presence of airborne corpuscles, Piattoli attributed asphyxiation to the mechanical actions of air (its elasticity), and Vicq d'Azyr located the dangers of gases in their chemical properties, even though the precise nature of their operation remained controversial.[45] "There is no agreement about the nature of the gas given off by the putrefaction of animal substances," Vicq d'Azyr wrote.

> Some physicians have believed that it was fixed air. Others, following Mr. Priestley, have thought it to be phlogisticated air. It is known that a certain quantity of inflammable air also escapes from animal substances in putrefaction. Mr. Volta has noticed that more of this kind of gas has been removed from ponds at whose bottom the remains of aquatic insects are decaying. It seems that these three kinds of gas are produced by animal putrefaction, but at different moments of its development. One would need many experiments to clarify this point of doctrine, which has so far only been adumbrated. Whatever the case may be, it is incontestable that the air from putrefaction is harmful to animals and cannot serve combustion.[46]

Vicq d'Azyr's principal contribution to this debate was his attempt to reconcile the competing theories by synthesizing them: the air produced by putrefaction probably contained all three of the noxious gases that investigators had recently isolated plus an "odorous vapor that affects the nostrils in a most disagreeable manner." These substances were, he speculated, released in sequence as decomposition progressed, and while the gases killed immediately, the vapor acted over time on the nervous system and animal fluids. The distinction is instructive, for while the nonodorous components are incapable of blending with life and kill on the spot, the one that smells seems able, despite its ultimately deadly nature, to insinuate itself into the organic processes of the body and to mix with life. "[I]t is quite likely," he wrote, "that to its action are due the dangerous nervous fevers, to which are subject those who practice dissections too assiduously, gravediggers, etc."[47]

When the chemist Antoine-Alexis Cadet-De-Vaux was commissioned in
1783 to study the hygienic conditions in the houses surrounding the Saints-
Innocents cemetery, he essentially repeated the same investigation that had
already been conducted in 1737, but his theoretical presuppositions and his
perceptions were strikingly different from those of his predecessors. Before
arriving on the site, he was already well aware that if corpse gas combined
with mephitic vapors it created one of the most toxic substances on earth, a
"poison that bears on all the organs, on all of the animal economy, and which
corrupts all the bodies united in contact with it."[48] He also knew that the
vapors of the dead combined with organic and inorganic materials, passing
easily from one to the other to spread pestilence. "Suspecting that the small
area of dampness on a surface of the cellar's wall was infected," Cadet-De-
Vaux wrote, "I advised that it be avoided."[49] This suspicion was given sad
confirmation when a mason recklessly placed his hand on the spot in question
and then refused to follow the doctor's advice to wipe his skin with vinegar.
Within three days his forearm had swollen into an oozing mass of pustules.
Similarly, the wine in bottles whose corks had touched a cellar wall abutting
the cemetery was found to be entirely decomposed.[50] One resident protested
that he and his family enjoyed splendid health, but the doctor noted, somewhat drily, that "the man had obstructions of the liver, his wife a disease
of the chest, and his daughter pale colors."[51] In particular, the "cadaverous
miasmas" given off by a common grave choked with some 15,000 to 16,000
bodies had become so virulent that food in the adjoining houses began to
putrefy as soon as it was cooked.[52] To a specialist, the physical dangers of the
dead could be seen everywhere: in smells, foods, wines, the humidity of cellar
walls, the pus flowing from a swollen arm, the complexion of a young woman.

From the late eighteenth century up until Louis Pasteur's breakthroughs
in the 1860s, scientists and educated people in general took these dangers as
a given. In 1784, Bernardin de Saint-Pierre wrote of the harm caused by
corpse gases and argued that cemeteries should be moved into the countryside.[53] In 1821 the doctor and naturalist Hippolite Cloquet described his concerns about the "odor that emanates from the putrefying corpses of animals."
"Everyone knows," he observed, "how dangerous these sorts of animal exhalations are. They become veritable poisons that spread through the atmosphere and whose first effects are directed toward the organs of olfaction,
although they seem nonetheless to debilitate the entire nervous system with
lightening-like speed."[54] These concerns also expressed themselves in practical applications. Claude Lachaise's 1822 *Topographie médicale de Paris*, for

instance, recommended a certain site for a graveyard partially because "its raised position . . . permits the prompt dispersal of miasmas."[55] He further advised against the practice of stacking tombs vertically to create a back wall in funerary chapels abutting hillsides, because "this arrangement can . . . become dangerous since, no matter how carefully the free side of each coffin is cemented, the corpses will transmit too directly into the atmosphere the deleterious miasmas that result from their decomposition and that lose the largest part of their activity by saturating the earth when it surrounds them on all sides."[56] Incidents in cemeteries continued to corroborate the findings of earlier researchers like Cadet-De-Vaux. In 1832, when a common grave in Angers was reopened only three years after having been covered, it let off "a cadaverous gas, a very subtle poison: of all the emanations that contaminate the air and menace the health of the inhabitants, there is certainly none more dangerous than those which are exhaled by the graves of the dead."[57] In 1849, responding to incidents in the Montmartre cemetery, Augustin Pellieux undertook an investigation of hygienic conditions in the crypts, concentrating on one tomb in particular, which had been signaled to him as among the most dangerous. "[U]pon penetrating inside," he wrote, "one perceived only a simple cadaverous odor. Although it had been open for twenty-four hours, a lighted candle, lowered to the depth of about one and a half meters, took on a ruddy glow and suddenly went out. Our attempts to get it to burn at a greater depth were futile. A bird lowered to the bottom of the vault was asphyxiated after a few seconds at most."[58] The virulence of these miasmas could further be judged by the fact that "these gases, of a highly deleterious nature, as has been seen, do not affect only the gravediggers employed in the vaults; they also exercise a pernicious effect on the persons who come to pray upon the tomb of their family members or friends."[59] In the same year, the chemist Henri-François Gaultier de Claubry was still forced to acknowledge that despite all of the progress made in isolating and identifying noxious gases, "up until now, chemistry has been powerless to recognize the products that, under the name of *miasmas*, obviously exercise such a great influence on the animal economy. This is no reason, however, not to make new attempts, which will ultimately lead to useful results."[60]

The Metamorphoses of Infection

As important as it was in discussions of urban hygiene, air pollution was, however, only one element in a larger and more complicated picture. Eugène

Belgrand, the *inspecteur général des ponts-et-chaussées* (Inspector-General of Bridges and Roadways) for Paris, would look back in horror, some hundred years later, at his city in the late eighteenth century. Everywhere his imagination lighted it recoiled in disgust at the human filth that the citizens had inhabited. To his mind, the invisible virulence exuded by the capital not only spread through the air, but it also penetrated into the soil below, creating a vast, subterranean reservoir of disease.

> Up until the end of the last century, no measures were taken to protect the general salubriousness of Paris. Fecal matters were held in permeable cesspools [*fosses*], and collected garbage was deposited at the city gates, close to the ramparts. Cemeteries surrounded churches; sewers were simply open trenches [*fosses*], whose waters leached into a permeable soil. The street gutters were in the middle of the pavement so that any vehicle that passed necessarily ran its wheel through them. As a result, the paving was always in a poor state of repair and a thick layer of mud, which some of us have still seen, lingered on the public thoroughfare, moved down the holes in its paving, and slowly penetrated into the subsoil, extending to the right and left beneath the houses. Our ancestors gave the names *crotte* and *gadoue* to this black mud, which was a most powerful fertilizer, highly prized by farmers, and which was, consequently, heavily impregnated with organic materials.[61]

Given the gravity of such problems, it was imperative that city leaders take urgent measures to combat them. Two of the principal solutions proposed were to encourage the movement of air and to remove the sources of infection. As Jacques de Horne wrote in 1788: "One of the principal points of salubriousness for a great city such as Paris is to encourage the free circulation of the air that is breathed in it by gradually destroying all the obstacles that can obstruct it . . . and by moving away from the dwellings all concentrations of dirtiness and corruption."[62] These, of course, were enormous undertakings and would demand the removal of buildings from the bridges crossing the Seine, the opening of broad avenues through warrens of little streets, the removal of cemeteries outside the city walls, and the establishment of an effective waste management system. But despite the delays that frustrated reformers like Claude Lachaise, the will seems to have been there.[63] The buildings did come off of the bridges, allowing air to circulate more easily, avenues were built, and an elaborate sewer system was constructed at enormous expense of energy and treasure. And this commitment to hygienic improvements reached into the most hidden corners of the city. Belgrand observed that by the turn of the nineteenth century, "the Parisian Administration was highly concerned by the general state of infection in the city's subsoil, and the most vigorous measures were taken to combat this evil. A royal ordinance of September 24, 1819, required all property owners to make their cesspools [*fosses*] impermeable, and the Prefecture of Police organized a system of oversight that still exists today."[64] Starting in 1830, a drainage network was created to replace holding tanks and to protect the Seine from toxic runoff, the open sewers flowing down the middle of streets began to be replaced by crowned paving, the gutters were flushed with water, and "the mud, removed every morning, ceased to infect the subsoil."[65] In general, a system of hermetic barriers was being set in place to separate the salubrious from the pestilential and to flush the latter out of inhabited areas.

These measures received a powerful new impetus in 1832, when a cholera epidemic swept through Paris, killing some 18,000 people during the period from March 26 to October 1 and raising the city's annual mortality rate to 44,463, up from 25,996 the year before.[66] The disaster came on the heels of a decade-long debate that had divided the Parisian medical community over whether diseases were communicated by contagion or by infection. Ultimately, the commission appointed to study the epidemic attributed its origins to the physical conditions of Paris itself, thus siding with the infectionists.[67] This explanation seems to have resonated throughout a broader public of nonspecialists as well, for it recurred one year later in Balzac's novel *Ferragus*. "The narrow north-facing streets, where the sun comes only three or four times a year," he wrote, "are murderous streets, which kill with impunity."[68] In thus ascribing a lethal force to confined spaces and the absence of light, Balzac was appropriating the infectionist beliefs about urban epidemiology that were beginning to prevail among contemporary hygienists. These beliefs were also documented in a detailed study of the epidemic published by Dr. François-Marc Moreau in the same year as the novel, and his findings offer a glimpse into the physical world of disease that was emerging in the medical imagination of the time.[69] Moreau examined the conditions in one street in the northern section of Paris that had shown a particularly high incidence of mortality. He focused on two environmental factors, the lack of light and the quality of the air, but also discerned other contributing forces. Among the various professions, for example, he found that *concierges* or doorkeepers suffered the third highest rate of mortality. "Everyone knows," he wrote,

> the insalubrity of their dwellings, so aptly named *loges*, and which, situated on the ground floor, damp, dark, and deprived of sunlight, though often insufficient to lodge an individual, nonetheless contain a whole family, sometimes with their animals. In these close and unhealthy quarters, where the air is constantly vitiated by

emanations of every sort, there vegetates an entire population, scrawny, etiolated, scrofulous, predisposed to all diseases, and whom the cholera will not spare.[70]

Hidden away from the salubrious effects of sunlight and sunk deep in a pool of stagnant air, the inhabitants of the *loges* were forced to imbibe the effluvia exuded by various waste products and their own bodies. Moreau went on to note that rotting foods, feces, and even flesh had similarly infected the most deadly of the locations under study, where the rate of disease was 1 out of every 4.85 inhabitants and the incidence of mortality 1 per 15.2:

> The Saint-Laurent market, once the meeting place of high society, the Palais-Royal of the day, is now a sort of *Cour des Miracles*, a receptacle of poverty and vice. Successively, over the course of several years, a portion of the constructions built in this enclosure have been knocked down, but, as the grounds they occupied were neither sealed nor paved, they have become muddy cloacae, impassible not only for pedestrians, but also for vehicles. What is more, the inhabitants and passersby have transformed them into public latrines, a little neighborhood garbage dump, and one can say without exaggeration that in many places the soil is so covered with fecal matter that it is no longer visible. . . . [T]he inhabitants, almost all of them rag pickers, sort the products of their daily searches then pile up in all the corners of their rooms and even under their beds old bits of cloth soiled with mud and bones to which strips of putrefied flesh often still cling; so there continuously escapes from these heaps of filth fetid miasmas that turn the bedrooms into constant breeding grounds of infection, especially in winter, when the closed doors and windows block all ventilation.[71]

The problem, once again, lay in the absence of hermetic separations between human beings and the environmental forces that undermined their health, for Moreau attributed the degeneration of the Saint-Laurent market to the fact that the grounds on which it was built were not *clos* or sealed. The conclusion was unstated but clear: to avoid further outbreaks of disease, the city must be articulated in such a way that its inhabitants were at all points isolated from infected substances or the permeable materials they might contaminate. And once again, the forces of disease were polymorphous and labile, creating a vast network spreading through forms of infection that included mud, feces, rags, bones, and putrefied meat.

For Balzac, the streets of Paris seemed to take on a human life and will, turning not merely deadly, but criminal. For Moreau too, parts of the capital had become vaguely animated, imbued with a certain, mysterious agency. His Saint-Laurent market had its own almost Balzacian history of splendor and decadence and now seethed with a pestilential activity that permeated the ground, polluted the air, and reached even under beds to infect every detail of the buildings. For Moreau was categorical: cholera was not a contagious disease that spread from individual to individual, but was an infectious condition arising out of environmental conditions. If members of the same family fell ill in rapid succession, that, he argued, could be explained by the fact that they lived in the same rooms and were exposed to the same influences.[72] But for Moreau, like many of the hygienists influenced by Louis René Villermé, the conditions in the Saint-Laurent market represented a larger social problem. If the defects of the street were the cause of the cholera that devastated its inhabitants, those defects were in large part artificial. While certain locations, such as bogs, were naturally mephitic, that was not the case of this particular neighborhood. Instead, it was the shape and placement of the buildings combined with the behavior of their occupants that created the disease. And the single most powerful factor in that creation was indigence. "The affluence of the inhabitants noticeably attenuates the effects of insalubrious locations," Moreau observed, "while on the other hand poverty destroys the advantages of a healthy dwelling."[73] Some eleven years earlier, Claude Lachaise had advanced similar arguments about the relations between social conditions and disease. While he noted that "in general the mortality rate seems to be in direct relation to the narrowness of the streets, the elevation of the buildings, and the crowding of the inhabitants," this principle was complicated by the activities of the people in a neighborhood.[74] What were then the eighth, tenth, and twelfth arrondissements of Paris, for instance, all suffered mortality rates that could not be explained by their physical conditions alone. The eighth, he observed, "contains workers who toil at the most difficult labors along with individuals who commit the greatest dietary excesses," while the tenth housed an abundance of charitable institutions. "In short," he concluded, "the excessive mortality of the twelfth is explained, on the one hand, by the insalubrious workshops that it encloses and, on the other, by the defects specific to the location itself, and by the extreme indigence of the inhabitants who occupy certain parts of it. No one even questions that this last cause is the most significant of all."[75] As for Moreau, the most powerful among the artificial determinants of disease was poverty. Driven by its imperious rule, the working classes and the destitute were forced to create the conditions of their own mortality. In a more general way, however, these hygienists were discovering that the city itself was toxic, a repository of human wastes that constantly threatened its inhabitants with illness.

Behind this notion of environmental infection, a more subtle but more significant belief guided the hygienist imagination. This belief held not merely that environmental factors—such as weather or light—could weaken animal bodies, leaving them more prone to illness or failure, but that disease itself was physical, an element or property that could be situated in certain precise locations, like the Saint-Laurent market, the feces that covered its pavement, or in the flesh clinging to discarded bones. Two of the most dangerous and frightening of the places in the city were, according to this thinking, among its most common: toilets and graves. The two went together, moreover, for one of the most important metamorphoses of filth was the one that linked dead bodies to human excrements, and this connection was reinforced in both the popular and scientific imaginations by the fact that corpses seemed to share many of the noxious qualities of excrements. Even the word *fosse* was ambiguous, designating both the grave and the latrine. Human waste was, in Emile Trélat's words, "contrary to life."[76] Or as a group of scientists led by Cadet-De-Vaux had put it a hundred years earlier: "Happy the cesspool cleaner who, in the theater of his labors, does not open his own tomb!"[77]

The sources of infection were multiple and varied, reaching from rags and feces and corpses to more intangible conditions like miasmas, darkness, and poverty. Still, underlying all these different forms was a single force, a fungible operator that united these disparate entities as vectors of contamination in much the same way that physical symptoms were unified as the multiple expressions of a single underlying lesion in the body. The nature of this force was elusive, however. Pasteur's discoveries were still several decades away. The work of chemists and gas theorists had produced remarkable discoveries about the nature of air and its effects on animal organisms, but even they failed to explain the malignancy of urban life. The miasmas that polluted the city seemed to function according to some other principle, whose workings remained mysterious. "In recording the purity of the waters of the Seine, wherever it was drawn," Lachaise wrote in an 1822 study that echoed the hygienists' frustrations, "we have given only the results of the chemical analysis; but we are convinced at bottom that this analysis is as inadequate for detecting the mephitic principle that the water drawn downstream from the city might contain, as it has been for discovering the material cause that makes the air breathed on the banks of certain swamps . . . so promptly deadly for those who are exposed to its action."[78] The shadowy double of Paris, the abject other that expressed itself through a network of organic contamination, was held together by a single, noxious force whose nature still escaped satisfactory explanation. Increasingly, however, as attention focused on the link uniting feces with the dead, that force came to be identified with the processes of putrefaction, which accordingly moved to the center of discussions about public health, in both scientific literature and the popular imagination. In the next chapter, I will therefore turn my attention to the question of decomposition, examining the ways in which the relation between death and decay was theorized and the implications of those studies on the conceptual division between the living and the dead.

FOUR

Death Comes Alive

Among the more remarkable aspects of the environmental approaches to public hygiene that arose in the early nineteenth century was their tendency to view pathogens as elements with an objective presence in the physical world. In the form of germ theory, this has become conventional wisdom in post-Pasteurian societies, but that should not numb us to the strangeness—in a strict sense—of this perspective, for it was a conception of health that went beyond not only the problems of the individual but also of the animal body itself to view illnesses as potentially independent agents, with their own, autonomous existence. Sickness, by such reckoning, was not merely an alien force, it was a localizable entity. And as hygienists increasingly identified the environmental causes of disease with miasmas, the latter assumed a more expansive significance in medical thinking. They started to be treated as a latent form of disease itself, a noxious agent that could infect material objects and then, under the right circumstances, transfer itself into living organisms. To theorize this noxiousness, hygienists focused on the processes of putrefaction and decomposition, which came to be understood in terms of life and

death. The result was that death itself seemed possessed of a material existence. This belief had broader implications for the conceptualization of
society and urban space—not only from the objective viewpoint of the
hygienists, who treated death as something present in the physical environment, but also from a subjective angle, since the agency of death seemed to
be endowed with a certain sentience and, therefore, something approaching
a consciousness. This decomposing "subject," as I shall subsequently argue,
fascinated the scientific and popular imaginations of the early nineteenth
century. In that role, it acted as an irrational and largely unspeakable force
motivating the hygienic reforms that would transform Paris both physically
and conceptually.

Rotting Waste

As François Moreau's 1833 description of the Saint Laurent market made
clear, a particularly virulent source of infection could be found in the human
wastes that accumulated daily throughout the city, and their management—or rather mismanagement—provided a constant subject of concern
among the more progressive members of the population. Already in the
1780s, Sébastien Mercier had remarked that "each person has in his home
storehouses of corruption; this multitude of cesspools (*fosses d'aisance*) exhales
an infected vapor. Their nightly emptying spreads that infection throughout
an entire neighborhood, costing many unfortunates their life."[1] The deadly
properties of human waste moved throughout the city, not merely from the
isolated points of latrines, but by a generalized pollution of urban matter.
Seeping everywhere, human feces forced their pestilential effects into the
hidden, subterranean sources of life, contaminating the soil and from there
entering the water supply in a vicious circle of poisons. Mercier conjured up
a horrifying picture of this invisible and toxic Paris:

> Often poorly constructed, these cesspools [*fosses*] allow their materials to escape
> into neighboring wells. This does not stop those bakers who are in the habit of
> using well water from continuing to do so; and the most ordinary foodstuff is
> necessarily impregnated by these noxious and mephitic parts.
>
> The cesspool cleaners as well, to spare themselves the trouble of transporting
> fecal matter outside the city, dump it at daybreak into sewers and gutters. This
> frightful sludge makes its way slowly down the streets toward the Seine river,

infecting its edges, where water carriers every morning fill their buckets with the water that the unmindful Parisians are obliged to drink.[2]

In Mercier's view, the city's population was forced to breathe, eat, and drink its own feces, which were able to insinuate themselves everywhere throughout the capital. This, then, was the enemy: deadly, invisible, secretly oozing through every substance with which city dwellers came into contact. The force of such images was such that they troubled the hygienic imagination well into the nineteenth century. Hippolyte du Roselle would still worry in 1867 that the contents of the city's latrines were polluting its wells. "I shall not speak," he wrote, "of the purposes to which households might put that [polluted] water; fortunately, it is often used before the necessary heat has produced . . . the mephitic gases that are so harmful and so deadly to men and animals."[3] These fears survived even the Pasteurian revolution, when they merely adapted to a new vocabulary, replacing miasmas with germs. In 1882, Emile Trélat, a partisan of the *tout à l'égout* or "everything to the sewer" approach to urban waste management, worried about the pestilential materials that flowed through the city's underground canals. Feces could not, of course, be left above ground, he observed: "You might as well lay out the contents of our ten thousand cesspools before our eyes and spread their odious tapestry down the length of our streets, literally poisoning the atmosphere of the entire city."[4] But even in their subterranean channels, these poisonous substances still threatened to infect inhabitants, since "there is a constant exchange of air between the sewer and the atmosphere of the street."[5] In winter, the normally invisible action of these contaminants could actually be observed: "There is not a single one of us who has not seen, in cold weather, a sewer grate vomiting out vapors that condense in the cold outside. One cannot therefore doubt but that the dust and germs that have settled on the sewer walls detach themselves and float along the public way and into houses."[6] The circulus of deadly filth that Mercier saw flowing through the wells and underground water sources of the capital yielded, in Trélat's writings, to an image of interwoven threads, a texture of abjection at once blanketing the city and knitting it together. Or again, for Trélat, Paris could be thought of as a body belching up the contents of its intestines onto its inhabitants, and its anatomy that of the citizens, enlarged into monstrous but not incalculable proportions: "Two million two hundred thousand Parisians ingest for their daily sustenance three million kilograms of alimentary substances," he wrote. "Each day, they release two million five hundred thousand kilograms of exhausted materials that have been transformed by digestion. These remains, incompatible or contrary to life, are naturally expelled from the body. But they compromise the health of the inhabitants if they are left in their vicinity."[7]

As corpses decayed, they became increasingly like feces to the hygienists who studied them. It was not uncommon during this period to speak of graveyards as cloacae and to lump them together with latrines among the various factors believed to contribute synergistically to the production of the most virulent miasmas. Vicq d'Azyr's 1778 preface to Piattoli's *Essai sur les lieux et les dangers des sépultures* (Essay on the Placement and Dangers of Sepulchers), detailed some of the problems arising from the Saints-Innocents cemetery: the rotting vegetables from the adjacent market and the human excreta from the open sewers that surrounded the cemetery combined their deadly effects with the decaying bodies inside, whose gases stagnated in the enclosed space between the neighboring buildings.[8] While studying the seepage of toxic substances from the Saints-Innocents into adjoining basements some years later, Cadet-De-Vaux remarked that the effects he observed were similar to ones he had already encountered in latrines and mephitic wells.[9] In 1821, Hippolyte Cloquet wrote that the "myriad insects in animal corpses" were not, as had previously been believed, "the product of corruption," but rather developed out of eggs deposited by vermin that had been attracted to the smell of decay, whether that of corpses or of fecal matter. "*Bousiers, sphéridies, escarbots*, etc. come from all parts toward the remains of digested foodstuffs," he wrote. "*Necrophores, dermestres, sylphes*, and *ptines*, etc. attack and destroy cadavers."[10] Cloquet's juxtaposition of corpses and feces united them as different forms of an underlying process that could be detected by certain insects. In 1852, Ambroise Tardieu published a lengthy monograph on the handling of corpses and feces in urban zones. "The connection made here between garbage dumps and cemeteries," he wrote, "sufficiently indicates that these two great centers of animal decomposition must be studied from the perspective of those putrid emanations that they both exhale and from the point of view of their common influence on the health of the populations in whose midst they are located."[11] Even as late as 1884, Félix Gannal still spoke of tombs as "cloacae" that emanated deadly gases capable of penetrating and crossing the porous stones enclosing them.[12]

Fecal matter and corpses were thought to be deadly or "contrary to life," and their noxiousness was believed to result from putrefaction. This was the great fear that haunted hygienists and that insinuated itself into all the dominant theories of life and death during this period. As early as 1745, Porée had observed the deleterious effects of decomposition on the air we breathe and seemed to think that the process of rotting converted any organic substance into poison. "Everywhere there are animals, fish, and insects that corrupt and putrefy," he wrote. "Even vegetables spoil, rot, and exhale putrid particles. How many contagious illnesses have been caused by heaps of insects that people have neglected to burn?"[13] Similarly, in 1786, the abbé Bertholon recorded that "we have seen villages struck by epidemics that were entirely eradicated by filling in certain sewers where manure had been left to rot."[14] Several decades later, in 1858, Emile-Louis Bertherand stated explicitly that it was not fecal matter in itself that was insalubrious, but the effects of its decomposition. In proposing improvements to the system for emptying the latrines in Parisian buildings, he observed that "the frequency with which they are cleared . . . [can prevent] the materials from remaining in them long enough for the gases produced by fermentation to become so concentrated that they are perceptibly noxious."[15] By the second half of the nineteenth century, the connection that Bertherand observed between fermentation and putrefaction seemed to cast an important new light on the dangers created by decomposition and moved them increasingly toward the center of discussions on urban hygiene. In an 1867 pamphlet about the waste management system in Amiens, Hippolyte du Roselle spoke of the odors that emanated from sewers and continuously threatened to "decimate" entire populations. He approvingly cited a recent report by Lord Ebrington, a member of the London Sanitary Committee, who signaled "the regrettable effects on human life produced by the pestilential gases that are emitted by materials stagnating in sewers," and vaunted the merits of a new ovoid sewer system. By removing fecal matters "before their fermentation and putrefaction," Lord Ebrington wrote, "[this system] prevents them from producing the fevers and illnesses that afflict humanity."[16] Although the relations between rotting, fermentation and disease were unclear, they nonetheless helped explain the dangers of certain previously recognized urban problems, such as open sewers. The new scientific imagination revealed these to be constant sources of hidden fermentation, for when household waters "laden with highly putrescent vegetable and fatty matters" were thrown into the streets, du Roselle noted, they "make their way through the gutters. The water, which tends constantly to purify itself, deposits these matters into the gaps of the pavement. These materials ferment, then putrefy, whence the pestilential miasmas that escape from even the best-maintained gutters."[17]

The Pasteurian revolution of the 1860s eventually put an end to miasma theory, but the processes of rotting and putrefaction, which were central to that theory, also played a key role in Pasteur's work, for his discoveries began in an attempt to understand the workings and deleteriousness of fermentation. He wanted to explain why some barrels in a brewery produced alcohol and others lactic acid, and although his findings would lay to rest theories of spontaneous generation of life, which were still being debated in the Académie des Sciences, and eventually open the way to the modern science of microbiology, they left many significant ambiguities and questions.[18] He argued that the germs of contagious illness were carried by microorganisms and that these microorganisms, because they were living beings, obeyed certain natural laws governing life and generation. "Thus," he wrote, "when a ferment such as beer yeast is not susceptible to *direct transmission*, when it does not give birth to a germ that is resistant to the various causes of destruction, it will be affected by putrefaction just like all living organic matter. But this will not be the case when the ferment gives birth to a germ that is able, in an appropriate environment and after a long period of inactivity, to determine the development of new generations of ferments."[19] Pasteur's reasoning would suggest that putrefaction was destructive to all forms of life, including yeasts, but the picture was more complicated, because he also argued that decomposition could actually aid the activity of certain microorganisms. This could be seen, for example, in the propagation of typhus:

> clinical experience and medical observation teach that, in order to create a typhoid fever, one needs: . . . a breeding place [*foyer*] made of decomposing organic materials, whether they be ordinary fecal matter or the dejections from typhus sufferers. The distinction is of little importance in Paris, where one can be certain that fecal matter, collected in cesspools [*fosses*] and other hotbeds [*foyers*] of putrefaction, has so many opportunities to receive the seeds of typhoid fever.
>
> How do these germs propagate? If these fecal matters foul the water that we drink, they will be able to spread typhoid fever.[20]

Putrefaction destroyed life, but at the same time it provided a nurturing environment for certain living organisms, such as typhus germs. These dormant seeds entered into rotting substances, where they awaited the arrival of "an appropriate environment"; once such a "milieu" had appeared, the germs would be reactivated and give birth to further generations of disease. Rotting was thus ambipolar. Until Pasteur, this most reliable sign of death was still believed capable, even by members of the Académie des Sciences, of giving birth to new life, as if some occult vital force dwelt in the matter of death itself. Pasteur's theories of germs still retained this ambiguous core of putre- faction, although they displaced it slightly, replacing the notion that life sprang from rotting materials with the argument that its seeds were nurtured in it.

Indeed, studies on fermentation amounted to sustained reflections on the boundary between life and death, pitting materialists such as Justus von Lie- big against vitalists such as Pasteur. As François Dagognet has written about Pasteur's research on yeast and alcohol, "it is . . . a sort of Manichean vegetal- ism that opposes life and matter, agricultural production and chemical prod- ucts, nature and artifice."[21] While Liebig had argued that fermentation resulted from chemical reactions that had nothing to do with life, Pasteur's studies formed part of a larger project to define what the author himself described as "a chemistry of dead nature and a chemistry of living nature."[22] In fermentation and putrefaction, however, those two natures joined into a close and interpenetrating relationship, whereby inert or dead matter sus- tained the processes of life and the latter, in turn, transformed the chemical structures of the former.[23] Rotting thus condensed two opposite tendencies, one toward the destruction of life, the other toward its preservation and propagation. Putrefaction was a sure sign and cause of death, but of a death that now seethed with animate drives, and as Pasteur's careful original dis- tinctions between seeds, ferments, and decomposition blurred in the hygienic imagination of authors like Trélat and du Roselle, for whom fermentation and putrefaction were treated as identical, his concept of a life *in* death started to blend into that of a living death. In a telling example of such confusion, Louis-Auguste Cadet reversed the terms of Pasteur's universe, describing the cadaver as "the germ of death," rather than the seed of life resting latent in the realms of death.[24] It was difficult, even in the aftermath of Pasteur, to dispel the notion that in miasmas and putrefaction it was death that labored and not life, that death itself was somehow physically present in rotting matter.

Even for Claude Bernard—after Bichat and Pasteur, probably the most important medical theorist of the nineteenth century—putrefaction remained a mysterious process, but central to the understanding of life and death.[25] On the one hand, he observed, it was long established that animal bodies begin to decompose at death and that, as a subcategory of fermentation, putrefaction was one of the three ways in which organic matter could be destroyed.[26] On the other hand, for Bernard, all life involved the systematic destruction of its own material organization, and so it seemed possible to him that fermentation could be a necessary aspect of vitality. "Such is the current state of our knowledge about putrefaction," he declared in 1876. "Can similar actions with identical processes occur in the living organism and destroy its organic matter [?] . . . Chemists, skilled experts in such studies, do not hesitate to answer in the affirmative. I have long heard Mitscherlich say: 'Life is nothing but rotting [*une pourriture*].'"[27] Bernard sided with Mitscherlich's astonishing assessment, holding that fermentation was unique to animate matter, indeed that it "characterizes the chemistry of the living."[28] It would be difficult to overestimate the strangeness of Bernard's position, for it reversed the previously established terms that had long separated the living from the dead.[29] It is little surprise that figures such as Trélat, Du Roselle, and Cadet were confused.

Rotting was the primary source of concern for urban hygienists, since it seemed to be the root cause of key environmental problems such as miasmas and infection. At the same time, however, to identify rotting as the primary culprit in public health issues opened the way to deep theoretical difficulties, for under scientific scrutiny, fermentation revealed itself to be a mysterious process that raised fundamental questions about the border between life and death. To clean the city was thus to enter into a sustained meditation on the nature of those two states. Indeed, it raised the specter of a possible confusion between them, a zone that constituted a life in death or a life of the dead.

Living Death

Michel Foucault observed that "in the medical thinking of the eighteenth century, death was at once an absolute fact and the most relative of phenomena," for on the one hand "it was the end of life, and the end of disease as well, if the latter happened to be fatal." On the other hand, death represented a force of disaggregation that continued the processes of disease itself, so that the difference between illness and demise was one of degree rather than of kind.[30] This ambiguity reached deeper, however, in the years that followed, for confusion arose about the differences not just between death and illness, but between death and life. This confusion emerged, in precise and crucial moments of what was probably the most important field of medical inquiry in the early nineteenth century. That field was physiology, or the study of living organisms and their various parts, and its most significant advances were made through pathological anatomy.[31] Erwin Ackerknecht summarized the significance of those advances by remarking that for the first half of the nineteenth century, all the various "warring factions" among the medical scientists "had a common ground in pathological anatomy."[32] The defining figure of this new movement was Xavier Bichat, whose *Recherches physiologiques sur la vie et la mort* appeared in the last year of the eighteenth century and established the general framework of clinical medicine for the next fifty years. For Ackerknecht, Bichat's central role in physiology, and therefore in medicine as a whole, was symbolized in a monument that was erected after his death in 1802. He noted that a statue of Bichat stood in the courtyard of the Faculté de Médecine in Paris, "at the spot which, for one hundred and ten years, was the center of Parisian and of French medicine and, for fifty-five years, the center of world medicine."[33] Bichat's own colleagues and successors recognized, in other words, that he was at the center of the center.[34] Now, somewhat unexpectedly, the question of death and the possibility of identifying and defining it were key aspects of physiological research during this period, a fact to which the very title of Bichat's volume attests. So, not only was the principal work on death being conducted by physiologists, but death was at the core of the most important field in the early history of modern medicine.

The relations between materiality, sentience, and death came under scrutiny in the physiological studies of the late eighteenth and early nineteenth centuries, and out of that scrutiny there arose images, often discredited and repressed, of marginal ontological and biological states that blurred the boundaries between the living and the dead or the organic and the inorganic. Bichat attempted to isolate the processes of death in the animal body, to chart its progress through the different systems, their interactions as one or another of them failed, and the precise moment at which life ended. He concentrated on three organs in particular, the lungs, the heart, and the brain, observing their reactions as the links between them were severed in living creatures. In short, he instrumentalized death, using it as a means to reveal the relations among the different bodily parts, their various needs, and the limits of their resistance.[35] These horrifying vivisections, often performed on stray dogs, led Bichat to conclude that life could be divided into two sorts, the animal (or thinking) and the organic (or plant), which consisted in the assimilation, circulation, and excretion of nutrients.[36] Life, unknowable in itself, could only be defined, according to Bichat, in relation to its opposite.[37] "Life," he wrote, "is the set of functions that resist death."[38] As I have already observed, this formulation was harshly criticized, most notably by Bichat's cousin F.-R. Buisson, who argued that it amounted to circular reasoning, or a *cercle vicieux*, but such an objection is valid only if one views life and death as abstract theoretical principles with no objective, physical existence—which is exactly what Bichat seems to attribute to death here.[39] Death, for him, existed in the material world and attacked the vital functions, while these could be perceived, in turn, as a constant effort at self-preservation in face of such attacks.[40] Despite his insistence on the antagonism between the two states, however, Bichat's meticulous clinical studies on the process of demise led him to identify a liminal state between the animate and the inanimate. "Natural death is remarkable," he wrote, "because it almost entirely terminates animal life, long before the organic one ends."[41] His scalpel and clamps had shown that individual organs could continue to function even after the individual as a whole had succumbed and that they retained sensitivity to stimuli within an otherwise dead body. There thus existed, for Bichat, a realm caught between two deaths, where creatures were neither alive nor dead but bound to an existence of animal reactions and sentience without thought, a curious, vegetative state in which animation was reduced to its purest, most minimal residue, still locked in a struggle to resist the encroachments of inorganic matter.

As early as 1802, Buisson took issue with Bichat's findings in his *De la division la plus naturelle des phénomènes physiologiques* (On the Most Natural Division of the Physiological Phenomena). His first objection was that his predecessor had distinguished between animals and plants but not between animals and human beings, and this criticism formed part of a larger attempt on Buisson's part to create more definite separations between the animate and the inanimate—to erase, as it were, the indeterminate zone between life and death, matter and sentience, that Bichat had opened up.[42] "I see in man," Buisson wrote, "a being that *thinks*, that *wants*, and that *has the means to execute its will*. An irresistible feeling [*un sentiment irrésistible*], that is common to me and all the universe, teaches me that *thought* and *will* cannot be the attributes of matter, and I know that the being who possesses them is designated by the name of *intelligence*."[43] He is marking a critical point—indeed *the* critical point—in his thesis about the nature of life, and yet the reasoning drifts away from clinical observations and deductions to something vague and almost mystical: the justification for this absolute division between intelligence and matter is a transcendental, emotional insight. As the case is put here, the limits of intelligence are not knowable through intelligence, that faculty that allows for analysis, linguistic articulation, and communication, but rather through some other, lower form of awareness that is shared not only with other animals but with the universe as a whole. According to the terms of this passage, this subintelligent, subhuman, indeed subanimate intuition was the source of Buisson's central insight into the living world, and so it was an inanimate force that did the thinking—or rather nonthinking—central to his theory. And Buisson's attempts to justify the sudden absence of "intelligent" reasoning from his argument are still more revealing. "I will be permitted not to accumulate proofs here," he writes. "They can be found in the writings of all true scientists [*savants*]. Only bad faith [*la mauvaise foi*] can deny them. And it is not on a truth so unanimously recognized that I shall expect to hear objections as shameful for the mouth that utters them as for the heart that formed them."[44] At what should be the core of his theory of life, proof is replaced by the same sort of circular reasoning that Buisson had denounced in Bichat, for he cites as support for his position the writings of "true scholars," but the only apparent characteristic that distinguishes these scholars from others is the fact that they believed as Buisson did. The truth that should have motivated his belief is thus simply the sharing of that belief. Buisson's reference to *mauvaise foi*, takes on a strange—lucid but displaced—appropriateness here, for it seems to summarize not only his approach to truth but also his own decision to employ the term *mauvaise foi* at all, as if he were at once signaling and denigrating his own self-awareness of his polemical strategy. Argument yields to indignation, while reasoning, at the theoretical juncture between thought and matter, is replaced by some other motivation, involving shame and dishonor. It is not particularly interesting to say that Buisson was engaged in simple *mauvaise foi*, with the belittling implications that would have for him. It is more helpful, and revealing, to understand that *mauvaise foi* to mean that he was thinking *more* than he could bear or accept, that his thinking—which he himself describes as a strange subanimal intuition—exceeded its own self-imposed limits.

Similar excesses reoccurred in works by other writers. Some ten years later another physiologist, César-Julien-Jean Legallois, published a monograph that continued Bichat's investigations into the nature of life but concentrated on the heart and circulatory systems.[45] Like Bichat, he instrumentalized death in his experiments, vivisecting rabbits and guinea pigs to observe which functions continued, and for how long, after others were arrested. Although Legallois, like Buisson, refused to define life and argued that there was an infinite distance between it and death, his observation that isolated organ systems could continue to function after the death of the body as a whole was very similar to Bichat's notion of a postmortem organic vitality.[46] In the thirties, another disciple of Bichat, François Broussais, studied the principle of irritability, or the capacity of living tissue to react to stimuli, and attempted to explain psychological conditions such as madness through this function.[47] As the most primitive form of sentient activity that could be perceived, irritability represented an intermediate zone between thought and matter, even more elementary than the isolated organ functioning observed by Bichat and Broussais, and it would later be picked up by Claude Bernard as one of the distinguishing features of protoplasmic life. Francisque Bouillier, in 1862, identified the vital principle with the soul, seeing in it an organizing force that combated decomposition and joined the various bodily parts into a whole. He recognized the continuation of certain activities in isolated organs or amputated members, but argued that these were not in fact life, since they did not involve the soul.[48] Understanding the term *animate* in a strict, etymological sense, he described irritability and contractibility as "vital processes" but attributed them to dead matter, furthering the confusion between life and death by creating the notion of an inanimate vitality, or living death, as the unwanted theoretical by-product of an attempt to limit the meaning of life to a higher faculty.[49]

With Claude Bernard, this confusion was repositioned onto questions about the nature of fermentation and putrefaction.[50] For Bernard, life itself could be neither perceived nor defined, and instead he described two inseparable but antagonistic forces in living beings, one that created and the other that destroyed biological organisms.[51] The former he identified with life, the latter with death, seeing in this division the basis for all physiology.[52] Earlier theorists, such as Dumas and Boussingault, had maintained that plants were structurally different from animals in relation to the processing of nutrients, with the former synthesizing vital forces into materials like fat, albumin, and starch, and the latter capable only of converting those bound forces into energy and activity, through processes like combustion and oxidation.[53] But Bernard himself had already demonstrated, some thirty years earlier, that animals were able to create their own sugars and, later, their own fats, thereby weakening the great divide that separated the two kingdoms of living organisms.[54] Conversely, plants could be shown to oxidize nutrients through respiration.[55] But there still remained the old argument, dating back to Linnaeus, that while minerals *are*, and plants *live*, animals alone *feel*, which was further developed by subsequent theorists, who also noted that plants' immobility distinguished them from animals.[56] Bernard quickly dismissed this distinction by drawing on the notion of irritability, which had been developed by earlier scientists such as Broussais, and observing that plants too can feel and react to stimuli. "If plants do not present locomotive functions comparable to those of animals," he wrote, "they nonetheless possess a kind of sensitivity, which is the *primum movens* of every vital act."[57] In place of what he called dualist theories of life, Bernard offered the notion of a single, amorphous protoplasm that formed the elementary stuff of all living creatures.[58] And while this "living matter" had no particular form in itself, it could be poured into particular organisms like cells, organs, or individuals.[59] It thus flowed from being to being, reaching across time from no determinable origin, an elementary substance that could be grasped by neither vitalist nor purely materialist theories but that combined principles of both, embedding the living, in its most primitive and pure manifestation, into physical existence.[60] Life is a formless, sentient matter. It is inextricably bonded to this world. It uses individuals to perpetuate itself and then abandons them to death. And we, as human beings, are elaborations of the principles encoded in this protoplasm.

Now, it would seem that despite Bernard's demurrals about being able to define life, he did just that, but the terms of his argument shifted over the course of the lectures I have been discussing. I have already shown how this happened in relation to fermentation, which was treated ambiguously as a force of destruction—or death—and as the principle of life itself. A similar situation arose in Bernard's identification of life with a creative force, since in one of his last lectures he proposed a related but significantly different concept of animation, describing it as the interaction between two opposing forces. "Life," he wrote, "is a conflict. Its manifestations result from a close relation between the *conditions* and the *constitution of the organism*."[61] Life was, in this sense, the protracted struggle between an organism and its material environment. This struggle was, in turn, a slow form of demise, for "when a part, such as the muscles, glands, nerves, or brain, functions, the organ consumes its substance and destroys itself. This destruction is a physico-chemical phenomenon and most often the result of combustion, fermentation, or putrefaction. At bottom, it is really the death of the organ."[62] In this later view, which seemed still under elaboration in Bernard's final days, life would not simply be embedded in dead matter, but would actually *be* in part dead. And this death was, moreover, an active agent that was most often produced by the processes of rotting.

Repeatedly, in these various texts, the ongoing argument that there is an infinite or absolute difference between life and death falters, leading to the possibility that the two states are in a continuum or, worse, indistinguishable. The notion of a vague, material sentience that informed the physiologists' studies on life seems to have taken shape and found an emblem in certain, lower-order animals, and prime among these were the mollusks. They were not frequent figures in discussions of pathological anatomy or vitalism, but they did embody a certain idea of life in its most primitive aspect, and perhaps because they were not often cited explicitly in these discussions, mollusks attracted judgmental reactions that indicate some of the irrational and emotional investments that these debates aroused. George J. Romanes's 1882 *Animal Intelligence* described some of the observations and speculations that had recently been made on subhuman minds and offered insights into the state of the field on both sides of the English Channel. Of the mollusks, Romanes wrote that "it is not to be expected that the class of animals wherein the 'vegetative' functions of nutrition and reproduction predominate so largely over the animal functions of sensation, locomotion, etc., should present any considerable degree of intelligence."[63] These creatures thus represented a realm in which the lowest biological functions prevailed but mixed with sentience and even some dim level of thought. As such, they offered a glimpse into the relation between matter and intelligence that Buisson had so flatly rejected. To indicate that such lowly creatures were, in fact, capable of thought, Romanes quoted from a manuscript of Charles Darwin, who wrote:

> Even the headless oyster seems to profit from experience, for Diquemase . . . asserts that oysters taken from a depth never uncovered by the sea, open their shells, lose the water within, and perish; but oysters taken from the same place and depth, if kept in reservoirs, where they are occasionally left uncovered for a short time, and are otherwise incommoded, learn to keep their shells shut, and then live for a much longer time when taken out of the water.[64]

The key term here is, of course, *learn*, for it indicates that mollusks are capable of thought, memory, and judgment. Apparently the intellectual capacities of shellfish were common knowledge among the purveyors of seafood to the

French capital, for, in something like an oyster version of *L'éducation sentimentale* or *Illusions perdues*, Romanes described the training that these animals underwent before shipment. In a footnote to the Darwin quotation, above, he observes:

> This fact is also stated by Bingley, *Animal Biography*, vol. iii. p. 454, and is now turned to practical account in the so-called "Oyster-schools" of France. The distance from the coast to Paris being too great for the newly dredged oysters to travel without opening their shells, they are first taught in the schools to bear a longer and longer exposure to the air without gaping, and when their education in this respect is completed they are sent on their journey to the metropolis, where they arrive with closed shells, and in a healthy condition.[65]

The chapter goes on to describe other evidence of intelligence among slugs, snails, and cephalopods, and Romanes was led to marvel at these capacities, which even seemed to involve relations of empathy and altruism between members of the same species.[66]

But not all commentators were as sympathetic as Romanes, and for the most part oysters and other invertebrates were treated with revulsion. In the medical literature of the time, the mollusk became a figure of abject sensitivity. In 1849, Dr. Amédée Latour, the editor-in-chief of the *Union médicale*, drafted the following description of the human mind: "In imposing limits on human reason, you limit the power of God. God made man free and perfectible. If he attached the oyster eternally to its rock, he gave to the human soul activity, spontaneity, liberty, the imperious desire to know and understand, along with the means and instruments to acquire and enjoy."[67] Embedded in its physical environment, the oyster represented, for Latour, the antithesis of freedom. The latter, according to contemporary theories of the sublime, was peculiar to human beings, since it existed on the level of reason alone. And if freedom represented the sublimation of the imaginable world, the mollusk, it would seem, conversely represented the desublimation of consciousness, its subordination to the powers of the physical, rather than intellectual, world. Palpitating slowly, its entire being one viscous mass of tender organs in an infinite and grotesque nudity, the oyster had become, among both doctors and the broader public, a figure for the horror of idiotism and death, the organic realm of abjection from which humanity must detach itself. Elsewhere, an anonymous manual of hygiene from 1840 observed that "the oyster is the only animal that man eats alive."[68] Although not true, this perception is revealing, for the alimentary practice it describes recognizes in the mollusk a unique intermediary status between life and death: normally one eats what is dead, except in the case of the oyster, which consequently is treated as dead even when alive. In the same brief section on mollusks and crustaceans, the author also remarks that "the slug, for which many persons feel an insurmountable repugnance, was the favorite dish of the Greeks and Romans."[69] In a long chapter on the hygienic properties of various comestibles, this is the sole point at which the author speaks of aversion, much less disgust, toward certain foods. The invertebrate is not merely associated with an ambiguous biology, it is also the only nourishment notable for its repugnance. Once again, in a medical document, these creatures group together revulsion, horror, and the notion of an indeterminacy between the living and the dead.

The indeterminacy of life and death expressed itself in certain animals, in foods, and in other aspects of normal life, such as rotting. It surfaced as well in concerns about the treatment of corpses. The delay before inhumation, which was lengthened during the nineteenth century to allay growing fears about premature burials, led to extended vigils by the dead.[70] Clinical and common experience showed that putrefaction forced the individual back into the strange animation of the inorganic, the breakdown and activity of the corpse, its weird semblance of life. As the physician Félix Gannal wrote in 1868:

> Who has not seen a beloved person that, but a few moments earlier, was still alive, now laid out in dreadful immobility upon a bed? They are no longer anything more than a corpse. . . . Later, the members regain their suppleness and the temperature rises once more, but it is not life that is returning, it is decomposition that has begun. Fetid gases escape from the mouth, the belly distends, the chest swells, and the face, which until then had kept an expression of calm, alters in its turn: the eyes bulge, the eyelids puff out, as do the cheeks. Family and friends withdraw so as to avoid seeing more of the horrible spectacle that *putrefaction* will present in its rapid progress.[71]

The author was explicit, as if there could be some confusion in this crisscross of physical demise: this is not life returning, it is decomposition beginning. So close was the resemblance between living and rotting. And this false life, with its quick, determined step, seemed fantasmatically to be endowed with its own vague consciousness. That was the lesson of the oyster. But the triumph of the modern city is unknowingly heralded in the first words of this passage: "Who has not seen . . . ?" How strange the question now sounds to the inhabitant of an occidental capital. Today it has become: who *has* seen this horrifying spectacle?

For the physiologists, who were at the foreground of studies in biology, death and life were seen as inextricably interconnected, but the influence of another, more radical paradigm can be detected in their writings, a theory holding that there was not an absolute difference between thought and matter and that matter was or could be sentient—and not just any matter, but explicitly dead matter. The authors attempted to reject this possibility, but the arguments and science did not always support those attempts, as in Buisson, or they ended up contradicting themselves, as with Bernard. So there was an unexplained, almost emotional need for the distinction between life and death to be maintained beyond the scientific evidence. And from these studies there appeared *nolens volens* an image of death as an objective, physical, and even living entity: living in the sense that it was active and sentient, dead in that it was embedded in its environment, formless, and destructive to organized existences. A benign if repellent form of this existence was expressed in oysters and other mollusks. But it was also expressed in the fear that motivated the hygienic reforms of urban space, in the belief that death was physically present in the city and perhaps even dimly conscious. This might appear to be no more than a form of materialism, which would consider animation to be the result of chemical or other physical processes rather than of a separate vital force, but all of the theories I have discussed viewed death as corrosive to life, even when intimately joined to it. Life was a battle against death. Consequently, up until Pasteur's discovery of germs, waste and feces were considered to be dangerous, inanimate matter, but inanimate in a way that did not necessarily exclude sentience and possibly consciousness. And, as I shall argue, it was considered possible to inhabit the viewpoint of the dead—not merely through thought experiments or observations of lower life forms, but through certain sense experiences. Principal among these was the experience of smells.

The Smell of Death

Stimulated by new theories about gases, a subtle but far-reaching shift occurred in the relation between smells and death during the period when miasma theory prevailed. The idea that dead bodies gave off a peculiar odor yielded to the notion that death itself had a characteristic scent. "The wolf is often alerted by his nose even before he can see," Cloquet had observed. "The smell of carnage attracts him from more than a league away. . . . After combats, they have been seen hurrying to battle fields and unearthing the corpses."[72] Other animals seemed to share this special gift: vultures and condors, crows, flies, and sharks all seemed capable of sensing the presence of death—or even its mere immanence. He wrote that sharks "are attracted at a distance of five or six leagues by strips of rotting flesh and follow vessels where someone is on the point of dying."[73] Cloquet was not describing the smell of blood or some specific disease, since the odor was unaffected by the particular cause of demise. He was writing, instead, on the smell of death itself, and the latter emerges from these passages as an autonomous entity or condition, a tangible thing with its own characteristics. Cloquet did not treat it as some abstract category such as the absence of life, but as a presence in its own right. And what is particularly remarkable here is that death could make that presence felt even before declaring itself fully, could enter into the body even before the body dies. In a similar vein, he also noted that doctors considered "cadaverous stools" or ones of "a cadaverous odor" to be a very ominous portent in the semiotics of various illnesses, as if death could insinuate itself *as death* into the functioning of a living being.[74] Similarly, in 1849, when Eugène Bouchut described the means for differentiating between true and apparent demise, he isolated putrefaction as "the most certain of all the signs of death," an opinion corroborated in 1868 by Félix Gannal, who wrote that among the indicators of death, "only one is certain in itself, which is to say that it is sufficient to characterize death, and that is putrefaction."[75] Only the dead putrefied, and only putrefaction revealed death. But putrefaction itself could be hard to identify, since its own signs could sometimes be mistaken for bruises or gangrene and vice versa. For Bouchut, it was smell alone that allowed the observer to distinguish among these various conditions. "Putrefaction," he wrote, "can only be confused with gangrene or with a violent contusion followed by bruising. But with contusions there is no putrid odor. With gangrene, it is true, there does, in fact, exist a disagreeable odor, coexistent with the more or less pronounced softening of the tissues, but this characteristic odor differs from that produced by putrefaction."[76] No one appears to have argued that death had its own feel or taste or look, and even a symptom like the death rattle operated differently in the medical and popular imaginations, since it never cohabited with the living or lingered by the deceased, but simply marked the moment of transition between two states. And it was not merely that death, like almost everything else, had its own odor; among the five senses, smell was the one most intimately tied to it. There seemed to be some special bond between the two.

For Cloquet, smell "gives rise only to material sensations." Odors in themselves were "in some way more material" than the objects of other senses and seemed to maintain only the feeblest connections to intelligence and social existence.[77] In fact, for Cloquet, smell marked the divide between the intelligible and the sensuous, since "an individual deprived of the sense of smell could not acquire certain kinds of physical knowledge, but he would still keep all his essential prerogatives, since his intelligence would still have all the means necessary to develop and act."[78] Scents were also more sexual than the objects of other senses, more closely linked to the genital organs, and had the capacity to evoke, instantly and vividly, the most troubling memories.[79] Indeed, they seemed to create a peculiar relation to time itself, since they lingered in a way that other sense stimuli did not. Most quadrupeds, according to Cloquet, have such a refined sense of olfaction that "they smell things at greater distances than they can see them; and not only are they alerted from far off to bodies that are currently and actually present, but they even recognize their emanations and traces long after they have gone away and are absent. Accordingly, Buffon considered this sense to be for them like an eye that sees things not only where they are, but even in all the places where they have been."[80] The reasons for this distinction between the eye that sees and the eye that smells are not clear. Certainly, there are visible traces that indicate past events, but somehow, for Buffon and Cloquet, these were different from odors, in that the mind perceives the olfactory object as still present, whereas it recognizes that the cause of a visual trace has disappeared. There was only, by this reasoning, a present tense for the sense of smell: the past lingered in it without passing.

Cloquet's arguments built on more detailed studies of the relations between matter and consciousness in the previous century. The philosopher Etienne de Condillac, in particular, had tried to imagine how intelligence could emerge out of an individual's relation to the sensuous world by carefully constructing an elaborate series of thought experiments, which he published in 1754 as the *Traité des sensations* (Treatise on the Sensations). In this work, Condillac imagined a sort of human statue with absolutely no knowledge whatsoever, and to it he successively granted the different senses while trying to determine what sorts of ideas and functions his creature would be capable of at each point in its development. Smell is the first of the senses that Condillac attributed to his statue, who, in its earliest moments, simply identifies with the objects of its perception. Presented, for example, with a rose, "it will be in respect to us a statue that smells a rose, but in respect to itself, it will be only the odor of that flower."[81] Thus at first, the statue makes no distinction between itself and its surrounding world and consequently has no notion, no impression even, of a self. Because it is incapable of making comparisons, it is incapable of perceiving time—and "whole years will disappear in every present moment"—or of generating abstract concepts, since for it, each odor is singular and incomparable.[82] All of this changes, however, under the influence of memory, although it is unclear from what source the statue derives this faculty. It is not possible for memory to come from outside, since smells in themselves are timeless, but if it is innate, there is no explanation of why it should not operate from the beginning. Still, Condillac is categorical. At first he asserts that "forever limiting its attention to a single manner of being, the statue will never compare two such objects nor ever judge the relations between them: it will enjoy or suffer without yet having either desire or fear."[83] Then, some pages later, he declares that "being endowed with memory, there is no odor that does not remind the statue that it has been another one," and he immediately draws some of the consequences of this new capacity to make comparisons: "This is its personality, for if it could say 'I', the statue would say it at every moment of its duration, and each time that 'I' would encompass all the moments stored in its memory."[84] Although at this point Condillac is circumspect about the origins of language, separating it from the ability to compare with the contrafactual "*if* it could say," in the very next paragraph he inexplicably abandons these hesitations and identifies comparison as itself the source of language. "Insofar as it does not change, it exists without any reflection on itself, but as soon as it changes, it judges that it is the same as the one that had previously existed . . . , and it says 'I.' "[85] Thus the 'I' and language are both immediate results of an ability to perceive continuity in change.

The "I" arises from the recognition that it is different from particular sensuous experiences and, indeed, from sensuous experience itself, since sense stimuli change and it remains. The subject's separation from the material world is thus a product of the perception of time and its simultaneous negation through memory, even if any explicit reference to negation is absent from the *Traité*. And Condillac insists on the permanence of the "I" by distinguishing between its perishable qualities and a more enduring element, which would be something like a subject:

It is not the assemblage of qualities that makes a person, for the same man, young or old, handsome or ugly, wise or mad, would be so many distinct people; and whatever the qualities one loves me for, it is still me that they love, for these qualities are only different modifications of me. Were someone, having stepped on my foot, to say: "Have I hurt you? No. For you could lose your foot without ceasing to be." Would I be convinced that I myself had not been hurt? Then why would I think that, because I can lose my memory and judgment, I am not loved, when I am loved for these qualities? But they are perishable: so what? Is the "I" then a thing that is necessary by its nature? Does it not perish in animals? And is its immortality in man not a favor from God? In Pascal's sense, God alone could say, "I."[86]

A different sort of reasoning has entered obliquely into the argument, subtly shifting its register, which might explain why Condillac buried this passage in a footnote. It is the permanence of the "I" that separates it both from sense experience and from the various qualities that might modify it, and it is memory, in turn, that supplies that permanence. But memory, as Condillac treats it here, is itself only a quality of the "I" and as such can be separated from it. This contradicts everything that has preceded in the main body of the text. And so, with this apparently offhand observation about memory, all justification for the existence of the "I" evaporates, and we are consequently thrown back into a world of sheer sense experience. It is perhaps for this reason that after having dissociated the essence of the "I" from its memory, Condillac dissociates the "I" from itself, allowing that it too might be, by its own nature, impermanent, like the consciousness that inhabits other, lower life forms. By this reasoning, it is God alone who has an "I," in the sense of a self-sustaining negation of time. The continuity of the self would thus derive from God, an explanation that Condillac seems to borrow not from Pascal, but from Descartes, who argues, in the *Méditations*, that if the subject persists, not only in death but at all moments, it is because of divine intervention. And, indeed, the main question in Condillac's footnote is not so much about the immortality of the "I," as its existence at all. The possibility that one could lose one's memory opens the way for a sentience without a subject, a consciousness imbedded in the sensuousness of the material world. Such an existence would be, in Condillac's terms, to continue, after one's own perishing, in a kind of living death. But—in the most indirect way, it is true—he allows the possibility for another, nondivine source of the subject's continuity. "Why," he writes, "would I think that, because I can lose my memory and judgment, I am not loved?" Even if it appears that one is loved for one's qualities, the self can lose its memory and yet still be loved. Its continuity here comes not from God, but from the amorous gaze of another, who sees in the "I" what the "I" has forgotten and therefore lost: itself. Even in a godless world, the subject would seem to be maintained by the play of interpersonal memory, by the very fabric of the social itself.

Indirectly, through the hesitations and inconsistencies that trouble the reasoning of an author like Condillac, or in the theories of a hygienist like Cloquet, the contours of another consciousness dimly took shape. It is an awareness directly attached to the sensuousness of the material world, a thinking that vanishes with its surroundings and has no idea of itself as a discrete entity. It lives in a world without self, without others, without love, and its permanence, such as it is, is maintained instead through the durability of its material composition. The moment that dissolves, consciousness disappears too, and so it exists only insofar as it is poised on the verge of nothingness, a dim mirror of its environment, like an oyster in its murky bed. The principal opposition in these texts seems not so much to lie between life and death, between matter and thought, or the organic and the inorganic, as between this figure of a material sentience and a social, ethical, amorous world—between, in other words, consciousness and subjectivity.

It is true, Cloquet will argue that smell creates a sort of sympathetic bond among animals, since members of a species "are obviously drawn toward beings of the same or other species by the odorous emanations that mark their passing," but sympathy, as he understands it, has no moral or social component.[87] It is, instead, a purely physical relation, and, in fact, he uses the same term to speak of "that sort of sympathy that exists between the sense of smell and the intestinal tract."[88] In the world of smell, animals are drawn to each other as they are drawn to their food—simply as the satisfaction of a bodily need. And so Cloquet is explicit: "Olfaction is quite different from sight and hearing, which are necessary to the social state and without which that state could not continue to exist. Smell gives rise only to material sensations, it establishes no intellectual connection between a man and his peers."[89] And because this is a world without others, it is also, according to Condillac, a world without mortality. As he puts it: "Ultimately, it is not by reflecting on the succession of our ideas that we learn that we have begun and that we will end, it is by the attention we give to beings of our own species, whom we see come into life and die. A man who knew only his own existence would have no idea of death."[90] So it is that animals, which have no idea of death, live nothing but death. They lack that intellectual power that makes of death a concept, a nothingness always yet to come, utterly separate from life. If they live without the fear of their own mortality, they also exist without a sense of life. This is part of the fantasy of their materiality, their sympathetic embedment in the sensuous world.

Condillac's human statue is an imaginative construction, a philosophical monster designed to reveal our relation to the material world, but it was also understood to constitute a real and ongoing aspect of human consciousness, a part of ourselves so hidden by successive layers of consciousness and experience that it can only be isolated and recognized, like the German bacteriologist Robert Koch's anthrax spores or the chemical composition of air, through a rigorously controlled series of experiments.[91] By its location at the beginning of the statue's sensuous education, smell lies at the juncture of the presubjective (or animal) and the subjective (or human) worlds and is the sense most closely attached to materiality. Smell, in this way, is shorthand for an elaborate fantasy, that of a material sentience melting at the limit not between the human and the animal, but between the animal and the inorganic, somewhere in the zone inhabited by the oyster and the corpse. But because they persist, odors are also especially potent remnants of the past, sorts of memories embedded directly in matter itself. Smells, as Cloquet and Buffon observed, have a peculiar power to remain and collapse time. The "I," in this regard, operates like an odor: it persists over time, negating it. Indeed, in its earliest moments, Condillac's statue so purely identifies with what it smells that it is no more than an odor that perceives, a conscious scent. The only difference between smells and subjects seems to be that the former are not aware of the difference between the passage of time and themselves, that they cannot conceive what they are not. Smells would thus seem to offer the possibility of a purely material subjectivity—a subjectivity without subject—for the realm of odors is a world without negativity, an existence of pure plenitude.

The Smell of Time

Miasma theory produced the notion that death was somehow materially present in smells. Studies about olfaction, on the other hand, offered the model of a sensuous and material subjectivity, one that existed in odors themselves. Work by the German philosopher and literary critic Walter Benjamin indirectly suggests that these two positions go together imaginatively and conceptually, so that smells can represent a state of subjectivized death, a state that was characteristic of urban—and especially Parisian—experience in the nineteenth-century. In a study on Baudelaire's depictions of urban space, Benjamin offered an intriguingly inconsistent analysis of the relation between smell and self-identity. He began by citing the famous madeleine scene from *A la recherche du temps perdu* (In Search of Lost Time), in which Proust concluded that the past is "somewhere beyond the reach of the intellect, and unmistakably present in some material object."[92] Benjamin then contrasted this *mémoire involontaire* or involuntary memory, which lay outside the control of the intellect, with voluntary memories, and he made this opposition the crux of a general distinction between information and experience—a distinction that had produced, according to him, the defining trauma of the nineteenth century.

This trauma was, in essence, the loss of experience to information, and the distinctive character of the former was, for Benjamin, its capacity to be assimilated by a subject. Now, by assimilating something Benjamin meant integrating it into one's personal history, the way that a story does not simply convey information, but instead "embeds it in the life of the storyteller in order to pass it on as experience to those listening. It thus bears the marks of the storyteller much as the earthen vessel bears the marks of the potter's hand."[93] The subject, then, creates an image of itself and fashions itself *as subject* through this process of assimilation, this work of converting information into experience. Involuntary memory, as Benjamin understood it, was thus the persistence of subjectivity over time, a persistence that slowly organizes information into something personal and emerges, like a story, not under the compulsion of a preconceived and rational plan but from the hidden impulses of an individual life. At first, he cast this process in visual terms, speaking of the subject's dependence on involuntary memory to create an "image of himself" and thereby "take hold of his experience," but he subsequently reformulated it in reference to another sense. "The scent," he wrote several pages later, "is the inaccessible refuge of the *mémoire involontaire*. It is unlikely that it will associate itself with a visual image; of all sensual impressions it will ally itself only with the same scent."[94] Some of the difficulty of this passage stems from the fact that Benjamin seems to be getting his bearings even as writes, to be discovering something as it appears, hesitantly, on the page: what is at first explicitly an image is then unlikely to be an image and then can only be a scent. And smell seems to emerge here as the final refuge of subjectivity largely because Benjamin, like Condillac, Buffon, and Cloquet before him, detected in odors a unique power to obliterate time. "If the recognition of a scent is more privileged to provide consolation than any other recollection," he wrote, "this may be so because it deeply drugs the sense of time. A scent may drown years in the odor it recalls."[95] The problem that this observation created for Benjamin was that the persistence of smells might not merely provide the stimulus for self-recognition but constitute *in itself* the continuity of subjectivity, and if this were the case, then subjectivity could be objectified and alienated. Now, Benjamin had earlier rejected just such a possibility. He had observed that since Proust considered true memory to lie in material objects beyond the control of consciousness, it was "a matter of chance whether an individual forms an image of himself, whether he can take hold of his experience." Benjamin, on the other hand, had argued that the aleatory quality of self-identification was not an essential characteristic of memory itself but a contingent historical development, the result of a fundamental change in the social world that took place in the nineteenth century. "Man's inner concerns do not have their issueless private character by nature," he wrote. "They do so only when he is increasingly unable to assimilate the data of the world around him by way of experience."[96] The relation between memory and scent undermined this argument, however, since it placed the key to self-identity not in the dialectical process whereby an individual at once narrativizes events and creates him- or herself as narrator of them, but rather in an unchanging and nondialectical odor. It seems, therefore, no accident that at this point Benjamin switched the object of his analysis from smells to something else, namely festivals.

A comparison between the two is revealing, since it illustrates both the fears that a smell-based identity could provoke and the radical measures that might be taken to counteract them. After commenting on the unique persistence of odors, Benjamin remarked that a similar collapse of time was codified at certain points on the calendar. "Even though chronology places regularity above permanence," he wrote, "it cannot prevent heterogeneous, conspicuous fragments from remaining within it."[97] These discontinuous fragments were holidays, during which "the places of recollection are left blank" and "there is experience in the strict sense of the word," since in the repetitive, communal nature of rituals and festivals "certain contents of the individual past combine with material of the collective past."[98] Through holidays, the subject was able, in other words, to resist the rationalized organization of temporality into an endless stream of information and, in doubling back on itself against the passage of time, to reaffirm both itself and its capacity to experience. Conversely, however, the person who lost that capacity would be troubled by the feeling of having been "dropped from the calendar."[99] Benjamin cited as an example of this detemporalization the Sundays of the city dweller, for whom such ritual moments have lost their canonical significance and have become instead episodes of spleen, in which he senses the loss of experience.[100] Unlike these vacant moments, what Benjamin called "genuine historical experience" was built up from the ability to stop and assimilate events into a subjective negation of time, and by piercing through time, genuine (as opposed to splenetic) holidays thus functioned like smells: they were models of subjectivity.

Although they performed analogous temporal and subjective functions, holidays differed from odors in that the former were social and immaterial while the latter were asocial and material. These differences derived, however, from a more fundamental divergence in their relations to mortality. This becomes apparent when Benjamin compares his notion of history with Henri Bergson's concept of *durée* or duration. "The fact that death is eliminated from Bergson's *durée*," he argued, "isolates it effectively from historical (as well as prehistorical) order."[101] Presumably, by "prehistorical" Benjamin means "proto-historical": in other words, this deathless existence was, for some reason, incapable of providing a basis for the faculty of experience that would subsequently collect time into history. Whereas Bergson's *durée* was not even prehistorical, spleen was, so to speak, posthistorical and postsubjective, the conceptual space from which the subject looked back on its own demise. Through the dull emptiness of urban Sundays, one sensed the collapse of something crucial to experience and the world's simultaneous reversion to an earlier, presocial state: "*spleen* . . . exposes the passing moment in all its nakedness. To his horror, the melancholy man sees the earth revert to a mere state of nature. No breath of prehistory surrounds it."[102] The world returns, in such moments, to a previous, nonexperiential and, therefore, nonsubjective condition, an impasse that seems to bear no promise of historicity. Now, why this should be so has to do with Benjamin's conception of mortality. "The *durée* from which death has been eliminated has the miserable endlessness of a scroll," he wrote. "Tradition is excluded from it."[103] Death, in a word, was the thin line against the horrors of subjectlessness. Holidays, those hollow interruptions on the calendar that allowed time to accrete and organize into experience like crystals forming on a substrate, must derive, in some way, from the atemporality of death.

Odors were, for Benjamin, a form of subjectivity, a continuity that could underlie the information flooding through an individual and convert it into individual experience—but they could do so only through the intervention of mortality. It was death that mastered the atemporality of smells and holidays, that converted them from ahistorical states into proto-historical ones. Without an awareness of death's finality, consciousness, according to Benjamin, would be trapped in a state of nature. Although he did not explain this term, the tradition seems to speak for him. It is the prepolitical human condition, the life of those without a city. When, in his second *Discours*, Rousseau described human beings in the state of nature, he imagined their earliest form of consciousness to be just the kind of impersonality that haunts Benjamin's reading of Bergson. "Such was man's condition at birth," Rousseau wrote, "that he lived as an animal limited to pure sensations."[104] That state was, then, a sort of animal sentience. In the vacancy of spleen, in the listless *dérive* of a Sunday on the broad avenues of nineteenth-century Paris, the Parisian could, according to Benjamin, feel the persistence in him of a being without death, a consciousness without history, identity, humanity, or even life—the dull sentience that we have already seen emblematized by oysters. The melancholy urbanite was not *only* this state, but he did, in some way, recognize it in himself, for he was conscious of his own loss of subjectivity, aware, on some dull level, that he was living on after his own fear of death. Benjamin's melancholy urbanite was like an oyster that knows it is an oyster, that senses it has lost something it can neither identify nor define. Melting into its surroundings, the mollusk is permeated by its environment, the way that the body is permeated by smells and miasmas. The Sunday stroller knows, in contrast, that he once had a self, can intuit it somehow, and so feels the loss of his subjectivity as he dissolves into an environment of meaningless information, into a world in which not only the stones and buildings and mud are senselessly material, but also the texts—for, according to Benjamin, it is only the physical layout of a newspaper's pages that gives a semblance of coherence to its contents. In other words, Benjamin argued that existence without the concept and fear of death created a splenetic, subjectless experience. On the other hand, to the extent that smells both efface the notion of death and create a form of material subjectivity, the subjectivity they create is inevitably, by his reading, a subjectivity *of* death. And according to Benjamin this subjectivity was both new to and characteristic of urban experience in nineteenth-century Paris.

With Pasteur, a period drew to an end, a period when the world seemed different and smelled different, when individuals had, in some general way, another sort of affective relation to their material surroundings. It was an aesthetic period, in the sense that it was defined by the way things felt: the relation between the intellectual and physical worlds, between the intelligible and the sensuous, had a certain, cultural specificity that appears to have translated into actual, individual experience. And indeed, culture is perhaps itself the translation of experience into thought, since communities as such never directly feel, but always depend, instead, on the organs of their constituent individuals—insofar as a "we" feels, it does so only in a mediated way, by sharing information through some sort of language. Still, the triumph of the city was not altogether complete. Some aspects of the pre-Pasteurian world did not vanish afterwards, or at least not entirely. Its fantasies of abjection were born out of Enlightenment theories—what Foucault called its episteme—that are still prevalent in our respect for reason, our allegiance to scientific authority, and in our very notion of human progress. The sanctification of death as a defining absolute for subjectivity and history has only gained in force and clarity over the intervening years, as is attested not only by Benjamin, but also in larger currents of twentieth-century thought, such as Martin Heidegger's philosophy.[105] In a more obscure, subterranean way, nineteenth-century fantasies of the abject have persisted as well, although mostly in their inverse, marked by the countless, unthinking gestures with which our contemporary existences hold them at bay. We probably do not believe that we will fall sick and die from the smell of rotten meat, but still, in our very revulsion toward the putrid some dim world is conjured up, a world whose contours momentarily flashed up in the early nineteenth-century medical imagination. And every time we wash our hands, we check our vigilance against that world and reaffirm our allegiance not only to science and reason, but also, perhaps, to subjectivity and to death: not the death of swollen bellies and rotting faces, but the clean and terrifying death of thought itself.

The city, according to Rousseau, can never exist except in a republic. It is only when the people themselves are sovereign that the town, transformed into a place of justice, earns this higher name. "The true sense of this word has almost entirely disappeared among the moderns," he wrote. "Most of them mistake a town for a city and a townsman for a citizen. They do not know that houses make a town but that citizens make a city."[106] It is the engagement of the inhabitants in the political order, their acceptance of the rights and duties of rule under the social contract that so transforms the space in which they live. Paris, in this sense, became a city only under the Revolution, and before it had been something less. It became a city, in other words, when its people joined in a contract of reason to expel the unclean from their midst and to remember its exclusion with horror.

The difference between life and death was crucial to nineteenth-century medical theory and it troubled the popular imagination but it was also impossible to identify with any conceptual clarity. It seemed clear enough, however, that death related somehow to putrefaction and its whole gamut of cognate states, such as miasmas, rotting, and fermentation. And in those states, death appeared to take on an objective, material existence. More disturbingly, inanimate matter seemed, in those states, also to enjoy some of the qualities that were thought to characterize life, including some form of sentience. Individuals could experience this inanimate sentience, not only through thought experiments, such as Condillac's treatise on sensations, but in certain of those sensations themselves, notably smells. Death, in this respect, was not outside of individuals, but formed a part of their life, and indeed, as Walter Benjamin's writings on the Paris of the nineteenth century show, it could even be thought to form the crux of their individuality as a forgotten—or perhaps repressed—continuity underlying their conscious identity. Death—not as an absolute limit, not as the isolating and untransferable threat of mortality, but as an ongoing experience—could be imagined to form the source of individuality. In this sense, when the hygienists set to work on clearing Paris of its rotting mud and evil smells, they were also beginning to clear it of a prehuman aspect of themselves.

FIVE

Pleasure in Revolt

Corpses and feces were linked through the notion of putrefaction, which led hygienists to conceptualize them as eternal opponents to the living, noxious elements that must be excluded from the city. Still, pre-Pasteurian theories of fermentation and decomposition revealed that the distinction between the forces of life and death was more difficult to define formally than it was to intuit, and this difficulty created a significant ambiguity about the relations between the two principles. That ambiguity appears to have reached out in other, more emotionally charged directions, for the abject and the dead also aroused a curiosity that sometimes bordered on fascination, an interest that seems, in the words of Peter Stallybrass and Allan White, to have borne the impress of desire.[1] I will try to expose that desire in this chapter, to show how the enemies of life and the city exercised a disturbing allure over the scientific imagination. In what follows, I will first discuss the ways in which the dead were viewed as productive and even creative elements in the cycles of natural life and artistic invention. From there I will look at utopian projects for harnessing the latent powers of fecal matter for the redemption of humanity and the strange effects that those powers had on such basic concepts as time and the body. And finally, I will consider a social category that was closely assimilated in the hygienic imagination with feces and death: the prostitute. From this particular perspective, concerns about the sex trade in nineteenth-century Paris reveal how hygiene as a whole—or at least its central concerns about putrefaction—was saturated by unspoken and displaced erotic longings.

The Fertile Dead

I have already discussed Hippolyte-Louis Royer-Collard in the preceding chapter, noting that as the occupant of the chair in hygiene at the Faculté de Médecine in Paris he was probably the foremost figure in his discipline at the time. In his first course at the Faculté, in 1845, he laid out his vision of hygiene's importance and its role in society. To do so, he took a broad perspective, conjuring before his students the image of a marvelous continuity linking all creatures together. From the lowest animalcule up to human beings, we are all, he told his audience, composed of the same basic stuff. "If we cast our gaze on the whole of nature's beings, what do we see?" he asked. "An innumerable crowd of individuals who differ among themselves and in whom the same matter constantly circulates from one to the other, transforming itself from one into the other and thus offering us the uninterrupted spectacle of an eternal metempsychosis."[2] The passage of time revealed to Royer-Collard the boundless creativity of the physical world, the invention and destructiveness that belie the underlying unity of its various expressions. An outside observer might note, however, that as perceived by the hygienist's timeless gaze, animals as a whole bear a striking resemblance to the swarming creatures that horrify the civilized imagination: joined by a common substance that relentlessly asserts its dominion over particular manifestations of consciousness, individual blends with individual in a vague mass of sentience whose elements can only fleetingly be distinguished from each other. All animals, when seen from this perspective, pullulate like vermin. But in this constant flow of forms, nature, according to Royer-Collard, endlessly strives toward a higher perfection, moving inexorably upwards "from raw, elementary matter all the way to man," and in so doing, summarizes every previous step in the subsequent ones, so that each animal encapsulates in its being the phylogeny that preceded it. "Man, who stands on the highest rung of this ladder," Royer-Collard concluded, "therefore contains in himself all the substances and attributes of the beings below him."[3] Human beings thus retain a physical memory of creation as a whole, an ineradicable persistence of all that is subhuman, down to the lowliest manifestations of sentience, and even beyond, to darker, inanimate processes. Because of our bodies, we are still part oyster and membrane, dimly aware of our liminal status at the verge of the unthinking earth, where a primitive aspect of our being attaches us to the abject.

The hygienist described this idea—that the most elemental processes persist in higher life forms—as "no less fecund" than his observation about the circulation of matter.[4] These thoughts about the swarming of life and our own attachment to the abject are, it would thus appear, fertile, somehow engaged in a process that mimics those of reproduction and agriculture. "It seems to the physiologist," Royer-Collard continued, "when his analysis decomposes this immense and harmonious work, that all the parts of creation are, as it were, just the separate elements, the scattered organs of the human body."[5] The human body stretches, in this way, beyond itself, fading off into the distance of the material world. And this continuity reveals itself through a process that the hygienist called decomposition. The word operates in this context as a synonym for analysis, but it also suggests that the disintegration of the human body in death reveals something of its attachment to the larger world, that in putrefaction we are confronted by an image of our incorporation into an inhuman, indeed lifeless, environment. Death, in this sense, is a heuristic for the conceptual instrument that is analytic thought. In the very way that he presented his ideas, in his choice of vocabulary, the doctor revealed a continuum between the abstract processes that govern how we think about matter and the behavior of that matter itself: decomposition is analysis, ideas are fecund. The intellectual approach he proposed was thus based on material functions—or vice versa. In either case, the human mind is attached to the world in the very modes of its thinking: thought putrefies and fertilizes like the human bodies that sink into their physical environment at death and thereby reveal their continuity with it.

Through the process of decomposition, the dead themselves are thus caught in the cycle of renewal that is, for Royer-Collard, one of the most basic and fruitful principles of hygiene. His idea was not entirely original, for one already discovers similar scientific theories in the early modern period. Despite a general wariness about falling prey to superstitions and popular credulity, seventeenth-century doctors devoted lengthy passages and even books to describing the behaviors characteristic of dead bodies, passages in which they treated the corpse as an object of medical interest in itself and not merely for its diagnostic value in relation to illness, as would later be the case.[6] While L. C. F. Garmann equivocated on whether cadavers maintained some dim ability to perceive the world around them and remained skeptical that murder victims could react to their killer's presence with profuse bleeding, as was commonly believed, he did accept that some vestiges of animation continued after death. Hair, fingernails, and teeth continued to grow, he observed, the body still sweated, the penis could swell to erection, but all of these activities were transformed in quality and meaning at the moment of demise. The touch and secretions of cadavers, for instance, acted unlike those of other bodies, for they exercised unique effects on the living. Through the forces of sympathy and antipathy they were often capable of healing illnesses or preserving against the effects of age and accidents. It was for this reason too that the earth of graveyards had therapeutic value and encouraged the growth of vegetation. According to both the medical and popular imaginations of the time, as Philippe Ariès puts it, "corruption is fecund, the earth in which the dead are buried is, like death itself, the source of life: *exquisitum alimentum est*. The idea will become a commonplace in the eighteenth and early nineteenth centuries, up until the Pasteurian revolution."[7] Death itself is food, but made exquisite and strangely powerful by its difference from life.

And yet, despite obvious similarities with later theories about fertilizers and soil supplements, the seventeenth-century literature does not think of death as caught up in a cycle of decomposition and renewal or argue that matter will be released and transformed by the process of decay. Writers such as Garmann and Paul Zacchia imagined instead that bodies acquire a sort of ontological power by dying, so that their passage into another category of being altered the sense of everything they did, lending it what appeared, in the unscientific understanding at least, to be a miraculous potency that lasted until the corpse had entirely broken up. The idea that there is a material continuity between the living and the dead or a mutual exchange of substances between the two states did not really emerge until the following century, when figures such as Holbach and Diderot justified the need for mortality by arguing that there is an unvarying amount of matter in the universe. For creation to be possible, these *philosophes* reasoned, it must be offset by an equivalent destruction, and so each new life demanded a corresponding amount of death.[8] Enlightenment thinkers considered death to be part of a closed system of material vicissitudes in which inanimate bodies provided the space and stuff for other beings.[9] The deceased were, in this sense, not merely the excrement of an entire life, they were also fertile, the raw material for new existences. The vital powers of the corpse did not therefore derive, as earlier doctors had believed, from its *continuing* to act as a body, albeit transfigured by death; instead, its fertility came from its *ceasing* to be a body, from its dissolution into more primary elements and its return into an indeterminate material potentiality.

These ideas percolated through other segments of the educated classes, and by the latter part of the century some of the most progressive architects of the period had begun to translate similar beliefs about the fertility of death into vast new projects. Inspired by Newton's descriptions of physical laws and by recent writings on the sublime, Etienne-Louis Boullée and Nicolas Ledoux drafted plans for buildings that were intended to reveal the secret truths of the universe through physical structures and to reconcile social behaviors with the deepest laws of nature. "In funerary monuments," Boullée wrote, "I have undertaken to inspire the horror of death and thereby to lead men back to moral ideas."[10] He understood his creations to be instruments of social improvement and he took his inspiration not from previous artists but by returning to a meditation on the surrounding world itself. "Man," he argued, "can advance in his art only by studying nature, . . . it is by her that one can learn the poetry of architecture."[11] Although he described the influence that long theoretical investigations had exercised on his aesthetic approach, Boullée's idea of nature was a profoundly physical and emotional one. His most basic principles for funerary monuments, for example, came from effects of moonlight and shadow he had observed while walking in the woods and from the deep sadness that they had inspired in him.[12] It was through these observations, both of the world around him and his own sensibility to it, that he was able, as he put it, to "put nature to work [*mettre la nature en œuvre*]."[13] As an artist, he was, therefore, a *metteur en œuvre*, one who did not so much describe as do what nature does. And in his funerary monuments, he consequently strove to emulate that nature, to find the salutary sadness of death that speaks through shadows and half-light and to bend it to the shaping of a better, a morally superior individual.

It is not by accident that Boullée should have devoted so much attention to funerary structures, for the notion of death itself played a pivotal, if untheorized, role in his conception of human creativity. This sort of building represented for him, in some unspecified way, the essence of his discipline, for it "requires more particularly than any other the poetry of architecture."[14]

Of all the arts, it would seem, architecture is the one most adapted to expressing death, and death, in return, allows architecture to express itself most fully. Now, the purpose of funerary edifices, Boullée observed, is to perpetuate the memory of those for whom they are erected, and the most basic of the functions that they must perform is, therefore, to "brave the ravages of time."[15] They are, in this respect, buildings that step outside of time, and in so doing they are able to articulate some unvarying truth about nature: by their very essence, they speak of what is immortal in the physical world, of its underlying laws and secret workings. The cemetery, as Boullée conceived it, makes matter intelligible, although not in an intellectual way; instead, among the tombs of the dead, nature speaks out about itself in tangible forms, in rock and dirt, light and shadow. The problem was, of course, to find the moments in that language when it could become comprehensible to the human spirit, and Boullée's solution seems to have come to him out of nowhere: "there came to me an idea as new as it was bold," he recounts, "which was to offer the spectacle of a buried architecture [*l'architecture ensevelie*]."[16] Enraptured by the genius of his own discovery, he did not, or perhaps could not, explain why such an approach would be effective or how it was supposed to reveal the essence both of natural law and architecture, and so one must try on one's own to imagine what it represented for him. In describing his cenotaphs, Boullé spoke of the need to give them "squat and sunken proportions," so that "the spectator might presume that the earth had hidden part of them from his view."[17] By thus suggesting that the construction extended out of sight, the proportions of such buildings would seem far greater than they actually were, and so one would be able to create an architecture of almost infinite dimensions.

Rather than intimating a grandeur that could only be grasped by reason, the way that the pyramids did in theories of the sublime, however, Boullée's monuments sank into the ground, losing themselves not in the purity of mathematical thought but in the materiality of nature.[18] Death is pictured here as a return to the soil, and that soil itself is imagined to be fertile. Boullée spoke of a "naissance à ras de terre [*ground-level birth*]" to describe the way his forms emerged from the earth, as if the memory of the dead was to be understood as part of a process of renewal and life.[19] Similarly, in a description of his project for a model cemetery, Boullée's contemporary, Nicolas Ledoux, spoke about the creative forces of death, although in more ambivalent terms. "Is this a new world arising from the disorder of chaos," he asked, "or are these the catacombs of the universe?"[20] In the very notion of chaos itself, especially in the way that Ledoux used it, there is the suggestion of an immensely greater death, a breakdown of the laws of nature themselves, in which the world as a whole might end or be reborn. Individual demise would seem to be an image of this cataclysm, in which nature itself is reinvented or destroyed. For Ledoux, the fear of radical change seems to be that it might result in nothing at all, that in returning to a *tabula rasa* one might never get any further. But even annihilation itself seems to be a form of death's creativity for Ledoux, one of the infinite potential variations that it holds locked up in a dark latency. And if funerary architecture plays a central, although untheorized, role in Boullée's aesthetic program, it is because of the importance of death for his understanding of the universe. He argued that the arts must find their inspiration and guidance in nature. Nature, according to contemporary theorists, expressed its own creativity in death. Death was the power of transformation, the key that unlocked the dynamism hidden in matter itself. Death turned the potential into the real, made the earth move, and thereby animated nature. And it was in death that nature revealed itself as both mother and artist, as paradigm for the architect. This, I think, is the meaning of "naissance à ras de terre"—as imagined by Boullée, death's creativity was not merely a biological principle or the forerunner of such twentieth-century concepts as eco-systems; it was also a model for shaping aesthetic projects, for orienting their goals, and for justifying their value.

The belief in the fertility of death was eventually justified on the basis of chemical reactions, but it found its roots in a vaguer, more mythological notion of nature's creativity. And even before the connection between decomposition and soil nutrients was scientifically analyzed, this more informal, but still powerful, conviction was embodied in projects to combine cemeteries and plantings. The historians Richard Etlin and Thomas Kselman have both recently detailed the rise of the Elysian cemetery in late eighteenth-century France and the increasingly important role of vegetation in funerary architecture during the same period.[21] What Boullée had sought to capture through the play of light and shadow and the immensity of geometrical solids, younger artists tried to express through woodland parks and Arcadian settings. Rather than isolate the formal, even geometric, principles of the material world in their workings with death, this new generation preferred to integrate the deceased into actual landscapes. Mortality was thus ideologically subordinated to a larger and more reassuring principle, that of an undying nature. But the recycling of matter was often confused with the persistence of consciousness and individual identity, so that the laws of nature that indicated the necessity of death seemed at the same time to promise an escape from it. As a certain "citizen Légouvé" wrote in the November 2, 1796, issue of the *Moniteur Universel*:

> In the flowers, in the woods, dodging fate's blows,
> Our parents come back to converse with us.
> Reassured, our soul will see their shape in everything;
> And the fields, peopled by them, will become Elysian.

> Dans les fleurs, dans les bois, du sort trompant les coups,
> Nos parents reviendront converser avec nous.
> Tout rendra leur aspect à notre ame appaisée;
> Les champs, peuplés par eux, deviendront Elysée.[22]

Now the *Moniteur*, which transcribed daily sessions of the French legislative bodies and published accounts of the political scene in foreign capitals, was more given to reports of official business than to poetry. In all of 1796 it published only ten poems, and they tended to hew closely to the political and ideological functions of the paper as a whole. The first verses of the year, for instance, were an allegory of the state, entitled "Fable. Les Passagers et le Pilote [*Fable. The Passengers and the Pilot*]."[23] Easter was marked by "La Pâque naturelle: Hymne à l'usage des Philosophes [*Nature's Easter: Hymn for the Use of Philosophers*]," which sought to dechristianize the holiday by construing it as a celebration of the sun.[24] Within this context, Légouvé's verses represent something like an officially sanctioned attempt both to appropriate All Saints Day and to reconceptualize the notion of dead bodies themselves. Légouvé imagined that through the forces of memory and sentimentality the dead could be reintegrated into the plants around them, infusing them with their thoughts. For much of his poem he carefully avoided falling into a genuine animism, arguing that in Elysian graveyards "we believe" that the dead are still present, and that to mourners "it seems" that the flowers growing there still embody the essences of the departed. But in the lines quoted above that caution disappears, and the fantasy is embraced as a reality—the dead *are* still present in the plants growing above them and through that presence they *are* able to communicate with us. A similar slippage occurs in an article by A. Jourdan from the July 6, 1796, issue of the *Moniteur*, in which the author militates for the right to bury one's dead on one's own property. "For pity's sake," he writes, "do not force me to surrender my father's remains, to be profaned by your indecency, irritated by your brutality."[25] The idea that the dead could be irritated by impious handling could be read as a metaphor for our feelings toward them, but the choice of the verb *irriter* is significant since, as I have argued, irritation will subsequently be theorized by physiologists as the most primitive level of animal sensitivity. What begins, in both of these writers, as a conscious projection of feelings onto the deceased becomes a less controlled fantasy about sentient matter. A material metempsychosis underlies Légouvé's vision of the dead: they do not disappear but return instead under other forms, and the soil of the tomb creates a continuum between human and vegetable lives, so that sentience itself is caught up in the recycling of raw matter, as if it lingered, somehow lambent, in the processes of the physical world. The earth is memory, fertility, and the transformation of the deceased into new existences still dimly conscious.

Others, such as Athanase Détournelle, imagined the synergy between death and vegetation in more practical terms and proposed reclaiming burial grounds for agricultural uses by tearing down the walls once a cemetery had been filled and sowing the land with crops.[26] Despite the differences in their approaches, both he and Légouvé saw a physical continuity between the deceased and plants, the integration of the dead into an unconscious life that in some way they were able to nourish. Even late into the nineteenth century, writings about cemetery planning were still haunted by a confusion between agricultural and burial grounds. In a tract against the practice of interring the indigent in common graves, for instance, Jacques Fernand moved so smoothly between the ideas of the land a peasant cultivated and the graveyard where his ancestors lay buried that the two places started to fuse. "The Man of the fields is more fortunate than the beggar of the great cities," he wrote. "If his sweat has moistened the furrows where his food . . . his bread . . . that sacred viaticum . . . sprouts, then he is certain to be untroubled in the field of rest . . . where his mother lies in perpetual sleep along with all those he has cherished" (suspension points in original).[27] Despite all its interruptions, the syntax itself establishes a causal relation between the field where food grows and the graveyard in which the laborer is finally put to rest: if that, then this. The two plots of ground are thus joined in a balanced cycle of taking and giving: whoever cultivates and eats the fruits of the soil, the author promised, will return at death to the earth. The laborer's body thus establishes an equivalence and a cyclical continuity between cemetery and field. In its very physicality, in the sweat that pours from it, it becomes the *alimentum exquisitum* that makes growth possible. It is then consigned fully, at death, to the ground. The idea that his corpse in turn nourishes the field and becomes food is never stated as such, but this last link in the circle between field and tomb is hinted at in the use of the term *sacred viaticum*. By referring to the peasant's daily bread in this way, the scene of his labors is shifted into death, for the viaticum is the food of the dead, the nourishment given for their final, endless journey. With the use of that one word, the peasant is consigned to the eternal task of making the fields bear fruit, only he does it now in rest and with his whole body.[28]

Waste Redemption

Such fantasies of death's fruitfulness haunted the imagination of the Enlightenment and its aftermath. They shaped behaviors not only on the individual level, as in artists such as Boullée and Ledoux, or in carefully delimited discursive spaces such as Royer-Collard's lecture hall, since these imaginings also influenced social projects and urban planning. Because of the fungibility between feces and corpses in hygienic theories, the relation between life and death was also expressed through the interactions between the body and its excrements. The latter were, consequently, the object of a deep and ambivalent fascination that involved a positive, indeed jubilant, component.

Probably the most adventurous—although one of the least appreciated—theorists of fecal waste in the nineteenth century was the utopian philosopher Pierre-Henri Leroux, who, despite his irrepressible eccentricity, served in the national legislature and became intimate friends with leading literary figures such as George Sand and Victor Hugo, both of whom took his work seriously and sought to popularize his ideas. To understand the significance of Leroux's writings on waste, one must, however, place them in the context of Robert Malthus's economic theories, which they sought to refute. In 1798, Malthus published the first edition of his famously unloved *Essay on the Principle of Population* and by 1817, when its fifth edition appeared, he had become one of the most prominent and controversial economists of his period. His *Essay* was intended to debunk some of the basic political theories of the French Enlightenment: the tract's first paragraph cited the "great and unlooked for discoveries that have taken place of late years in natural philosophy" and "the French Revolution, which, like a blazing comet, seems destined either to inspire with fresh life and vigor, or to scorch up and destroy the shrinking inhabitants of the earth."[29] Those recent discoveries in natural philosophy revealed to Malthus, however, something very different from what they had shown to figures like Jean-Jacques Rousseau, who had been a personal friend

142 Pleasure in Revolt

of Malthus's father: basing his arguments on two fundamental "laws" of human existence—"First, That food is necessary to the existence of man" and "Secondly, That the passion between the sexes is necessary and will remain nearly in its present state"—Malthus concluded that poverty was ineradicable and that the poor, or at least considerable numbers of them, were forever doomed to perish from starvation.[30] "Population, when unchecked," he explained, "increases in a geometrical ratio. Subsistence increases in an arithmetical ratio."[31] The only realistic conclusion from this inherent discrepancy between population and the means to nourish it was, he concluded, that some must die. Misery and starvation were thus necessary companions of the human condition. "The natural inequality of the two powers of population and of production in the earth," he wrote, "and that great law of our nature which must constantly keep their effects equal, form the great difficulty that to me appears insurmountable in the way to the perfectibility of society."[32] The great law of nature, the force that reconciled this otherwise insuperable contradiction, was death, for famine would constantly prune away the excess members of humanity. Society, according to his reasoning, was not perfectible, indeed, the plight of its underclasses could scarcely be improved, since they were doomed by an inexorable mathematical formula inherent in nature itself, much like the laws of physics that Newton had isolated. Kant, drawing on the experience of the French Revolution and the principle of a disinterested moral interest in the fate of humanity, had argued that history was a process of progress and improvement.[33] Malthus, on the other hand, turned to the laws of material nature to argue instead that society could not better its lot, or at least not without imposing checks on its own fertility. To contemporaries, and apparently to Malthus himself, it was the entire Enlightenment and the legacy of the Revolution that were on the line in his theory, their sense of rational optimism in the fate of mankind, their reasoned conviction that basic injustices could be mastered and abolished.

In 1849, one year after another revolution that was expected to transform Europe, Pierre Leroux published a book-length refutation of Malthusian economic theory. In it, he attempted to resolve the crushing logic of necessary starvation that seemed to block the way to social renewal. Leroux was one of the great optimists of the nineteenth century, and his writing was at times feverishly exalted, drawing on evangelical notions of historical progress and redemption. His refutations themselves appear to be driven by an underlying sense of moral responsibility, the need to give hope, regardless of its justification or rationality—and there is, perhaps, something not entirely unreasonable in that attitude, since hope that is fully justified is not hope, but mere calculation. "Political economy," he wrote, "robs us of salvation and, in the same stroke, destroys Faith, Hope, and Charity."[34] Without the promise of salvation—a force beyond economics and beyond reason—all that is good in humanity falters and fails, and so, if there was to be any possibility of improvement in the human lot, history must be thought of as an irrational gesture of faith toward the future, a throwing oneself onto the unknown in goodwill, charity, and love. Leroux saw in history, especially the revolutions of 1789 and 1848, the sign of humanity's higher vocation, the proof of its ongoing progress toward its own betterment, and the promise of a second coming of divine justice. As his brother Jules put it in his preface to Pierre's book:

> It has been scarcely sixty years since that revolution became reality: that was in 1789, and behold how in 1848 an entirely similar revolution is breaking out, not only in France, but in Europe, overthrowing in its turn the regime of the triumphant bourgeoisie and founding, amidst its dusty rubble, the final reign of man, the reign of liberty, of fraternity, of equality, and of unity, that Jesus so often preached.
>
> What a spectacle to be admired! The endearing reversal of the lowly world! Adorable and divine justice!
>
> For the people, since 1789, have not let up their attack against the ephemeral bases of the bastard government of the rich and the bourgeois, who make common cause with the mutilated debris of their victims, the priests and kings, their former enemies.
>
> For the people, in their turn, have taken over history, science, morality, politics, political economy, and religion.
>
> It has washed them, purifying them of the gross and godless ignorance with which the bourgeoisie fouled them, like Homer's winged monsters, who soiled the foods that they touched.[35]

For Malthus, the masses would have borne the weight of starvation. For Jules Leroux, they bore the promise of redemption: by seizing what was rightfully theirs, they brought about the fulfillment of God's covenant and the advent of messianic time. Jules understood that new revolution, of which the early ones had been only incomplete premonitions, as a cleansing of ancient sins and injustices, while for him the social systems of the past, the ones that had locked humanity into a cycle of misery and despair, had behaved like the harpies in the *Odyssey*—the monsters who repeatedly befouled with their excrements the tables of food that Odysseus and his companions had been on the point of eating. The second coming was, as he described it, a form of hygiene, a washing away of the feces that had blocked humanity from consuming the food that it needed to survive. While keeping the same key terms, his brother Pierre himself conceived of the situation in a somewhat more complex way, however. His notion of redemptive hygiene was not merely metaphorical. And it did not seek to wash away excreta from the food supply, but rather to integrate them into the cycle of production.

"Political economy orders us to kill the children of the poor," Pierre wrote, somewhat inaccurately, of Malthus's followers, "the Gospel orders us to save them."[36] Against the Malthusian theory that it was structurally impossible to feed all the poor without imposing some limits on human reproduction, Leroux opposed what he called the "increase of sustenance" by man, who, "with his very organism, reproduces sustenance."[37] The redemption of humanity, the messianic revolution of history, was contained, for Leroux, in the human body itself. "One needs only man's excrements to answer Malthus," he wrote, for with them, we are able to give back to the earth the fertility it needs to produce food:

> Nature has established a *Circulus* between production and consumption. We create nothing, we annihilate nothing; we effect changes. With the seeds of the air, the earth, and the water combined with manure, we produce foodstuffs to nourish ourselves; and in nourishing ourselves, we convert them into gas and manure that can produce yet others: this is what we call consumption. It is the goal of production, but it is also its cause.[38]

The thrust of his proposal was simple: collect human excrements and use them as a fertilizer to produce food. The more food that was consumed, the more excrements would be produced, which, in turn, would guarantee yet more food. Since human feces were found to be especially dense in nitrogen, which was believed at the time to be the principle element in soil fertility, they would, according to Leroux's estimates, return to a piece of land more nutrients than they had cost it. In this way, he reasoned, human beings create a potential surplus of food every time they eat and defecate. His ideas—if not their implementation—caught on. Nine years after Leroux published his refutation of Malthus, Emile-Louis Bertherand used the exceptional properties of human urine as the rationale for a vast project to reform urban hygiene and agriculture. "Has Professor Schubler not proven by experiment that a soil watered with human urine produces *twice as much* as when it is fertilized with manure from stables," Bertherand wrote, "and *almost as much* as when it is enriched with fecal mater or blood from butchers' shops?"[39] Hippolyte du Roselle went even further, drawing up a table to show the relative density of nitrogen in the feces of various animals. The list began with cows at the bottom and made its way up through pigs, horses, and sheep, to human beings.[40] Or as Leroux himself reported: "Messrs. Payen and Boussingault have found that, in respect to nitrogen content, the ratio of human urine to cow's urine and animal dung in general is 23 to 3. Guano, which you now seek out in the farthest corners of the world, rates a mere 15 on their charts, in respect to its nitrogen content."[41]

Once it had been established that human waste was the most potent of soil supplements, the question became how to exploit the immense riches it represented. "The interests of agriculture, hygiene, and commerce," Bertherand wrote, "vigorously demand that we seek effective administrative measures to harvest urine distributed on the thoroughfares of our cities, in factories, prisons, hospitals, educational establishments, and barracks, and in the vicinity of railways, monuments, edifices, etc."[42] In a neat inversion, Bertherand spoke of "harvesting" urine for use in agriculture; the human body was, in this sense, analogous to the sown field in that it produced a valuable crop to nourish its counterpart. He imagined, moreover, an entire urban landscape transformed by this principle: wherever people urinated, even in the streets or along train tracks, a system of plumbing would be in place to gather up their precious wastes and return them to the fields. Instead of disappearing uselessly into the ground and poisoning the watersheds, human excretions could thus be turned to the profit of humanity. Similarly, a few quick calculations showed du Roselle that "an individual's fecal matter amounts to 750 grams per day, or 275 kilograms per year," and that, with a network in place to collect these wastes and indemnify their producers, "the urban homeowner should be able to extract 15 francs per year from his cesspool [*fosse*], enough to pay his water bill, the upkeep of his cesspool, and the constant disinfection of its contents. In this way, without opening his purse, he would have fulfilled all the conditions necessary for an altogether salubrious house."[43] Benefits would thus accrue even on the modest level of the single home, for once an appropriate system of collection had been set up, individual families could capitalize on the riches that they produced daily to offset the costs of their basic needs, entering into a sort of domestic circulus.

Leroux himself, however, nurtured much grander schemes. Exiled by Napoleon III, the philosopher moved to England and then Jersey, where, perhaps out of gratitude for the haven offered him, he drew up detailed plans to collect human excrements and then redistribute them as fertilizer throughout the island. "On Jersey," he wrote, "everything is already done or is easy to do."[44] During an earlier stay in London, Leroux had been impressed by the recently adopted system for distributing clean, flowing water throughout the city, which he contrasted with the more expensive and less reliable manual system in place in Paris, where supplies were brought into the capital by cart and then sold for two *sous* per bucket. Were the English system to be adopted, he calculated, with the turn of a tap, any domicile—even on the top story of the highest building—could enjoy an unlimited amount of fresh water at the rate of a penny per hundred, two hundred, or even more buckets. "Will the distribution of *liquid fertilizer* be any more expensive?" he asked. "Not at all."[45] He observed that the citizens of Jersey had already spent roughly five hundred thousand francs to create a drainage network to bring sewer waters from throughout the island to a single point, where they were dumped into the ocean.[46] But in casting its waste into the sea, the island, according to Leroux, was systematically impoverishing itself. "You have thrown your very riches to it," he wrote. The solution, to his mind, was clear: "All you need is to distribute this river of liquid fertilizer throughout your island, by the same means that are employed in London to distribute water to houses."[47] After a long series of minute calculations involving pennies per foot and the relative values of different fertilizers, Leroux came to the conclusion that "it would require but a twenty-fifth of what it cost to build the *Regent* fort to organize your *entire* island according to this method, so that there would be everywhere a tap for fresh or sea water and a tap for liquid fertilizer."[48] In this way, with an organized circulation of water and feces connecting every dwelling throughout the island, consumption and production—city and countryside—would be linked together through the bonds of circulus. Society would finally express the natural law of material redemption and lift the death sentence that Malthus had placed across it.

Probably the best known of Leroux's proponents was Victor Hugo. The two men had shared not only a passion for social reform, but had passed together through many of the same experiences as elected representatives of the French people. Both had sat on the Constituent and Legislative Assemblies in the aftermath of the 1848 revolution, both had subsequently denounced Louis Bonaparte's *coup d'état*, and both had figured among the sixty-six deputies driven out of France in 1853 by the new emperor. The two spent time together while in exile on Jersey, a period that Hugo largely devoted to table rapping and conversations with the spirit world, while Leroux drew up his project for transforming the island. Although they occupied themselves in two very different worlds, Hugo seems to have been deeply influenced by his friend's reformist ideas, for when he published *Les Misérables* in 1862, the novel clearly bore their stamp. "After long groping in the dark," he wrote, "science is now aware that the most fruitful and effective of all fertilizers is human fertilizer."[49] This unexpected revelation comes at one of the key points in the novel's narrative, the moment when, trapped behind a barricade and seemingly on the point of death, the protagonist, Jean Valjean, catches sight of a manhole cover and realizes that he might be able to escape through it. As Hugo structures it, the hero's salvation mirrors a larger one, that of society itself, for the sewer not only provides Jean Valjean the means of deliverance from his own fate, but also promises to save humanity as a whole from starvation. Once the protagonist opens the cover and disappears below, and as the sounds of the final assault on his former position wash over him, the story pauses to reflect on the meaning of sewers in general and to sketch out utopian projects that clearly reveal Leroux's influence. "Each year, Paris casts twenty-five million [francs] upon the water," the narrator observes in language that echoes Leroux's words about flushing sewer waters into the sea: "it is your very riches that you have thrown away."[50] Hugo went on to develop this idea over several pages, calculating the losses, marveling at the stupidity of them, and imagining the brilliant future for mankind if they were to be reversed. In the course of these meditations, he proposed adopting a system supposedly already in use in England and very similar to Leroux's project for Jersey: a "double tubular apparatus . . . that . . . would be sufficient to bring into cities the pure water of the fields and send back to our fields the rich water of the cities, and this easy back-and-forth, the simplest thing on earth, would keep at home the five hundred million that we now throw away."[51] Again, the very language itself seems to maintain, in its careful symmetry of expenditure and loss, the notion that there is an unvarying amount of matter in the world, and yet, at the same time, the author promises a future of unlimited advances in production, an endless story of progress similar to Kant's notion of history in the *Conflict of the Faculties*. When fertilized with human wastes, Hugo remarked, "Chinese wheat yields as much as a hundred and twenty times the grain that was sown."[52] Like Leroux, Hugo sees in the idea of circulus the end of starvation, for the animal and human materials that are thrown into the sea are, by his reckoning, sufficient to feed the world.

Like Pierre and his brother Jules, moreover, Hugo seemed to view the question as not merely a material one, but as somehow moral as well, a proof of divine providence in the laws of nature, the sign of a hidden justice in the workings of the world. For the redemption of wastes, their transformation, echoed another transcendence:

> These piles of rubbish on the roadside, these mud-filled wagons that lurch through the streets at night, this fetid subterranean ooze that the pavement hides from you, do you know what all this is? It is flowering meadows, it is green grass, it is marjoram and thyme and sage, it is game and cattle and the contented lowing of great oxen at dusk, it is sweet-smelling straw, it is golden wheat, it is bread on your table, it is warm blood in your veins, it is health, it is joy, it is life. So dictates that mysterious creation that on earth is transformation and in the heavens transfiguration.[53]

These lines bear the traces of a negative theology, the distant memory of Nicolas of Cusa and the Pseudo-Dionysios, for according to them, it is through the most abject elements of creation that we find the most powerful intimations of the divine, since they are metaphors of our own relation to transcendence. The horrors of the sewer are in reality an eclogue, a jubilation in the powers of life, because in the mysteries of circulus there lies, for Hugo, an image of the conquest over death. And in evoking the particulars of meadow and sewer, in focusing on individual names and details, he enters into the materiality of the world, filling the page with an image of its endless plenitude; stupid as the thyme and sage and oxen may be, they are caught up, unwittingly, in a higher intelligence that is the law of nature, the principle of circulus. And this natural organization is mirrored in the writing itself, where the concrete images are subordinated to a higher, propositional argument about the future of humanity. Hugo's style is polemical, not merely in the sense that it persuades by appealing to the emotions, but, more importantly, by offering, in its very organization, a proof of what it wants to argue: that brute matter can be informed by an impersonal, transcendent spirit, even if that matter remains unaware of its self-transcendence. The words on the page, the scratches of ink on wood pulp, are themselves evidence that a will can enter into lifeless things. And if that is so, then buried in the abject refuse of the city there can be law and redemption.[54]

Leroux's notion of sewage on tap never caught on, but the basic principles of his scheme lingered in the urbanist imagination, although sometimes only as the vague nostalgia for a future that never was. After long hesitations and concerns over all the valuable agricultural supplements that would be lost, it was only at the end of the century that the French capital adopted a network to flush excrements from homes into sewers and from there out of the city. In an 1882 discussion of the issue among some of the principal urbanists and hygienists of the time, a certain Durand-Claye gave voice to some of the fears that slowed the adoption of this program. He recognized the tremendous value of the new *tout à l'égout* system, but nonetheless observed that "it would be a great mistake to believe that with the inevitable progress of decontamination, which is to say with the increasing use of water inside homes, matter from their cesspools will long remain valuable enough to be treated industrially."[55] Several years after he pronounced those words, a brief but intense epoch would have passed, a strange, utopian moment in which the salvation of humankind had appeared to be on the verge of realization, a salvation brought about by the fantasy that the city could feed the countryside—and itself—through the endless riches of its anus.

Leroux might have been an eccentric—his contributions to debates in the Legislative Assembly had little practical effect on urbanism and were frequently met by hilarity; his hairstyles alone were the joy of contemporary caricaturists—he nonetheless voiced in clear and powerful terms a fantasmatics of the abject. By attributing a previously unrecognized value to human refuse and attempting to reintegrate it into the fabric of society, Leroux tapped—in theory and practice—an aspect of human life that other thinkers, and particularly philosophers, had largely refused to consider.[56] It is, in fact, Leroux's eccentricity, his willingness to theorize what lies outside of established social discourses, that makes him significant for a reading of the city's relation to its exclusions, indeed for a larger conception of the limits of society. He offered, moreover, a vision of the future that had implications not only for the material aspects of society, but also for its ways of making sense. For circulus was not merely an economic or agricultural scheme, it was also an intellectual paradigm, a model for understanding the workings of the world and the role of humanity in them. On a concrete level, circulus functioned as an interpretive key that allowed one to understand social events and thereby transform them into history. This function can be seen in Leroux's reaction to the massacres of June 1848, whose "horror" revealed, to those able to grasp them, the deeper laws of nature.

> I shall cite again that wretched battle as the emblem of another combat just as deadly, though one sees in it neither cannons, nor rifles, nor sabers—an unrelenting combat that men wage in time of peace (as they believe), driven as they are

by indigence to war among themselves for a scrap of bread. This is the battle of the shops and workshops that has produced so much poverty in the cities and in the countryside, so many bankruptcies in industry, so many unjust prosecutions, so many crimes, so many prisons and labor camps, so many hospitals and so many diseases of all sorts, so many women sold into prostitution, and so many children abandoned! Yes, you can take the bloody battle of June as an emblem.

For what, after all, led to that uprising? Has it not been called the *insurrection of the hungry*? It was, in short, the result of poverty. And what is the cause, I ask you, of that permanent indigence from which it results that for every three inhabitants of Paris, one dies in the hospital, and that out of thirty-six million Frenchmen, there are eight million poor and beggared? What is the cause, if not *the violation of some natural law*?[57]

By describing the June insurrection as an "emblem," Leroux imagined it to have a meaning: it was a sign, a form of language.[58] Events were doubled, haunted by their significance. And what the insurrection represented, when deciphered, was a deeper, more obscure battle that divided society, a violence that expressed itself not in a single paroxysm but in the constant degradation of the lower classes and in a network of oppressive institutions. Society as a whole could be read through this sign, which revealed a constitutional crime, a usurpation and injustice at the origins of the political order, the city organized around a misconception: Paris, in Leroux's vision of the 1848 massacres, bore the abiding mark of its birth. Hunger, for Leroux, was the great motivating force behind the ills of modern society, indeed its very structures; and that hunger was, moreover, born from a misunderstanding of providence. The foundational crime of the city was, for him, an ignorance of the value of the anus. When viewed through the hermeneutic lens of circulus, the events of June 1848 revealed the mythic, violent origins of the city along with the possibility of its renewal in the purging of that violence. But circulus also had a broader historical sense, a larger significance that revealed that the *of* in "the history of the city" was not only a subjective genitive, or the history that explained the evolution of urban space, but also an objective genitive, which is to say the history that was produced by, that was made possible by the city. For circulus did not merely provide a model for integrating events into a preexisting notion of human time; it also offered a way to organize that time into meaning. By showing that nature was bent toward the improvement of the human lot and the eradication of misery, circulus justified nature, making its inner laws and logic conform to a notion of human justice according to which, and by a perhaps irrational optimism, it was wrong to visit suffering on the innocent. Circulus reconfigured the notion of time itself and redeemed it, for what might otherwise have been seen as a force of degeneration driving human beings to the tomb became, in Leroux's understanding, the engine of progress itself, a miraculous betterment that numerically exceeded the law of the conservation of matter. In thus redeeming time, in demonstrating that progress was possible and that society could be reformed, circulus intimated another, higher redemption, for as society improved, it pushed toward a utopian moment of perfection. History, in this way, was shown to be messianic, an ineluctable movement toward transcendence guided by an incalculable and irrational surplus of goodness; for even if it was given a numerical value, the one hundred and twentyfold return on grains of wheat exceeded the laws of conservation and became, in this sense, irreducible to their calculations. The gift of the anus was at once an act of grace and a theodicy.

By reconfiguring the relation between individual domiciles and the collective space that surrounded them, circulus also changed the way that dwellings expressed—and extended—the bodies that inhabited them. A home that flushes all of its excrements out is a very different imaginary space than one that has sewage piped in next to the fresh water and gas taps.[59] The *tout à l'égout* home spreads its inhabitants' bodies out in linear fashion, with their mouth attached to the water faucet and their anus to the water closet. Such a home faces one direction, condemning its waste to an invisible forgetting. A home as Leroux imaged it, on the other hand, is circular and therefore capable, in some sense, of looking at its own backside. And since it revisits and remembers its wastes, the circular home's relation to time is different. What it expels is not, by that fact, transformed into an alien and hostile past, the residue of a present that is forever lost, but is instead introduced into a cycle of endless return in which the present feeds the future through its past.[60] The circular relation to lost—or rather *suppressed*—matter treats waste as a productive, creative force, the stuff of the future; but as a concept, circulus itself was already experientially creative, since it transformed basic aesthetic relations to the environment.

In its relation to time, circulus not only affected dwellings, it also changed the ways in which bodies were understood and experienced. A different but equally profound imaginative transformation of the human body emerged in another aspect of Leroux's rhetoric, which indirectly, but radically, altered the notion of gender. As I have argued, Malthus and his followers had reduced the question—indeed the possibility—of social justice to a mathematical comparison between two types of fertility: the field and the womb. The fecundity of the latter vastly exceeded that of the former, and the difference was made up in suffering, starvation, and death. Leroux cited Destutt de Tracy on this point, alleging that he "is content to prove that 'man's interest is, in all respects, to reduce the effects of his fertility,' and therewith to place his trust in Mathus's great provost, Nature—or Death—who *will know how to carry out his orders.*"[61] From such a perspective, female fertility is paradoxically deadly, since it inevitably creates a mass of individuals—which Leroux calculated to be one third of the French population—that is doomed to misery and annihilation. Women, in this sense, give birth to death and suffering, and their womb represents an organ constitutionally hostile both to individual human beings and to the perfectibility of society as a whole. Arguing, to the contrary, that women's fertility did not, in fact, outstrip that of the earth, Leroux rejected this gynophobic conception of history, but he did so on the basis of a very unusual understanding of sexual difference. "Nature," he began, "is of an unlimited fertility."[62] For nature to attain this inherent fertility, however, and to act as the "good mother that she is," it was necessary, he reasoned, for mankind to come to her aid; for her to be as fertile as the womb, she must be nourished, and the nourishment that she needed was human excrement.[63] Because of human wastes, and only because of them, the earth could fulfill its role as provider and become itself, which is to say, "the good mother that she is." Feces, in this sense, provided a necessary supplement to nature, allowing it to balance the abundance of women.

Nature's maternity, like its bounty, was thus assured by the action of the anus, but in construing the fundamental law of nature's relation both to mankind and to providence in bodily and familial terms, in imagining them as interactions between metaphorical and literal human bodies, between the "good mother" and the real mother, Leroux produced a fantasmatic entity that, from the perspective of human sexuality, was authentically monstrous. "It is a chemically proven fact," he observed, "that man . . . can *nourish himself simply by his faculty of existence* and as a result of the reproductive powers of his secretions." From this he concluded that "to feed all of mankind, we must make use of the superior reproductive faculty that nature has given it."[64] Man, in other words, engaged in reproductive acts with the earth and guaranteed its maternal abundance through his special and innate powers. If earth is the "good mother," Man, it would seem, is the good father. There is a certain, unresolved ambiguity at work in this happy familial scenario, however, since in the Malthusian paradigm the survival of the species was at odds with that of the individual. By the economist's reckoning, semen, the substance that assured the continuance of the former, would do so only at the expense of the latter. Leroux did not dispute Malthus's fundamental notion that the powers of male sexuality needed to be balanced against the fertility of the earth, but instead of trying to reach that equilibrium through checks on the human body's fecundity, he proposed that that same force be used on the earth as well. It was, however, a different product of the body that was exchanged in this new procreative act, for in relation to the field, the substance of life was not semen but excrement. Indeed, the value of the penis in relation to the soil derived entirely from its urethral function, for on the basis of recent scientific findings (that seem, nonetheless, to contradict the importance attributed elsewhere to nitrogen), Leroux argued that "the goal of agriculture must be to give plants as much ammonia as possible, since the other elements, such as carbonic acid, are provided by their environment," and concluded that the most pressing agricultural question was therefore to find a reliable and abundant source of ammonia. Fortunately, that source lay close at hand: "there is only one fertilizer that really supplies ammonia," he wrote, "*human urine*."[65] With this insight, the twin wombs of woman and the earth that Malthus had set against each other were both satisfied and balanced by the dual excretory functions of the penis. Woman is impregnated by semen and the field is nourished by urine.

There was, however, a sort of cross-pollination in this symmetrical relation between two fertilities, since the excrements that nourished the field altered the significance of women's childbearing capacities. The new abundance of the earth tempered the excess of the human womb and thereby corrected it. Human waste transformed the latter, in this way, from an instrument of death into a source of life, and an androgynous, presexual body thus redeemed the gendered, sexual one in the closed economy of circulus. Even female breasts were partially replaced by other organs in this fantasmatic monster of salvation, for some of the functions that they normally performed were taken over by the urethra in Leroux's imagination. He observed that the distinctions physiologists drew between secretions and excrements were inconsistent and misleading, since they were based on the erroneous belief that there is an irreducible difference between substances, like bile and gastric juices, that the body produces to aid in its functioning and others that serve only to evacuate harmful or useless matters. Had they thought more carefully about milk, Leroux argued, such scientists would have realized that the relations between bodily wastes and secretions were more complicated. "What?" he wrote. "Here is a fluid that, just like sweat or urine, cannot remain in the economy for long without disturbing it to some degree or other. Would you dare conclude that this secretion has no other purpose than to remove *useless or harmful materials* from the being that produces it? Its purpose is obviously to feed what that being loves the most, its child, its offspring."[66] Noxiousness, according to Leroux, could not be determined on the basis of a given substance alone, but had to be gauged also on other variables, such as the length of time that it stayed in the body and its value to others, for the organism that benefits from certain animal products might not be the same one that produces them. In this sense, some secretions aid the body only through the mediation of other members of the same species. The milk that a woman produces, for instance, does not feed her directly but instead nourishes her children; but by nourishing her own offspring, a mother gives something essential back to her own kind and thus helps to sustain the larger organism that originally supported, and continues to support her own existence.[67] Secretions are, in this respect, some of the most fundamental and permanent bonds that join people together, and indeed they could be called the matter of collectivity and society itself, since through them individuals are brought together physically and imperatively, are forced to collaborate across such necessary differences as age and gender. This social body, moreover, can be seen as a response to and a manipulation of such apparently inflexible ontological conditions as time. To the extent that it indirectly nourishes the body that produces it, milk, for instance, must make a detour through other human beings in which it moves backwards against the passage of the years to a period in which the body needed what it could not yet produce. The mother, in this sense, furnishes milk for the child that she once was, and this manipulation of time's linearity is possible only through a larger organism in which the individual participates. Because of this tortuous temporality, however, milk is an excrement to the mother, a secretion for the child, and it is only through these different social and biological relationships that the polyvalence and fungibility of bodily products can be fully appreciated.

And once this has been understood in relation to milk, Leroux argued, the true value of other excrements would be understood better. "Wouldn't urine have a purpose analogous to that of milk?" he asked.[68] An excrement only when viewed from a single perspective, urine was in fact a beneficent secretion, like mother's milk, when it had travelled outside of the body and returned, transformed into food by its passage through the plowed field. What the mother performs through her breasts, mankind as a whole does through its urinary tract and the mediation of the earth. This was part of a broader rearticulation of humanity that evolved out of Leroux's economic theories, a rethinking of its organs until they became physically monstrous. This new person procreated through its anus, lactated through its urethra, excreted through its breasts, and killed through its womb and semen. A pre- or proto-sexual body thus redeemed the sexualized one and underlay the possibility of social and familial relations and even of gender itself. At the same time, it linked human beings to an inanimate world through the most primitive and powerful form of libidinal ties—the pleasures of an inquiring appetite for what lay beyond it and the creative drive to respond with its own inventions. This new body emerged out of a willingness to return to the abject, to revisit and reconsider human wastes. It was an object of ridicule on the part of Leroux's peers and other contemporaries. But this new body was not simply the product of a personal erotics. It was also the response to broadly recognized social needs, a scrupulously elaborated project for humanity itself.

As the notion of circulus transformed and then replaced gender relations with the fantasy of a monstrously androgynous body, it also affected other, equally primordial aspects of human existence, especially life and death. From the very start, the motivation for Leroux's refutation of Malthus had been his refusal to tolerate a certain, supposedly inevitable level of mortality among the poor, and this refusal was reinforced by his conviction that "if so many millions of our fellow men are indeed condemned to die, it is society that has condemned them, and not Nature."[69] Circulus represented for Leroux the struggle of life against death, and he treated these terms not as theoretical principles or even the relatively abstract forces described by Bichat and his followers, but instead as physical, almost tactile presences. He wrote, for instance, about "these eight million poor who are doomed to a ceaseless swarming [*à pulluler*] in the very heart of death."[70] Death was a place—or perhaps something more indeterminate, such as a state—a swarming of bodies. One could live in death—and millions did. Its image was the abject mass of impoverished humanity and all the social ills that accompanied it—the filth, the forced moral compromises, the ambiguous sexual and familial relationships, the sheer physical proximity.[71] And if it made sense to call this death rather than abjection, misery or poverty, that is probably because the most prominent scientific notions of death at the time were, as we have seen, extremely material. Leroux's conception of poverty as death was not, in this way, entirely metaphorical; it reflected, instead, the belief in a continuum of existence and even of consciousness between the animate and the inanimate. Within these more supple limits, he glimpsed the possibility of escaping from mortality—not just that of the poor, but even, it seems, of humanity as a whole. He observed that through the kind of physical interdependence manifested in the production and consumption of milk, "this [natural] cycle also constitutes the outer life of beings, joins them, and makes of them the links in a single chain, with each of them giving and receiving in turn." As a result, "this law is more generally true than the one that is universally accepted (namely that death sustains life, in the sense that beings are nourished by each other)."[72] It had seemed clear to generations of *philosophes* that within the closed economy of the material universe, old life had to give way to new, and that within this other *circulus*, corpses functioned analogously to feces, decomposing and enriching the ground that would provide food for future generations.[73] This was, indeed, the very nature of earth. "These soils," Leroux himself wrote, "come from the excrements and corpses of animals, which have been mixed and *chemically* combined with the debris from plants and rocks."[74] But Leroux believed that his approach was fundamentally different from that of his predecessors and contemporaries, since he viewed the role of death in this system as only secondary to a more basic and important force. He argued that:

> far from being the whole of the law, the principle that entities are nourished by the death of other entities is therefore only one aspect of a more general law, which is that entities are nourished by the life of other entities; and . . . nature, which seems, so long as this truth is misunderstood, to be a gloomy labyrinth where life and death struggle against each other, turns out in reality to be nothing more than a repeating network, filled with the infinite variety of bonds created by this single law: nutrition and secretion exist to serve the nutrition of other beings.[75]

For Leroux, death was not the defining limit or the fundamental term of animal existence, the way it was for Bichat, who described life as the *"set of functions that resist death."*[76] Instead, life was the underlying principle in his system, of which death was only an epiphenomenon. Life was not, moreover, an endless battle against some implacable enemy, but rather the law of circulus itself, the dynamic, material connection that linked organisms both to each other and to their physical surroundings. For life was not just lactating and urinating, it was lactating and urinating *for* another, the body caught up unselfconsciously in relations of community and care. It functioned, in this sense, as a material ethics of the other that predated and underlay the notions of death, being, and nonbeing themselves. It was for this reason that Leroux held society rather than nature responsible for condemning human beings to death—or rather, the fault lay with the refusal of society, with the withholding of milk, semen, feces, and urine from one's peers. Death was the forced weaning of an individual from this collectivity born in the flow of excrements, it was the swarming of a hungry mass severed from a vital liquid circulation, it was the expulsion of wastes from the community, the pathos of their endless alienation from the city, it was the linear body that consumed and forgot, sacrificing the needs of others to its disgust toward its own excrements. To be aware of the continuity that bound bodies together was, on the other hand, to feel alive, and to understand the law of circulus was to grasp the principle of vitality. But if for Leroux feces were life, others among his contemporaries viewed death itself as a productive, vital force, in which a creative impulse secretly operated.

Abject Desires

In his studies of how disciplinary practices transformed the body during the nineteenth century—and his analyses of the prison, the clinic, and the military in particular—Michel Foucault concentrated on how those practices became instruments to enforce a normative idea of human physical existence. And while hygiene performed a similar function, I am more interested in what could be described as the undisciplined or luxuriant body, the one that precedes or escapes normative strategies and that in arousing the need for a constant vigilance brings them into being—the cholera victim, the rag picker in her hovel, the imbecile, the corpse. Such individuals inhabit a body that is the unspoken object of those strategies—unspoken, because its importance lies in its exteriority, its alien hostility to such attempts at control, while the moment it can be identified within them it is reduced to an extension of their conceptual field. As indicated by its designation, even the "abnormal" body is construed in terms of deviance from a norm rather than as the potential marker for an entirely different conceptual system. It is a deficient form of what is already understood—or in the process of being understood—rather than an alternate model of understanding. The luxuriant body is not therefore an object of understanding but an abject of experience, something that betrays itself not to cool reasoning and sober analysis, but in the whiff of revulsion one detects even in certain medical texts, in the disgust it provokes, in a nauseous disorientation even within the protocols of a well-defined science. One catches brief glimpses of this body in the writings produced by and against the disciplinary structures of the nineteenth century. It is strangely different from an adult sexual person, and its main connection to the external world seems to pass through its anus. It transforms the other organs and orifices—or, rather, reveals them in a new light, showing a different meaning and directivity to their functions and connections. Pierre Leroux championed a form of this other body, calling it the salvation of humankind, but others rose up also on behalf of the abject, asserting the value of the sick, the filthy, the dead—as such. In his own way, Sergeant Bertrand testified in favor of the abnormal body. In his desire and in his actions he asserted the value of the dead as dead, even if that value could not be understood or explained to others. Indeed, in its very muteness, his passion bore witness to what one could call a value system so different that it could not even defend itself propositionally. Part of its fascination lay in that dumbness—like a language so foreign that it spoke only in acts.

Another sort of person came out on behalf of that deviant body, a figure less eccentric, indeed, almost central to nineteenth-century Parisian culture: the prostitute's client. Within the language of the hygienists and social reformers who studied and sought to control the sex trade, prostitutes were assimilated with sewers and the dead. This connection has been remarked on before, but a significant and somewhat shocking aspect of that assimilation has gone unobserved and uncommented: if prostitutes are identifiable, within such discourses, with sewers, that suggests not only that prostitutes are abject but also, conversely, that the abjection of sewers is somehow erotically charged and desirable.[77] Seen from this perspective, the figure of the sex worker is the translation of another, unspeakable desire, which would logically be directed toward the inhumanity of fecal waste and its cognate, the dead. If the hygienist Alexandre Parent-Duchâtelet was able to plunge into the sewers or taste fecal matters but could not bear to visit a bordello unaccompanied, it was, I would argue, because desire for the sewers could be hidden in plain sight: it was so repressed as to be unthinkable, whereas the desire for prostitutes was the basis for their social and economic existence. Recent studies have attempted to describe the sex industry in nineteenth-century Paris from the perspective of the prostitutes themselves and to invert some of the oppressive ideological structures that bore down on women during the period.[78] In what follows, however, I will focus instead on the repressive fantasies of the hygienists themselves in an attempt to understand prostitutes as displacements for another desire, which was oriented toward the abject itself.

In nineteenth-century Paris, the brothel became a staple of literary production and the focus of an elaborate police and hygienic apparatus. The prostitute might appear to represent the sexualized, genital body par excellence, but in fact the way that she was treated by government offices and in artistic representations reveals a very different significance to her behavior. And while the very extent of the control exercised over her would seem to integrate her into the social order, it represents instead the degree to which she threatened to escape that order, the menace that something about her body represented to another, dominant image of the city. For the authoritarian forces deployed against her were impressive. As Yves Guyot put it in his 1882 abolitionist bible, *La prostitution*, the inhabitants of state-sanctioned *maisons de tolérance* "feel over them the full presence of the social order, from the mistress of the house, who represents capital, through the police officers, who represent all the force of society, up to the doctor, in whom she glimpses only a sort of torturer and jail keeper."[79] The danger of the prostitute herself was legible in the sheer weight of the forces that were established to constrain her. Hierarchy, order, and control must be imposed at every point of her existence, because she, for her part, did not conform to those standards on her own.

The single most important name in the medical theorization of prostitutes is undoubtedly Parent-Duchâtelet, a social hygienist active in the 1820s and '30s whose research and beliefs marked studies on the sex trade throughout the rest of the century. For him, the goal was not to abolish prostitutes from Paris, since he considered them to be necessary and therefore ineradicable parts of human existence, but rather to control them.[80] Later accounts continued to view the situation largely in these same terms. As late as 1880, a report by the doctor Louis Fiaux, for instance, asserted that sexual needs functioned according to a fixed cycle—entering into a "procreative crisis" every three or four days on average, men regularly built up fluids and needed to discharge them. Women, on the other hand, had a cycle of approximately twenty to twenty-five days.[81] Like most physics problems, surplus sexual desire could thus be reduced to a mathematical formula. This excess male sexuality was, for the majority of theorists in the nineteenth century, a waste product that had to be disposed of in order for society to function. As a way to manage these wastes, prostitution was to be tolerated but tightly controlled by the *police des mœurs* or vice squad. To do this, the prostitute had to be separated from society at large, locked away physically and then subtracted from view. Cultural historians such as Charles Bernheimer have pointed to the central importance of invisibility in Parent-Duchâtelet's reglementary system, the need, for instance, to keep *filles publiques* enclosed almost permanently in special houses, whose windows and blinds would never open.[82] The historian Alain Corbin has listed numerous examples of this imposed invisibility, such as the fact that the closed carriage used to transport registered prostitutes in secrecy to their medical examinations predated even the *voiture cellulaire* of convicts.[83] But even when hidden safely out of sight, this class of women continued to disturb certain powerful elements of society, pitting the *réglementaristes*, who felt that the practice should be tolerated but controlled, against abolitionists, who were themselves split by seemingly contradictory interests. The faction headed by Joséphine Butler argued against prostitution on the basis of its immorality, and when she spoke of abolition, Butler herself seems to have meant nonprocreative sex in general. Yves Guyot and the liberal left, on the other hand, targeted the abuses of the *police des mœurs* as one of the most egregious examples of a pervasive social authoritarianism. That authority, Guyot and his followers observed, was exercised without constitutional basis, since prostitution was not, strictly speaking, illegal. While one faction of the abolitionists thus argued for the suppression of prostitution in order to *expand* personal liberty, another argued for its suppression as a means to *diminish* liberties. In a deft Foucauldian turn, however, Corbin has pointed out that the two sides can ultimately be seen to coalesce, even in questions of morality, since Guyot argued that greater individual freedom would lead to greater personal restraint and an internalization of those powers of control that the police had previously embodied. In practical terms, freedom and continence would amount to the same thing.[84]

Even those who argued for abolition as a way to temper the state's interference in personal matters thus considered that the prostitute represented a breakdown of discipline and order, and indeed this disorder seems to have been widely perceived as her defining characteristic.[85] Parent-Duchâtelet's 1836 monograph, *De la prostitution dans la ville de Paris* (On Prostitution in the City of Paris), contended that a woman succumbed to "public prostitution" only after a period of "debauch" during which she had "lived in disorder for a more or less extended period."[86] Indelibly marked by these conditions, which reached back through her earliest years into her prenatal family history, the prostitute herself personified "turbulence" and "agitation."[87] The social reformer and future legislator Alphonse Esquiros echoed these beliefs when he wrote, four years later, that the *"fille* remains for the State a lost being, or rather, a dangerous one, fetid and unfortunate. . . . Indeed, to our mind, all this is a sort of disorder."[88] This impression of the prostitute extended beyond the group of those who had a special interest— professional or otherwise—in public sexuality, as can be seen in contemporary responses to Edouard Manet's *Olympia.* When it was first exhibited in 1865, most viewers considered the painting's subject to be a courtesan, but published accounts of their initial reactions betray a high level of perplexity about just what it was they were seeing, as if the subject's very nudity was itself inscrutable or disorienting. Journalists described her as "formless," "inconceivable," "unqualifiable," and "undecipherable."[89]

   The most intractable problem in controlling the prostitute seems, in fact, to have been her indeterminability. Virtually impossible to identify in herself, she was always being mistaken for someone or something else: the courtesan could pass for a patrician, the *fille* for a working-class woman. This was the horror of the *réglementaristes,* and it was not unfounded, as is clear from perusing only some of the most scandalous cases of misprision from the late seventies and early eighties. In 1876 the actress Roselia Rousseil was roughed up and taken into custody while strolling down a boulevard in Paris.[90] There was the "Augustine B . . . affair," in which a worker was arrested on her way home from a day of labor.[91] Or the arrests of a Mr. Bonnefous and his niece on June 22, 1879, followed by that of an eighteen-year-old intern at the Théâtre-Français three days later.[92] On March 29, 1881, in a case that ended up involving the president of the house of representatives, Léon Gambetta, and eventually costing the prefect of police his job, a Madame Eyben was taken into custody for standing in the passage des Panoramas, where, it turned out, she was waiting for her children.[93] The journalist A. de Pontmartin summed up the situation of the courtesan: "in clothes, manner of speaking, curiosity, and pleasures, the demimonde draws close to high society; all of this helps to confuse two worlds that should not even recognize each other. . . . On the staircase of Worth's dress shop, the patrician lady from the faubourg Saint-Germain crosses paths with the decked-out girl from the Bréda neighborhood."[94] Since the prostitute was not entirely visible she could not be entirely hidden, and as a result she circulated out of control, obscuring and confusing class distinctions. And the more that the solution to her problem depended on identifying her, the more her inherent social ambiguity withdrew her from mastery, thus creating a vicious circle of anxiety.

At the center of the *fille*'s indeterminability lay her lack of an individual identity, for according to a perception that persisted through more than fifty years of hygienic studies on prostitution, her disorder reached down to the most basic structures of her person. As Hippolyte Mireur put it in 1888, she had "made the sacrifice of her personality."[95] Nearly five decades earlier, Alphonse Esquiros had written that "one of the feelings most absent from children and prostitutes is the feeling of an 'I.'" He elaborated on how this was possible: "Accustomed to living in a sort of bestial community, these girls scarcely distinguish among themselves morally. This absence of individuality helps prolong their stay in bordellos, for isolation frightens rather than attracts them."[96] The prostitute, in a word, swarmed. She was abject, animal, asocial, and impersonal, living in an indistinguishable mass with others of her own kind. The way to save her, for those who thought such a thing possible, was, therefore, to create in her a sense of personal identity. "One must," Esquiros asserted, "give them a larger idea of themselves than they generally have in their present state of abjection."[97]

The prostitute embodied a paradox: no one was there. She was no one in herself, but she was also there, insisting, unbearably, on her subjectless, formless, irrational presence. "It is difficult," Parent-Duchâtelet wrote, "to get an idea of the lightness and the inconstancy of mind that characterize prostitutes. You cannot pin them down, and nothing is more difficult than to follow the course of their reasoning, for the smallest things distract and fascinate them."[98] Rebellious to reason itself, the very bases of their intellectual identity, such as they were, seemed not merely to escape beyond the structures that underlay the social order and intelligibility, but also, somehow, to threaten them. "One would have to begin by reintegrating these girls into the state," Esquiros wrote. "Nothing good comes from outside society."[99] He explained what he meant:

> You should be aware that, in the present state of things, prostitution is a source of instability and disorder. Over the long run, it always becomes dangerous for a state to allow its members to break off in this way from the center. These are the fractured and external forces that, at a given moment, cause revolutions.
>
> This poor creature, that society pushes aside with disgust and horror, opposes that society with her resistance, her rebellion, and her hatred. Like all individuals who feel out of place or who are in pain, the prostitute dreams of uprisings and maintains all around her in the same rebellious spirit.[100]

The *fille* was not merely a necessary receptacle for men's excess sexual desires, she also represented the will and power to destabilize the state itself. For all her sloth, her mindlessness, her disorder and impersonality, she was revolution in person, restlessly awaiting her moment at the edges of a society that necessarily abjured her and just as necessarily depended on her. Her body evidenced an abiding animal irrationality. She was horror, she was disgust, but because she lived in the structures of procreative desire itself she was also ineradicable. Parent-Duchâtelet himself described the prostitute's relation to the state in terms that recall Robespierre and Saint-Just's denunciations of the king and Diderot's proposals for handling those who, by madness, bestiality or perversity, refused the social contract.[101] "So long as a woman keeps to the normal habits of life, the government can consider her only as a part of society; it owes her protection and devotes no particular scrutiny to her case," he wrote. "But her status and the government's actions change the very instant this same woman enters that state of scandalous bestiality whose excesses the authorities must repress."[102] The moment that she cedes to the animality of desire, a woman loses her membership in society and must be repressed. The historical resonances of such language were not lost on contemporaries, as when Guyot called one of his colleagues to task for his willingness to abandon whole classes of human beings to the needs of society as a whole. "Dr. Mireur has taken this theory to its logical conclusion [in maintaining that] no one would dispute society's right to sacrifice the interests of the few to the interests of the masses," Guyot wrote, and then concluded: "Marat said similar things. This is the theory of public safety [*salut public*]."[103] In his, perhaps inadvertent, play on the ambiguity of the word *salut*, Guyot conflated the hygienist's concern for public health with the notorious Committee for Public Safety, led by Robespierre and Saint-Just during the bloodiest months of the French Revolution. Against the horror of the abject and animal, against the disorder of the inhuman and irrational, the state brought the forces of terror to bear, not just on the person of the king and his supporters, but also on the body of the prostitute.

For in the hygienic imagination the prostitute *was* abject and horrifying. The individuals who studied her drummed relentlessly on this point, insisting on the revulsion she inspired. "The prostitute," wrote F.-F.-A. Béraud, "is, with few exceptions, a monstrosity. . . . A woman never completely escapes from that abject state to which prostitution reduces her."[104] Guyot complained that "police regulations place streetwalkers on the same footing as the heap of trash [*amas de boue*] that must be removed because it obstructs traffic," but even he referred to the *filles*'s "moral putrefaction" and spoke of their houses as "breeding grounds [*foyers*] of moral infection."[105] Less compassionate than Guyot, Mireur saw in the *fille* a concentration of the medical dangers that constantly threatened the healthy organism. If, according to him, a prostitute did not have the good fortune to die before the age of thirty from one of the many diseases to which her debilitating profession constantly exposed her, she was doomed to a pestilential afterlife at the edges of the city:

> Let them go now, since death refuses to take them, and populate the seamy bars at the city's edge, those loathsome pits of debauchery!
>
> Men devoted to the public welfare have dared go down into these places so they might study, in the flesh, this ulcer on society. Mastering their disgust, they have made their way into these repulsive dens, where the only air is the miasmas exhaled by foul and wine-soaked bosoms. In reading their descriptions of the horrors they have witnessed, who could but shudder at the thought that human creatures can fall so low into the abyss of degradation?[106]

This was the fate of those who had sunk so low that they were undesirable even to death, the great leveler of social classes and the guarantor of social order. They lived on, in this way, after their natural end in an ambiguous state between the animate and the inanimate, a wound breathing out miasmas.

The prostitute's disgusting abjection and her role as a conduit to remove accumulated human wastes from the body politic assimilated her, in the hygienic imagination, with the sewers that were simultaneously under discussion—and later construction—in Paris. The trajectory of Parent-Duchâtet's career itself, whose two principal foci were the removal of animal by-products from urban spaces and the control of prostitution, attested to this connection, as did the explicit statements of his colleagues. In 1840, at the beginning of the hygienic interest in the sex trade, Esquiros wrote, "every day you wipe away onto these poor creatures all the filth, froth, and foam in your soul." He imagined how the "poor girl who is beaten and never loved . . . had this morning—how well you know, oh Lord!—collected her part of charity in the sewer of her honor."[107] Forty years later, Guyot was less poetic: "In certain of these houses," he wrote, "each woman submits to fifteen, twenty, twenty-five daily contacts. They take numbers. Men line up. The woman is a sewer, she plays no other role."[108]

More surprising, perhaps, is the candor with which Esquiros assimilated prostitutes with another form of abjection: the dead. Not only did she personify the new hygienic programs that were transforming the physical space of Paris, such that her behavior and organs functioned as analogues to the new structures that were appearing throughout the city—as a subjectless but still sentient breeding ground of pestilence and putrefaction, her medical significance was cognate to that of a corpse, and in this respect Esquiros's recurrent references to a special connection between the *fille* and death were faithful to the logic of contemporary hygiene. It was not merely that she spread potentially fatal diseases, but that her "I," insofar as it existed, was dead. He spoke of prostitutes as "these specters of women that glide pitifully along the walls at night like the larvae of Virgil or the shades of Dante" and imagined that if, instead of misery, disease and opprobrium, "it is death who comes to them, then prostitutes hail her grimly as their sister."[109] This special status was also visible in the effects that prostitutes exercised over their clients, whom they contaminated not only with physical illness but with death itself: "these unfortunate men learn in these ill-famed houses to despise women," Esquiros wrote, "and when, later, once they are older and established, marriage comes to them, it finds almost all of them with a withered soul, a sickly body, their illusions dead and their heart extinguished—fitter, in a word, for the coffin than for the nuptial couch."[110] In the final pages of his study, Esquiros summed up the prostitute's condition, speaking of himself in the third person to explain the object of his work: "he would like," as he put it, "to pour out a little oil to rekindle the lamp that burnt out in the hands of the foolish virgins; he would like to shake the tablecloth of the rich so that from it a few crumbs might fall into Lazarus's hungry mouth."[111] The prostitute was, in the end, Lazarus, that strange figure of the unfinished dead that haunts European fantasies of death like a troubled sleeper.

With these assimilations, both structural and thematic, among sewers, cadavers, and prostitutes, hygienists revealed something strange but significant about the relation between the city and its abject. As if one had turned a prism, the prostitute exposes another facet of an unspoken fantasy hidden in the violence of disgust: miasma, putrefying, abject, and horrible, she was nonetheless an object of desire. She demonstrates that one can feel both disgust and desire for the same object and that the two affects are not therefore mutually exclusive. More significantly, if the prostitute was a sewer and a corpse, that meant, conversely, that sewers and corpses were somehow like prostitutes. Now, that does not necessarily mean that sewers and corpses shared all of the characteristics of prostitutes, and it is true that nowhere among the documents I have consulted does an author assert that he or she felt erotic excitement toward filth. That does not mean, however, that such an excitement did not exist in repressed or dissimulated forms. And while I cannot prove that the prostitute embodied one of those forms, I think that the evidence strongly indicates that she did. The resemblance among prostitutes, corpses, and sewers was too powerful and too frequently reiterated, the ambivalence she aroused too intense not to suggest that the fascinated revulsion evoked by corpses and feces comprised some element of desire. Certain truths cannot, perhaps, be fully demonstrated, but their validity can be judged by the explanatory richness that they allow. In this sense, what the prostitute reveals is that there was something erotic about the filth that had to be excluded from Paris, that everything horrible about the abject was also bound up with a dreadfully potent attraction.

If there was something marvelous and inexplicable in the hygienic fear that gripped Paris in the early nineteenth century, a fantasmatic and unavowable element in the drive to reconfigure the city, it was probably this: the heart of filth was an unacceptable longing. It was this desire that had to be cordoned off—not the prostitutes themselves, not the diseases that they might spread, not the miasmas that they exhaled. Throughout his career, Parent-Duchâtelet argued the innocuousness of putrefaction, so convinced of his own reasoning that he dared to defy contemporary wisdom by descending into the hold of ships laden with dried human excrements, tasting fecal ooze, and painting his workroom with a solution of rotting hemp.[112] But despite such dramatic refutations of miasma theory, the prostitute remained abject, precipitating fears and fascinations that reached down to the bases of the social order and the origins of the city. Other fantasies crystallized around the concerns she raised about the communication of syphilis, fantasies of disorder, infection, and disruption to the body politic that far exceeded notions of disease. If the prostitute was another face of feces and the dead, then the horror attached to these latter would have been a product of their desirability as well. The sewer and the cemetery wall would, consequently, have been protections not against waste and corpses, but rather against the city's own longing for its excluded. In the violence of the hygienists' horror toward the *fille* and the miasmas that pollute the capital, toward the death that seemed to dwell among its inhabitants, there was the urgency, too, of desire. And without that desire, the hygienic revolution is incomprehensible.

In their very abjection, the forces that can be glimpsed in these fantasies of the prostitute exceeded the closed economic system that reformers and the *police de mœurs* tried to impose on them. They exceeded, as well, the parsimony of the anal character as it was theorized by early psychoanalysts. Her body was disorder and excess, the breakdown of recuperative rationality, but it was also, fantasmatically, a form of selfless affection that bordered on the saintly. Those who studied prostitution generally agreed that it was not from lubricity that the *fille* entered her profession. "For the person who engages in it," wrote Guyot, "prostitution is the exact opposite of sexual satisfaction."[113] If she had no identity of her own, it was either because she had never progressed beyond a childlike indifferentiation or because she had, as Mireur put it, "made the sacrifice of her personality."[114] Innocent of the horror she embodied, the prostitute gave endlessly of herself in an infinite act of love. The *fille* blended with those around her, dissolving into an indistinct mass of femininity within the precincts of the *maisons closes*, offering an erotics without identity, an impersonal love in which the subject broke down and disappeared into the objects of its affection. "Mr. Arnould Fremy's notion of morality is based entirely on tolerance and charity . . .," wrote Esquiros approvingly. "He turns then to the courtesan and adds: 'Go, my child, you will be given much, for you have loved much!'"[115]

The prostitute's body was strangely different from the normative idea of a sexual adult body. Nonprocreative, her desire was effaced and her organs reconceptualized. Her sexual significance, even when physically genital, was anal in its meaning and function within the theoretical and police structures designed to control it. Semen was waste, analogous to feces, and the prostitute's sexual organs were reduced, in the hygienist imagination, to a cloaca. In her body one sees the coalescence of pleasure and disgust and the identification of the anus as a dominant form of erotism to which all others are subordinated. But her person became, at the same time, the instantiation of an impersonal form of love, which was only possible by embracing the creative aspects of the anus and the fecal, a redemptive agape that one also glimpses in the utopian projects of Pierre Leroux. By turning away from its more fundamental products, by turning its back on one aspect of its existence, society, according to Leroux, cut itself off from salvation, and, indeed, from life. Forerunners of the unconscious, of the abject drives that are suppressed by the socialized ego, as the great creative and destructive forces of the unsocialized, feces were a paradigm of the city's other. And the corpse was the feces of life itself, of the whole living individual, a gesture into the unknown, a self—or a part of the self—that, after years of subordination to the socialized subject, would eventually assume its own existence fully and become the other of the self: a nonethical other, another notion of life, of existence, of being. In the form of the corpse, abjection was thus an act of production concomitant with one's own extinction, an act of creation that absolutely exceeded, and in exceeding devoured, the creator. It was a paradigm of invention and loss, of creation and alterity, of the infinitely distant and infinitely close relation of the mind to the material world.

If, for Jacques Lacan, there is "no such thing as a sexual relation," that is because he understood sexual difference to be an absolute unknowable, in which each partner is faced by an impossible relation to a phallus whose significance infinitely exceeds him or her: the transcendence of that relation is coextensive with the difference between two subjective experiences.[116] In the imagination of nineteenth-century hygienists and social reformers, however, there was no sexual relation with a prostitute because she did not, as a human subjectivity, exist. She was, to borrow Jann Matlock's term, a fantasm. But Matlock understands that fantasm to be a "scene in which a man, prohibited from seeking satisfaction with prostitutes, sought to relieve his urges . . . [and] driven by desires beyond his control, . . . would begin to seduce well-bred daughters, to corrupt servants, and to lead working-class girls into the depths of depravity."[117] This would certainly seem to have been a fear on the part of bourgeois families, but it was, as Matlock herself documents, a fear that was abundantly represented at the time; for it to be a *fantasm* in a stronger, because unconscious, sense, that fearful scene of desire would need, however, to be inexpressible in direct terms. For that reason, if there is a fantasmatic component behind the male control of prostitution, it must be about something else than what Matlock describes.[118] That something else is, I have contended, a desire for abjection itself, and what this means, in the context of my larger argument, is that hygienic reform and the entire social discourse that it represented were driven, to some as-yet undetermined degree, by an erotic longing for the same sources of revulsion that the medicalization of nineteenth-century French society was simultaneously identifying and excluding.

SIX

Monsters and Artists

In the previous chapter I discussed an otherwise unstudied aspect of nine-teenth-century France's relation to the dead—the creative and erotic poten-tial hidden in concerns about putrescent matter. In this chapter, I will look at the aestheticization of physical death and the abject desires associated with it to see how that potential could be tapped by artists. I will concentrate on three examples of what one might call *medicalized* art, in which the physical properties of death were, on the one hand, treated as a material to be reworked imaginatively and, on the other, as the object of a sustained medita-tion. In each of these cases, the artists in question consciously entertained what one might call a diacritical relation to contemporary scientific thought, in that they reflected, from their own disciplinary perspective, on the mean-ing of what was happening in medicine—*diacritical* in the sense that those reflections inflected the significance of the scientific theories they drew on. These are not simply examples of artists borrowing metaphors or conceptual structures from the sciences, but rather evidence of artists bringing their own powers to bear on those imaginative aspects of scientific theory that I have

described in the preceding chapters. Conversely, each of the cases I will discuss also treats the materiality of death as a means to understand artistic
imagination and the physical aspects of aesthetic production, so that medical
thought must be seen as part of the process of creation. For Odilon Redon,
recent developments in biology and evolution offered insights into the plasticity of artworks and their relation to thought and sentience. For Balzac, the
dead and their abjection were a way to understand fictionality and, in particular, literary characters. Finally, for Flaubert, corpses became a means to conceptualize the relation between literature and historical narrative. A final
section will describe contemporary texts that reflected on the peculiarly intimate relation between language—especially writing—and the dead, and will
indicate why, in general terms, corpses should have had such importance for
Balzac and Flaubert. It should be emphasized, however, that these were not
attempts to "apply" medical theory to artistic production, but rather a continuation, by different means, of those irrational and imaginative aspects of
medicine that I have previously discussed. In this sense, Redon, Balzac, and
Flaubert represent an important extension of medical history, one which
opens the possibility of moving beyond simply recounting what happened in
these documents toward, eventually, lending them a meaning.

The Arts of Abjection

Given everything that has gone before, it might be easy to forget that despite
all the public outcries, the disgust, the transfer of cemeteries, and the general
exclusion of the deceased from the haunts of the living, nineteenth-century
France was a passionately and pervasively necrophilic society. In their imaginations, writers and the educated public embraced the inhabitants of the
tomb with an unusual enthusiasm. For Victor Hugo, the defining characteristic of the Romantic movement was melancholia, "a new emotion, unknown
among the ancients and singularly developed among the moderns," which
seemed to translate itself most frequently into an unrequitable longing for
the past and an obsession with the dead.[1] From their earliest writings, the
Romantics had attributed a central aesthetic and ideological role to the grave.
Lamartine's *Méditations poétiques* are widely credited as being the first
Romantic verses in French. The most famous and enduring of them—"Le
lac [The Lake]"—is an elegy. Chateaubriand placed a burial scene at the
dramatic heart of his seminal novel, *Atala*, and then, later in life, composed

memoirs imagining himself to be writing from "beyond the tomb."[2] Hugo
was so fixated on death and the dead that he spent years of his life in conversation with them, holding séances and then passing sleepless nights transcrib-
ing and deciphering their results.[3] Although his morbid fascination expressed
itself more discreetly in his writings, it still appears with a dissimulated
strangeness and power at key narrative moments: Jean Valjean, the hero of
Les misérables, must undergo a harrowing burial alive as part of his entry into
redemption, while *Notre-Dame de Paris* (The Hunchback of Notre Dame)
closes with the quick and oblique glimpse of a necrophilic scene, in which
Esmeralda's skeleton is found embraced by that of Quasimodo, who must
have broken into the vault and then died while clutching her cadaver.[4] The
second-generation Romantics shared this aesthetic pathology. The group of
so-called *bousingos* which included the writers Gérard de Nerval, Théophile
Gautier, and Petrus Borel, looked to the charnel house for the décors of their
parties and seductions, celebrating the gothic and drinking toasts from
human skulls.[5] In one of the few poems where he does not brood on questions
of nothingness and doom, the *bousingo* Philothée O'Neddy depicts a man
dancing with a corpse.[6] Several years later, Baudelaire picked up on this tendency in *Les fleurs du mal* (The Flowers of Evil), whose dark vision of human
erotics included scenes of a particularly violent necrophilia, as can be seen in
poems such as "Une charogne [*A Rotting Cadaver*]" and "A une madonne [*To
a Madonna*]."[7]

This aesthetic was not, however, the exclusive privilege of famous authors,
and two of the doctors who published on Sergeant Bertrand's case cited
Auguste-Hilarion de Kératry's *Les derniers des Beaumanoir* (The Last of the
Beaumanoirs), a novel whose plot centered on a scene of sexual intercourse
with a corpse.[8] The population in general seems to have gotten caught up in
the mood as well, not only consuming the literature of this period, but also
participating more actively in the rise of morbid sentimentalism and its
piously eroticized cult of the deceased. Less intimate expressions of this fascination with the dead could be found in the popular crazes of spirit-writing
and table rapping that were gripping Europe at almost the same time that
Sergeant Bertrand was beginning his nocturnal exhumations.[9] And by the
middle of the century, this intercourse between two worlds flowed out into
the streets, where it was enshrined in a new public institution that displayed
the dead for all comers on a site that had been selected precisely because it
was one of the busiest in the capital. By the last quarter of the century, the

morgue had become a leading Parisian attraction, drawing crowds of inhabitants and tourists, who sometimes formed lines as much as 1,000 to 1,500 people long outside the building.[10] Although this was never part of its official mission, the morgue seems to have promoted a public erotics of the abject: an element of its immense attraction derived from its peculiar and unprecedented combination of death and sexuality, for until 1877 bodies were exposed totally unclothed, making it one of the few, if not the only place, where Parisians of all milieus could view naked strangers. Children, ladies, *flâneurs*, they had merely to wait in line.[11]

The ambient necrophilia of the moment caught the imagination of authors and occasionally crystallized there with a jarring force. Emile Zola, in particular, tried to imagine the sort of erotic excitement the morgue might arouse as part of an attempt, in his first successful novel, to structure a work not merely around the psychological conditions of two murderers slowly driven mad by memories of their victim, but, more exactly, around the gruesome image that obsessed them: a decaying corpse laid out on a viewing slab. *Thérèse Raquin* recounts the story of Laurent and Thérèse, a young man and woman who decide to kill her husband in order to marry each other. After the crime has been committed, Laurent begins frequenting the morgue, waiting for their victim's cadaver to appear so that a declaration of death can be made. The details of these visits seem to obsess not only the criminals but the author himself and to infect descriptions throughout the work, so that the "yellowish," "blackish," and "greenish" tints of the husband's corpse, the "blafard" pallor and the "whiteness" of his body set the palette for the rest of the volume.[12] Even before the murder, the secondary characters who populate the young lovers' small social circle prefigure the scene at the morgue, as if their entire world had been reduced to the urgings of sexual desire and visions of material death. Zola depicts a typical weekly get-together with the husband's friends as a rendezvous of the dead, in which "old Michaud displayed his pasty [*blafard*] forehead blotched [*tachée*] with red, . . . Olivier, whose bones stuck through his cheeks, carried his stiff and insignificant head on a ridiculous body," and "Suzanne, Olivier's wife, . . . sat completely pale, with distant eyes, white lips, and an inert face."[13] The violence and the particulars of this description look forward toward the vocabulary of the husband's lifeless body, to the "nudities brutality spread out and flecked [*tachées*] with blood" that Laurent will discover at the morgue, to the skin that he will see being torn away from the bones on a drowned man's face, and in general to the pallor and hideous passivity of the dead he will encounter while looking for his victim's body.[14] Thérèse herself already decodes these anticipated references in the preliminaries to her eventual madness, when she explicitly sees in her guests an image of the living dead: "sometimes she was seized by hallucinations that made her think she had been locked in the bottom of a tomb amid a company of mechanical corpses."[15] Through these visions, Zola offers a key to decrypting the resemblances between the two sets of descriptions: the living have become doubles of the dead—and not the dead of reminiscences and nostalgia, but the material dead, the ones that turn color and rot away. Whenever the lovers try to embrace, the vision of the drowned husband rises between them, as if sexuality had fused with the imaginary of his corpse.

It is through this hallucinatory lens that Zola views his character's visits to the morgue. They are mixtures of revulsion and desire:

> These nudities, brutally spread out, flecked with blood, and pierced in places by holes, attracted him and made him linger. One time, he saw a young woman, who must have been twenty years old, a working-class girl, stout and strong, who seemed to be sleeping on the stone. Her fleshy body gleamed coolly with the most subtle shades of white; she half smiled, her head tilted gently to the side, and thrust her chest out provocatively. One would have taken her for a courtesan sprawled out on her bed, were it not for a black line that circled her neck like a shadowy collar. She was a girl who had just hanged herself out of despair for love. Laurent looked at her for a long time, letting his gaze roam over her flesh, absorbed in a sort of fearful desire.[16]

The character's lingering is echoed in the length of the description, which dwells indecently on the material particulars of a dead body in an attempt to evoke its erotic attractiveness. The morgue is a place of fearful desire, where images of sexuality blend with horrifying disgust. What is original in the novel is certainly not its plot, but rather the way in which a simple story of passion and murder is motivated by a psychological universe that derives from an experience with this new Parisian institution, this place in which naked corpses entered publicly into the urban experience. Zola's novel imagines the ramifications of that entry, the way in which necrophilia could shape the perception of human relations and social structures to the point that it obscured the difference between the living and the dead. The images are exaggerated, but they represent a sustained effort to acknowledge and, to some extent, understand the terrifying attraction of the dead. His novel does not delve far into the motivations or etiology of this pathology, preferring instead to depict its effects on the characters' impressions of their world. Zola does offer a glimpse, however, of a more restrained, a more socially adequate reaction to this new erotic encounter, a response that could have entered more durably into the fabric of daily life. One of the well-dressed ladies who frequent the morgue stops before the body of a "tall, strapping fellow." "Transfixed by the spectacle of this man, the lady examined him, as if turning him over and weighing him with her gaze. She raised a corner of her veil, looked again, and then left."[17] An act of exquisite intimacy is evoked in this brief passage; the lingering by the dead, the voluptuousness of time itself as the lady indulges the pleasure of an imagined physical contact, and then the discreet undressing on her part, in which she unveils her own sexual organ, the eye of the voyeur, and thereby reciprocates with the dead.

The morgue launched Zola as a novelist and social pathologist, whose express intention in writing fiction was to apply Claude Bernard's method of experimental medicine to an observation of human behavior.[18] If he abandoned questions of necrophilic desire in his later works, the morgue seems nonetheless to have been the original and subsequently sublimated model for his overall clinical approach to the novel. The strange attraction that is glimpsed only obliquely in the eye of his fashionable bourgeois lady can, however, be seen more clearly in the aesthetics of an earlier author. More than any other writer from the nineteenth-century French canon, Théophile Gautier devoted his talents, especially in *Spirite* and his short stories, to depicting an erotics that crossed the boundary of the grave. The majority of his tales took this transgression for their theme, as if the whole category of the fantastic were on the verge of shrinking to this single, necrophilic act. That act itself was, however, covered in veils of prettiness, for Gautier's style is light and gently ironic, and the scenes he evoked were filled more with the nostalgic delight of a Fragonard painting come to life than the grim physicality of decomposing bodies. Gautier's revenants possessed charms that far exceeded those of living women. "Never, even in a dream," he wrote in "La Cafetière [The Coffee Pot]," "had anything so perfect come before my eyes."[19] "Oh, how beautiful she was!" one of his characters exclaims in "La Morte amoureuse [The Dead Woman in Love]." "Even the greatest painters, when they seek out the ideal of beauty in the heavens and bring back to earth the divine portrait of the Madonna, do not come close to that fabulous reality."[20] Not only were the dead more beautiful, they could offer more as well, and the pleasures that they promised transcended those that could be shared with the living. "If you agree to be mine," one of these lovely ghouls promises, "I shall make you happier than God himself in his paradise; the angels will envy you."[21] The examples quickly accumulate, and in their exaggeration, in their repetitive assurances that the dead are vastly superior love objects to the merely living, they recall the words Sergeant Bertrand pronounced about his first necrophilic experience: "I cannot define what I felt at that moment, all that one feels with a living woman is nothing in comparison."[22]

For Gautier, the dead were somehow cleansed, their materiality sublimated by death and the passage of time, and this is what makes them, in his writings, so much more desirable than the living, who are burdened by their fleshy materiality. Octavien, the hero of the story "Arria Marcella," speaks of the revulsion that living women inspire in him: "By my disgust toward other women . . ., by that insurmountable reverie that drew me towards those radiant prototypes at the bottom of the centuries as if toward beckoning stars, I understood that I could never love [*que je n'aimais jamais*] except outside the limits of time and space."[23] As part of this sublimation of the deceased, in which the word *jamais* is hidden both conceptually and hypogrammatically in the pronouncement *j'aimais*, Gautier explicitly excludes the horrors of physical death and decomposition from the erotics of his short stories. The remnants of ancient tombs that line one of the streets of Pompeii in "Arria Marcella" elicit, for instance, a sharp distinction between two types of dead:

> The three friends followed down that road lined with sepulchers which, by our modern standards, would make for a lugubrious avenue in a city but which had a different meaning for the ancients, whose tombs, instead of a horrible cadaver, contained only a handful of ashes, the abstract idea of death. . . . [T]hose funerary monuments, so brightly gilded by the sun and set on the edge of the path, still seemed to be attached to life [so that they] inspired none of those cold repulsions, none of those fantastic terrors which our lugubrious sepulchers evoke.[24]

On the one hand, there is the death of abstract ideas that lies, like the women Octavien desires, outside of time and space. On the other, there is the "horrible cadaver" that inspires disgust. In their revulsion, Gautier and his character conflate the putrefying corpse with women in their physical sexuality. One consequently wonders what those terrifying fantasies are that the narrator mentions, that attach themselves to the flesh and cannot distinguish between the rotting and the living. Persistently excluded but only partially hidden from Gautier's necrophilic aesthetics is this confused idea of an eroticized corpse, an image of the horrible blended with a nonsublimated desire, something like the cadaver that haunts the criminal imagination of Zola's *Thérèse Raquin*. What emerges as the real object of sexual desire here, the one that must be explicitly rejected, is the material body, the one that does not lie in a *jamais* beyond time and space but expresses them in an aesthetic encounter that confuses cold repulsion and erotic passion. What is horrible, perhaps, in all of this is the image of the human condition as thinking, feeling flesh, the experiential deconstruction of the barrier between thought and substance, the horror of our embodied existences. In our sexual appetites, according to the logic of these fantasies, we become the dead, their bodies visibly worked by an inhuman and inanimate force. This is desire, the laboring of a speechless other on our very persons, the flesh communicating in its autonomous language.

Both ideal lovers and the bearers of transcendental truths, the dead held an appeal that the living could not always offer each other in early nineteenth-century France. They were pursued in narrative, in painting, in séances and even in the street, where they were badgered to give up their secrets and their goods. Zola and Gautier gave explicit utterance to necrophilic tendencies, working, from opposite directions, on the aesthetic possibilities and affective charge embedded in their abject material condition. Zola picked up enthusiastically on the most disturbing aspects of physical death, appropriating them for the substance of his imaginative universe in *Thérèse Raquin*, and then using Claude Bernard's medical theories as a way to conceptualize the function of literature itself. Gautier, on the other hand, labored to create an aesthetics of sublimation, in which death operated as the negation of materiality, but his efforts created a negative counter-image of abjection that seems to have exercised a more powerful effect on his imaginary world than the ethereal love objects that ostensibly interested him and his characters. Despite their differences, in both cases the erotics of abjection became determining, indeed crucial factors in literary creation. For Zola, moreover, this also involved an explicit engagement with medical science and an attempt to theorize literary practice as a medical procedure.

In more dissimulated, but also more searching ways, other artists of the same period were reflecting on the relations between aesthetic production and the physical aspects of death, thereby revealing other, more internalized ways in which medical theory had become a matter for creative invention.

Odilon Redon

When J. K. Huysmans's novel *A rebours* (Against the Grain) appeared in 1884, it thrust an obscure lithographer, Odilon Redon, before the public. For over two decades, Redon had been laboring quietly to define a personal style and thematic universe that seemed, when his astonished contemporaries finally took notice, to have virtually no precedents. Strikingly original and somehow intuitively coherent, his techniques and visual vocabulary nonetheless remained troublingly incomprehensible even to those most sympathetic to his work, with Huysmans himself commenting that "it would be difficult to define Mr. Redon's surprising art."[25] Later critics perpetuated this uncertainty. Some emphasized the dreamlike qualities of his drawings and engravings, while others argued that they stemmed, instead, from very concrete concerns about social justice or the folkloric traditions of the Landes region in the Médoc, where Redon had grown up. Some, such as Huysmans, pointed to the importance of contemporary scientific theories in Redon's imaginary, an approach that others, notably Jerome Viola in the 1960s, rejected on the grounds that the artist was really concerned with spiritual issues.[26] Such ambiguity, which affects the reception of all artists, seems, however, to have been an intentional aspect of Redon's work. The artist himself wrote that "the sense of mystery is to remain at every moment equivocal, to sustain double or triple appearances, or the impressions of appearances (images in images), forms that have yet to be or which will be, depending on the viewer's state of mind."[27] But although it produced images of oneiric plasticity and spiritual resonance, Redon's aesthetics of indistinction was not based on the free play of subjective fantasy, as such a quotation might suggest, or in the romantic movements of the heart. Instead, that indistinction emerged out of convictions about the nature of the material world and the role of consciousness in it, convictions that themselves were shaped by a life-long study of the sciences. Although he consistently rejected the importance of philosophical ideas in his art, Redon was nonetheless able to work through basic questions concerning the role of sentience and thought about the limits of life and death.[28] What marks the principal difference between his approach and philosophical inquiries on the same sorts of subjects is that Redon tried to address these questions not conceptually, but through matter itself.

Redon's sustained and conscious attempts to integrate contemporary scientific principles into his work belie, or at least complicate, his claim that his creations did not involve abstract thought. His interest in the sciences seems to have been inspired early on in life by his friendship with Armand Clavaud, a botanist some years his senior and who would later become an assistant director at the botanical gardens in Bordeaux.[29] A brilliant polymath, Clavaud kept abreast of the most recent developments in literature and helped orient his young friend's curiosity and readings. "Clavaud was extraordinarily gifted," Redon would later remember. "He was by nature as much a scholar as an artist (which is rare), always moved to pity by the revelations of the microscope . . . , he surrendered himself passionately to reading and literary research with an enlightened erudition."[30] What Redon saw in his friend is revealing, for Clavaud seems to have passed on to his protégé a conviction about the connection between the arts and the sciences and to have inspired Redon to see how their elements could fuse into something human and alive. The observation about the affectivity of Clavaud's gaze is significant as well. The botanist appears to have communicated to Redon some of the pity and compassion that he felt towards the revelations of the microscope, for the artist's drawings seem to find a sorrowful tenderness in the monsters they depict. That tenderness, as the brief description of Clavaud indicates, was part of how Redon himself imagined the human relation to the subvisible. And even though he rejected Huysmans's suggestion that his ideas stemmed from an analysis of the microscopic world, he seems really to have objected to a perceived criticism that he was simply offering illustrations of what could be seen through the lens.[31] Rather than transcriptions, Redon's *noirs*, as he referred to his black-and-white works in charcoal, etching, and lithography, were meditations on the significance of the universe that optics had disclosed in infinitely small things. They bespoke an interpretive rather than instrumental relation to the microscope, an attitude that might best be described, in a distant echo of his portrait of Clavaud, as pitiful or pathetic.

The fold took. After moving to Paris in the 1870s, Redon began to attend lectures at the Ecole de Médecine and to accompany the medical students he had befriended on their rounds at a local hospital.[32] He studied the skeletal remains of various life forms, current and extinct, in Georges Cuvier's osteology displays at the Muséum d'Histoire Naturelle.[33] He sent a copy of his lithographic series *Origins* to Pasteur along with a letter. Pasteur responded, praising the artist's ability to "give life" to the monsters of the natural world.[34] By the 1880s Redon had become familiar with the principal debates roiling the sciences of his time. He was knowledgeable about the positions held by the leading figures in evolutionism, including Cuvier, Jean-Baptiste Lamarck, Charles Darwin, and Geoffroy and Isidore Saint-Hilaire. He had studied osteology in courses at the Muséum d'Histoire Naturelle and probably at lectures by Marie Philibert Sappey. He was most likely familiar with Pierre Paul Broca's work on neuroanatomy and the nascent field of anthropology, and he had passionately followed the progress of Pasteur and his contemporaries in germ theory. If Redon's art seemed unprecedented to his audience of the time, it was probably because his sources were as much to be found in the amphitheaters of the medical schools as in the work of Goya and Gustave Moreau.

Indeed, the very idea of indeterminacy, which according to Redon lent their mysterious quality to his works, was more of an evolutionary and biological principle than an artistic one. Evolutionism had broken up the boundaries between various life forms, introducing the idea of movement among different species by arguing that they were constantly in flux. There were, according to these new theories, crossover beings, whose identity was caught in the fluidity of time, and scientists could point to specific examples from the present, to creatures who bore the stamp of ambiguity in their bodies and who expressed, in that way, the unfinished work of history. The mollusk, according to Lamarck and Geoffroy Saint-Hilaire, occupied a taxonomical zone somewhere between the vertebrates and invertebrates.[35] The most interesting of these biological indeterminacies for Redon seems, however, to have been the possibility of a middle ground between the plant and animal kingdoms. Again, the original impetus appears to have come from Armand Clavaud, who, according to Redon, "sought out—I don't know quite how to put it—at the borders of the imperceptible world, that intermediary life between plant and animal, that flower or being, that mysterious element that is an animal for several hours each day and only under the effect of light."[36] This, for Redon, is a source of mystery, and I would argue that he uses the word both to mean something incomprehensible or curious and in a more archaic sense to refer to a spiritual significance, so that the two schools of thought that would oppose those tendencies in his work are really separating concepts that for the artist himself would have overlapped.

Redon's friends and critics quickly perceived this biological aspect of his work. After the artist's second individual exhibition, for instance, Huysmans described his pictures in the following terms: "Some of the works in charcoal went even farther into dreadful, congestively tormented dreamscapes; this was a world of vibrios and volvoces, vinegar eels [*animalcules du vinaigre*] swarming in soot-stained glucose."[37] The vocabulary is revealing. Vinegar eels (*Anguillula aceti*) are among the first creatures that van Leeuwenhoek observed under his microscope, while vibrios are comma-shaped bacteria whose genus includes the cholera pathogen, which the German physician Robert Koch was to discover in the following year. Although similar figures do populate Redon's noirs, it was probably the choice of this particular word that provoked the artist's later dismissal of Huysman's review, since it seemed to reduce his work to the status of scientific plates, as if limiting his inspiration to an objective cataloguing of the visible world.[38] More suggestive, however, is the term *volvox*, a word that the critic Jean Lorrain also used in his review of "In the Primeval Slime" at the 1894 retrospective of Redon's work. It designates a microscopic alga that forms in pond scum.[39] Although now firmly classified as a plant, there was dispute about that point in Redon's time, for these organisms have flagella that allow them to move, sexual organs, and small eyespots that orient their motion toward light sources, attributes that led zoologists in the 1880s to include volvoces among the protozoa and, therefore, to classify them as members of the animal kingdom.[40] In perceiving what at the time were indeterminate life forms among Redon's figures, Huysmans and Lorrain thus indicated that they understood the artist to be exploring the ambiguity between plants and animals. The critic Emile Hennequin also picked up on this theme in his review of the same exhibition:

> Some of his works are as upsetting as the sensation produced by a sudden contact with a viscous object—his *Animated Flower*, among others, in which a short herbaceous stem rising from black soil supports in the shade a perfectly round calyx, a large yellowish face with dead eyes and a placid smile. Elsewhere, in *Muds*, infusoria—part vibrion, part aquatic cryptogram—emerge from a tenebrous background, presenting to the spectator the malevolent, malicious, perfidious, or ridiculous deformations of the human face . . .
>
> But Redon does not limit himself to the lower levels of life. He exhibits, in what might be called a heroic genre, *Etruscan Woman*.[41]

No picture with the name "Animated Flower" seems to have come down to us. Most likely, Hennequin was referring to a charcoal that would later be reworked into the lithograph entitled "The Marshflower: A Sad Human Head" (see Figure 1).[42] During the early 1880s Redon produced several versions of this image, showing a plant sprouting a human face, and some more distant variations on the same theme, such as his "Cactus Man," in which a blunt and thorny human head emerges from a flower pot, and "Spirit of the Forest (Specter from a Giant Tree)," which depicts a human skeleton with a fleshy, balding head apparently growing out of the branch on which it is standing.[43] Hennequin's reaction to the flower image indicates the accuracy with which Redon was able to communicate his concerns, even in his earliest public exhibitions. The very word *viscous* situates the relation between the critic and the drawings within the mysteries that Redon himself had

Planche II.

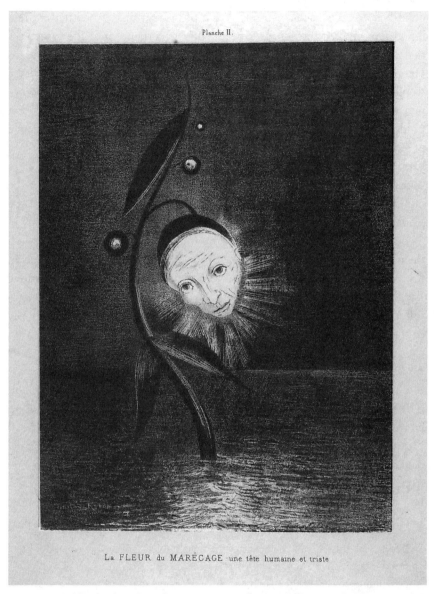

La FLEUR du MARÉCAGE une tête humaine et triste

Figure 1. Odilon Redon, French, 1840–1916, *The Marsh Flower, a Sad Human Head,* plate 2 of 6, 1885. Lithograph in black on ivory China paper laid down on ivory wove paper, 272 x 202 mm (image/chine); 441 × 306 mm (sheet), The Stickney Collection, 1920.1588, The Art Institute of Chicago. Photography © The Art Institute of Chicago.

described, for the viscous is itself a state of indeterminacy. Neither entirely liquid nor solid, it introduces a frightening uncertainty into the categories that would structure our responses to the physical world, "upsetting" us, as Hennequin says, and causing us to pull back in fear and disgust. As Sartre would write: "Viscosity is the agony of water; it presents itself as a phenomenon in the process of becoming, without the permanence in change that water has. Instead, it represents something like a slice removed from a change of state."[44] What oozes, for Sartre, is much like Saint-Hilaire's mollusk: a palpable attestation to the mutability of material things, a being caught in transition so long as to become perceptible—and even, in the case of the mollusk, to perceive. This oozing life, caught between the animal and the plant, was the universe of Redon's imagination.

But while Redon was concerned about the biological sciences and drew on their discoveries in his work, he was also fascinated by the physical aspects of his own artistic production. In this, he differed from his mentor, Rodolphe Bresdin, who obviously felt some ambivalence, if not outright resentment, toward his materials, or at least toward the large stones that he meticulously engraved, working on them over years and sometimes lugging them from continent to continent. He inscribed his frontispiece to Thierry-Faletans's *Fables et contes* (Fables and Tales) with the words "I've carried this stone for fifty years."[45] Redon, on the other hand, seems to have taken a tactile delight in the process of creation. Part of this may have been because the materials he worked with were lighter and less cumbersome, for it was only after Henri Fantin-Latour showed him how to transfer drawings from specially prepared paper to stones that he embraced lithography. His pleasure derived not only from an increased facility or a minimization of his contact with his materials, but from the secrets that those materials alone were able to reveal to him. Later in life he described his creative process in the following terms:

> Besides the aptitude that he acquires from the influence of the people and the places that surround him, the artist also yields, in a certain measure, to the demanding powers of the matter that he uses: pencil, charcoal, pastel, grease pencil, printing inks, marble, bronze, earth, or wood—all of these supplies are agents that accompany him, that collaborate with him, and that say something too in the fiction that he is going to produce. Matter reveals secrets, it has its own genius; it is through matter that the oracle will speak.[46]

His unusual approach to lithography—indeed his very choice of a medium that had found few practitioners among fine artists and had for the most part been relegated to mass production of posters and other ephemera—seems to have derived from this conviction in the meaningfulness of his materials themselves, in their ability to communicate to and through him mysteries embedded in the physical world. He tended to build up the black areas in his stones and then scratch them away to produce effects of light, and in this way he caused that light to emerge out of a primary dark, to create it by working with the blackness itself, as if the visibility and intelligibility of the images could not be dissociated from the substance of the ink itself. In describing his method of working, he wrote that he did not try to impose ideas on his materials and to fashion them according to a preconceived form, but that his images arose out of his contact with those materials, the grease pencils, paper, and heavy stones that he manipulated.[47] It is with this in mind that one should read Redon's many remarks about his physical relation to his works, as when he recalled the pleasures, during the year he studied sculpture in Bordeaux, of touching "that exquisite material, soft and supple, that is modeling clay [*la terre glaise*]," or when he wrote that if someone wanted to understand his experience, "it is . . . in painting, the act of painting; just losing yourself in the stuff [*la pâte*], a brush in hand."[48] He liked, however, the touch not only of paints or clay, but of the soil itself, for he recalled, late in life, the joys he felt when he sketched with hands stained by the dirt from his garden, that "sacred and silent matter, that reparative source" and exulted in "the contact with any other unconscious element."[49] The media of the artist were, for Redon, particularly eloquent versions of a more basic materiality that he understood to inform his work, the very earth itself, which he seemed to suck up into his being like a plant. Attached to the soil by "secret lineaments," the artist, according to him, was constantly receptive to his sensations and environment, while the changing seasons affected his "sap."[50]

Matter, even the dirt itself, had secrets for Redon, mysteries that it spoke through him in the visible darkness of his *noirs* and in the silence of unconscious things. Already, however, in speaking of an "unconscious element," Redon raises the issue of consciousness, as if inert matter were somehow deprived of it and defined by that lack. The inanimate is missing consciousness, but in Redon's universe, that missing, or *manque*, seems to have the dual sense of a lack and, paradoxically, an awareness of that lack, as when we say, "I miss you." The black of his inks suffers its stupidity, and this is part of the pathos of his works, which echoes in his description of Clavaud's attitude toward the discoveries of the microscope. It is aware of its lack of awareness. This pathos is betrayed in the upward cast that characterizes the eyes of

Redon's monsters, as in "The Marshflower" and "Eye-Balloon" (see Figure 2).[51] Like bubbles caught in a viscous liquid or the photosensitive spots on volvoces, they strive toward the regions above them but remain trapped in the darkness from which they only half emerge. These are figures of longing, of a desire to rise to the surface and to the light of thought, which lies somewhere beyond the upper edge of the paper, for the creatures always look outside the image toward something to which it can only allude. Another variation on this idea of a dim consciousness in the unconscious appears in a description of Bresdin's hands. "When he was working," Redon wrote, "his fingers stretched out as if extended by fluids that attached them to his tools. They were not 'prelate's hands,' as the saying goes, they were conscious, loving hands, sensitive to substances and without disdain for humble objects, but still finely tapered, elegant, soft, and aristocratically supple. Artist hands [*des mains artistes*]."[52] The fingers appear to blend with the materials they manipulate, as if they, like the skeletal figure in "Spirit of the Forest," had grown together with them. And they are not artist's hands, but artist-hands, in other words not the hands *of* an artist but independent and creative in their own right. Indeed, they, not the mind, seem to be the organs that produce Bresdin's lithographs, for they are the ones who feel, react, and love. They are, as Redon puts it, conscious. In unison with the tools and materials they touch, it is the hands that think. In general, by the sheer fact of adding a sense organ to his *noirs*, as in the eyeballs that recur throughout them, Redon attributes a sentience to their dark materiality, and when he gives faces to monsters he lends them a form of personhood, so that in this intermediate zone between animal and plant, between thought and matter, we can recognize ourselves. The effect of this recognition is not so much that the monsters argue for a personality among the infusorians of the microscopic world or that they enjoy human self-awareness, but that they remind us how, in our own persons, we retain an attachment to a lost epoch that still teems in mud and pond scum and that lives on even in our own hands.

Several titles from Redon's works indicate his concern with this penetration of matter by thought. An illustration for Flaubert's *Temptation of Saint Anthony* shows a snake-like body emerging out of darkness and ending in a head with closed eyes and wrapped in folds. The plate bears the title "Oannès: I, the First Consciousness of Chaos, Arose from the Abyss to Harden Matter, to Regulate Forms" (see Figure 3).[53] As represented in this lithograph, the power of thought had its own historical moment, when it first emerged and began to act on the material world, but this moment continues

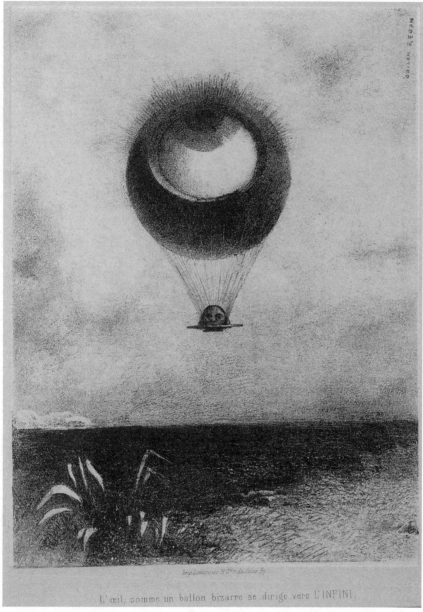

L'œil, comme un ballon bizarre se dirige vers L'INFINI.

Figure 2. Odilon Redon, French, 1840–1916, *The Eye, Like a Strange Balloon Moves Towards Infinity*, plate one from *To Edgar Poe*, 1882. Lithograph in black on ivory China paper, laid down on white wove paper, 263 × 198 mm (image/chine); 443 × 315 mm (sheet), The Stickney Collection, 1920.1570, The Art Institute of Chicago. Photography © The Art Institute of Chicago.

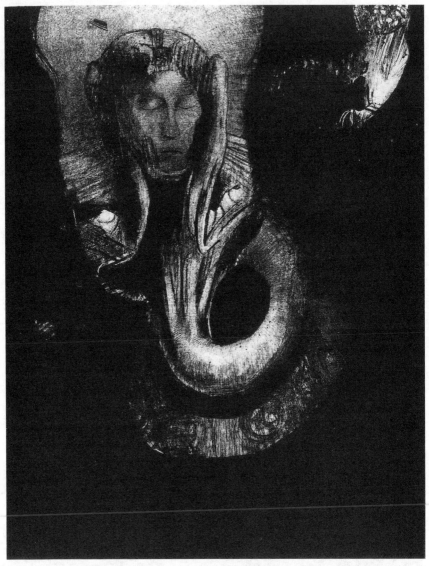

Figure 3. Odilon Redon, French, 1840–1916, *Oannes: "I, the first consciousness in Chaos, rose from the abyss to harden matter, to determine forms,"* plate 14 from *The Temptation of Saint Anthony (3rd series)*, 1896. Lithograph in black on ivory China paper laid down on ivory wove paper, 278 × 217 mm (image, overlaps chine); 451 × 360 mm (sheet), The Stickney Collection, 1920.1771, The Art Institute of Chicago. Photography © The Art Institute of Chicago.

to repeat itself endlessly throughout nature, and if it can be depicted, it is not so much in this one plate, with its specific features, as throughout Redon's opus, in the way his images preserve the process of their creation, the effect of thought on matter. In this respect, "Oannès" is the least representative of Redon's works, since it allegorizes all of the others, stepping back, one remove, from their embeddedness in their materials to think about the process of artistic thinking itself. If Redon's other works are aware, this one is self-aware. "When Life Was Awakening in the Depths of Obscure Matter," from the 1882 show at the *Gaulois*, catches a similar moment, when lumpy creatures, whose invertebrate bodies still adhere awkwardly to the ground, begin to stare out at the world through open eyes and bovine faces. One of the plates from his third series of lithographs for Flaubert's *Temptation of Saint Anthony* comments on the line ". . . And Eyes without Heads Were Floating like Mollusks" (see Figure 4).[54] It seems to focus on the tiny figures from the background of "When Life Was Awakening," as if peering into increasingly smaller sections of his own artistic world and tying his monsters into contemporary fantasies about oysters and other shellfish, atavistic life forms that were imagined to inhabit the regions between the animate and the inanimate.[55]

Here again, in respect to the possibility of a liminal zone between matter and consciousness, Redon's idiosyncratic aesthetic universe was shaped by contemporary developments in the sciences, especially among the evolutionists. A particularly telling example is the German zoologist Ernst Haeckel, in whom Darwin saw the most important of his potential continuators. [56] Perhaps because he was more marginal than Darwin, Haeckel throws an important light on the intellectual culture that surrounded the elaboration of evolutionary theories. He developed a mystical theory about the connectedness of all life forms and in one of the earliest evolutionary diagrams ever produced, he traced plants, protistae, and animals back to a single "radix communalis."[57] The sheer fact that in this document Haeckel represented the evolutionary process as a tree demonstrates the persistence of plant forms throughout the organization of living beings, since the structure of their structures can be depicted as a vegetal shape. In a similar vein, it was also Haeckel who devised and first promulgated the famous, if misleading, slogan "ontogeny recapitulates phylogeny." This theory held that all modern life forms retain the imprint of their evolutionary antecedents in the development and shape of their bodies. The importance of these scientific theories for deciphering the meaning of the world can be deduced from Haeckel's

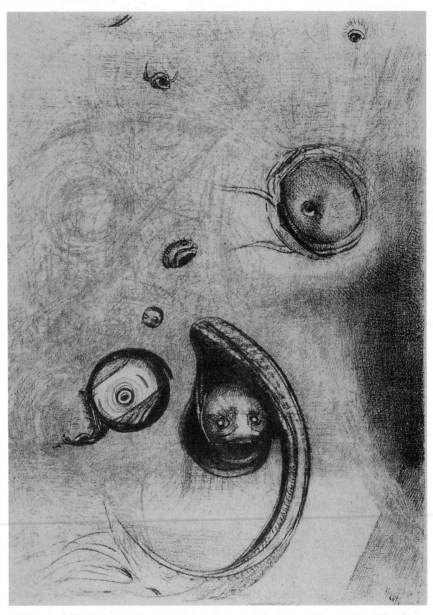

Figure 4. Odilon Redon, French, 1840–1916, *And that Eyes without Heads Were Floating Like Mollusks*, plate 13 of 24, 1896. Lithograph in black on light gray China paper
laid down on ivory wove paper, 311 × 226 mm (image/chine); 526 × 349 mm (sheet),
The Stickney Collection, 1920.1769, The Art Institute of Chicago. Photography ©
The Art Institute of Chicago.

own behavior and philosophical convictions, for he was a pantheist who believed that the physical universe was infused with some sort of intelligence. He wrote, in *The Wonders of Life*:

> As the object of this work is the critical study of the wonders of life, and a knowledge of the truth concerning them, we must first of all form a clear idea of the meaning of "life." . . . For thousands of years men have appreciated the difference between life and death, between living and lifeless bodies; the former are called organisms, and the latter known as inorganic bodies. . . . [M]odern science has shown that the sharp distinction formerly drawn between the organic and the inorganic cannot be sustained, but that the two kingdoms are profoundly and inseparably united.[58]

As with Claude Bernard and the physiologists that preceded him, Haeckel was drawn by his studies to question the very possibility of distinguishing between life and death and he thereby opened the possibility of an intermediary zone of inanimate sentience, which his zoological works would attempt to illustrate and define. Darwin himself seems to have been similarly seduced by the idea of a certain intelligence in inanimate life forms, writing on the "wonderful" sensitivity of radicles, the embryonic segments that develop into the main root of a plant. Their growth is influenced by gravity and light and they respond to destructive forces by slow but evasive movement. What particularly interested Darwin in these small bits of vegetable matter was their ability to communicate "an influence from the excited part to another which consequently moves."[59] The radicle, according to him, "perceives" certain aspects of its environment, such as humidity, and thus betrays something analogous to intelligence in animals, a dark awareness of its surroundings.[60] And Darwin points quickly to this possibility, although without attempting to elaborate it at length, by concluding his 1880 volume on *The Power of Movement in Plants* with the following observation: "It is hardly an exaggeration to say that the tip of the radicle thus endowed, and having the power of directing the movements of the adjoining parts, acts like the brain of one of the lower animals; the brain being seated within the anterior end of the body, receiving impressions from the sense-organs, and directing the several movements."[61] These are the last words in the book, as if the naturalist himself did not want to stray too far into the curious realms of sentience he was opening up. Plants have organs like brains that perceive what is around them and send that information to other parts of the body, thereby directing their movements. More remarkable and unsettling, perhaps, is the

obverse of that same observation: human minds are like plant radicles, groping tenderly in the darkness of their material world. The trees in Redon's
works, like "Day" from *Dreams* (see Figure 5), look in at the viewer with an
incomprehensible gaze that is nonetheless part of the human condition.[62]
They are, moreover, self-portraits in a very specialized sense: they reveal
the vegetal intelligence that lingers in human bodies, directing, among other
things, the movements of the artist's hand. The monsters in Redon's works
thus seem, in general, to figure a world in which, like plant-animals, creatures
are caught in a basic sentience and embedded in a material world to which
they give thought. They figure out, give intelligence to matter itself. At the
same time, they look upwards, almost always, as if in longing for the higher
regions of thought and of being, for subjectivity and humanity. Caught below
in the mud of materiality, they are reflections on our embeddedness in the
physical world and a sorrowful rejoicing in that state, a sad, if sometimes
bemused, acceptance of our lot rather than an abstract negation of it.

Redon's own interest in osteology and evolutionism derived, however,
from a deeper and more idiosyncratic concern about biology, in particular
about the difference between life and death. He used the terms bluntly in his
own writings on art, rejecting photography, for instance, because "the snap-
shot transmits only death," and praising Frans Hals as "the most powerful
man ever to translate animal life in its paroxysm."[63] His own *noirs* include
works entitled "Germination" and "Blossoming" and explore an imaginary
realm at the origins of life. He described nature as "a pure means for expressing our feelings and for communicating them to our fellow men, without
which our own ambition to create must remain a dream, an abstraction, and,
in some way, a simple palpitation of life that otherwise has no perfect organ
by which to appear in its full force."[64] Here the term *life* seems to have
replaced the vocabulary of sentience and consciousness that one finds elsewhere in Redon's writings and in the science of his times. But if he rejected
that simple palpitation of life as insufficient for art, he was nonetheless aware
of it and bore it in mind when thinking about the purpose of his creations.
And if this simple palpitation is not enough, that seems to be because it is
incommunicable. The artist's goal, according to this passage, is not so much
to escape from the lowest levels of biology but rather to find the means to
express them, even if that expression must necessarily transform them into
something different, into monsters aware of their own unawareness and possible only in the human imagination.

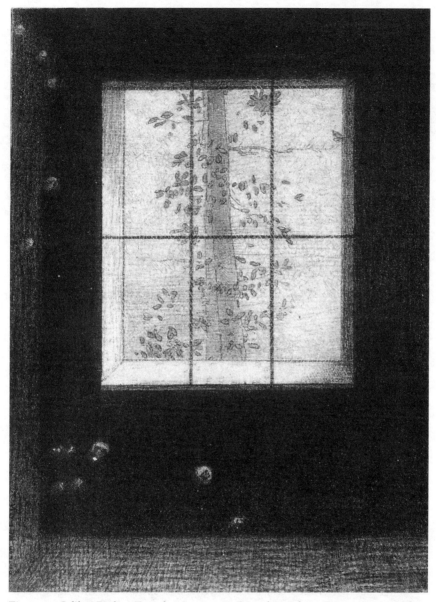

Figure 5. Odilon Redon, French, 1840–1916, *Day*, plate 6 from *Dreams*, 1891. Lithograph in black on ivory China paper laid down on white wove paper, 210 × 157 mm (image/chine); 440 × 316 mm (sheet), The Stickney Collection, 1920.1693, The Art Institute of Chicago. Photography © The Art Institute of Chicago.

192 Monsters and Artists

Redon saw his art works as life forms in a very literal sense, describing his creative process as a kind of fermentation: "Nature . . . becomes my source, my yeast, my ferment. On the basis of this origin, I believe that my inventions are true. I believe it of my drawings; . . . one could not bear their sight for an instant (for they are humanly expressive), were they not, as I say, formed, constituted, and built according to the law of life and of moral transmission that is necessary to all that exists."[65] Again, two elements seem to predominate in Redon's description of his own works: their expressiveness and their animation. Their truth and morality lie in their conformity to the principles that govern life. They are moral and they are true, in other words, because they are alive and because they make that life intelligible to others. And Redon seems to have taken seriously the idea that his creatures were alive, or at least could potentially come to life. His friend and biographer André Mellerio recalled a conversation they had had in 1891, during which the artist described how he had been influenced by the courses in osteology he had attended at the Muséum d'Histoire Naturelle and by the doctors who had overseen his studies there:

> It was in the Museum that he understood Cuvier's great law, the concordance of beings, especially among the vertebrates. "That was where I really got the idea for my monsters, and what is curious about them—and it's enormous—is that they could live. They are constructed according to laws for that. Consequently any exaggeration in respect to one part will lead to the reduction or atrophy of another. That is to say, the equilibrium is broken or it is replaced by another sort of compensation. So for an enormous head a little body, or vice versa."[66]

There is a literalism in Redon's approach to life that seems to astonish even him. His works, at least in this period, are not intended as depictions but rather as creations, unique beings so obedient to the laws of biology that they are on the verge of animation. And this concern about their conformity to Cuvier's principles of compensation expresses one form of a deeper, more generalized interest in the sources of life itself. Darwin and Pasteur had revealed that matter teemed with sensitivity, perception, and the vaguest consciousness, and Redon seems to have followed these revelations with an excitement that even decades later had not left him. He attempted to capture this life, this sentience, in his own pieces, and although he never says as much, Redon's writings on the process of his work indicate that there is some confusion as to where that life lies. It is not just in the monsters whose forms we grasp, but also, and more importantly, in the ink and paper themselves, in the sensitively erotic but unconscious way the artist handles his materials, and in the fruit of that encounter. And the impetus for that animation is the viewer's eye, which illuminates the darkness of a primeval world and which Redon obsessively inscribed within his *noirs* themselves. Somehow, for Redon, in that sensuous moment of looking, a transmission occurred between the consciousness inherent in his media and the human being that apprehended them. That was their truth and their morality.

His contemporaries picked up on these concerns in his works, but tended to grasp them along another, more forbidding register. Mellerio wrote that "with a Darwinian vision he embraced initial chaos" but found in it "minuscule insects" that bred "death and decomposition of the organism."[67] The Darwinian world was also, to the critic's imagination, the world of putrefaction, and this, as we have seen in earlier chapters, comprised the strange, transformative forces of death that labor and recreate the world in defiance of the struggles of living matter, the unconscious and inanimate works that blossom in the corpse. Hennequin saw this too in the 1882 show at the *Gaulois*, remarking about one plate: "Black moon dancing on top of a puddle of water, it seems to be the materialization of a miasma."[68] At this moment, even many in the scientific community did not seem to have appreciated the full significance of Pasteur's discoveries in germ theory and still confused the organisms that transmitted disease with the miasmas of an earlier period. But microbes, even if deadly, were alive, while the miasma was inanimate matter, often confused with death itself. It embodied death as a principle and a substance, death at work, not in the sense of Hegel's abstract force of the negative, but as an inanimate malevolence that made its way into the living body with a determination and quasi-intelligence that foreshadowed the sensitivity that Darwin observed in the tips of radicles. And by locating the origins of his own artistic creation in the "ferment" and "yeast" that nature represented for him, Redon choose those terms that most powerfully condensed the contemporary confusion between the order of life and the order of death, for fermentation was at once widely held to be the very essence of putrefaction and the stuff of life. At the same time it was the source of Pasteur's discoveries, for his isolation of pathogenic microorganisms had begun in his work on beer yeasts.[69]

For his own part, Redon reflected on death throughout his life in surprisingly consistent terms, describing it as a sanctuary free from the concerns and agitations of existence, but also in a strangely physical way. As a child he jotted down in a notebook: "I passed through the cemetery's cold and silent alleys and by the empty tombs. And I felt a calm of mind. O death! How great you are: in the calm that the thought of you gives me, what strength against cares!"[70] Many years later, a visit to another graveyard would inspire similar reflections: "Death, there [*là*], beneath my feet, in the dark graves, where friends and kin are resting, happy at last, because they feel no more. Death, . . . I saw it there [*là*]."[71] What predominates in these lines is the sense of peace, the absence of suffering, indeed of sensation, which would suggest that death, for Redon, represented a complete absence of consciousness and an absolute break with even the most minimal levels of sentience, such as can be perceived in the tips of radicles. And yet certain aspects of these descriptions belie that impression. Most strikingly, the insistence on the physical location of death, its presence *"là"* represents it as a material, rather than conceptual entity, a thing that lingers in the ground, like miasmas. Death is not nothing, it is there, beneath his feet. And although the dead themselves may be beyond feeling, perceiving, or caring, the use of the apostrophe in this and another, similar passage from elsewhere in the same volume presents death itself as something that can hear and that is endowed, therefore, with certain sense perceptions.[72] In fact, Redon represented death several times in his works, as in frequent images of skeletons and skulls. The third plate from the volume *To Gustave Flaubert* is probably the most famous of these and bears the title "Death: My Irony Exceeds All Others" (see Figure 6).[73] Redon produced a color version in oil of the same image several years later under the title "Green Death," and both variations bear an unmistakable resemblance to "Oannès: I, the First Consciousness . . ." (see Figure 3), which was produced in the interval between them. In fact, the resemblance is so distinct as to be necessarily intentional. In both cases, a powerful, serpentine body coils around itself in deep darkness and culminates in a human head wrapped in folds. The idea that death should be cognate to consciousness itself runs counter to the more quietist descriptions of cemeteries in Redon's writings, but it does confirm the suggestions of sentience and intelligence hidden in their use of the vocative. That more restless image of death, that notion of death as an entity endowed with some form of awareness borrows from the traditional personifications of mortality but under pressure from Redon's studies in contemporary science forces them in a new direction and toward new meanings. Death is less an anthropomorphic being for Redon than a force and lifeless will, similar to oysters and plants but even more closely attached than they to matter itself.

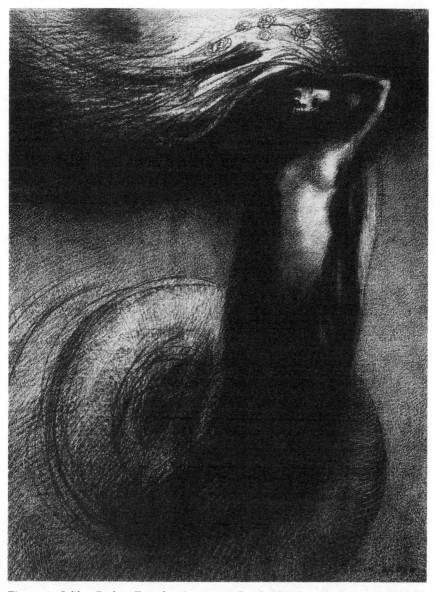

Figure 6. Odilon Redon, French, 1840–1916, *Death: "My Irony Surpasses All Others,"* 1888. Transfer lithograph in black ink on thin ivory wove paper, laid down on heavy-weight ivory wove plate paper (chine collé) , 261 × 197 mm (image); 347 × 452 mm (sheet), The Stickney Collection, 1920.1651, The Art Institute of Chicago. Photography © The Art Institute of Chicago.

Hennequin and Mellerio had perceived that physical death in Redon's works when they found depictions of decomposition and miasmas in them. Another friend, Jules Boissé, saw in Redon himself evidence of the belief in such a death, a belief that contradicted his more reassuring depictions of death as a haven. The artist described his last visit with Boissé:

> All that night, he seemed to worry about my motive for coming to be there with him. Although he was affectionate, he refused to believe that it was from anything but curiosity! "You've come to see me die," he said, when he saw me arrive. "It's not very interesting. You see, I still have my analytic consciousness"—those were his very words—"and I can follow the progress of the decomposition. I've got another six hours, for the unconscious molecules of my body are at work. This hiccup, I can't control it . . ."
>
> Whose turn is it now? Death has taken up residence in my mind because I *saw* it.[74]

Here again, Redon insists on the visibility of death: he has *seen* it. And death, as his friend describes it, is unconscious, like the beings that "feel no more" in the graveyard, but still it works in the molecules of his body, acting on the living and bringing them down. Boissé thought that Redon would be interested in that work of death, that physical performance that betrayed its activity and presence in hiccups and decomposition, that seized at the dying man's throat and spoke through it in involuntary and inhuman noises. And this belief is a testimony to the personality of Redon as he was known by those around him, a side of him that contradicts the more romantic raptures about cemeteries that fill his writings but that seems more consistent with his work as an artist. This was the work of death, its haunting language and presence. This was also a labor that the artist takes up again in inert materials longing with meaning and even in his own hands, for they too are unconscious but mysteriously active. In his *noirs*, Redon denies the absoluteness of death, arguing, in his silent way, that one can live in death, that nature itself and our material attachment to it constitute a way to escape the theoretical limits of mortality.

But Redon's works are incomprehensible without the thin, almost invisible lines that cover them, for the abstract line—the line so thin as not to exist physically—was what, according to the artist, gave meaning to his images. His thinking on this subject was, however, somewhat contradictory. He felt ambivalence about the notion of abstraction itself, referring to it sometimes as an impediment to appreciating the pleasure and sense of artworks, as when he said of metaphysicians that "their mind is too occupied with abstractions for them to fully share and taste the pleasures of art," or when he described nature as "a pure means for expressing our feelings and for communicating them to our fellow men, without which our own ambition to create must remain . . . an abstraction."[75] Elsewhere, however, he seems to have taken the opposite approach, seeing in abstractions the very possibility of communication. In a discussion of the "abstract line" from *A soi-même* (To Oneself), for instance, Redon writes that "suggestive art can provide nothing unless it draws solely on the mysterious play of shadows and the rhythm of mentally conceived lines." He adduces as an example the work of Leonardo DaVinci, where such mysteries reach their apogee and form "the roots for the words of his language."[76] They are the dim forerunners of intelligibility, the earliest probing of thought into matter. Or again, in describing Rubens, Redon writes: "he has a certain affinity with the English school. Like it, he never uses lines to generalize—indeed, he seems unaware of their existence. By line, I mean the straight line, that active and decisive abstraction without which forms, and paintings, have no organism."[77] The line generalizes and thereby renders communicable what is buried in the colors and textures of the artist's media, transforming them into a sort of thinking. The line, for Redon, is the intervention of thought in the materiality of his images and the source of his language. But it is also the line between life and death, the act of intelligence that illuminates unconsciousness to reveal in it a sentience that was already there but unaware of itself, like the groping of a plant's radicles or the effervescence of decomposition. In this respect, Redon's *noirs* are not about representing but about presenting. In them the abstract line instantiates and fixes consciousness in the materiality of the black. One can see this movement of thought in the thin tracings on their surfaces, down to the apparently offhand marks such as the scratchings around the serpentine coils in "Death: My Irony Exceeds All Others" (see Figure 6) or in the background of "And Eyes without Heads . . ." (see Figure 4). This is the flash of light in the darkness of Redon's *noirs*, the place and gesture that capture the eye of the viewer and transform their materiality into the first inklings of intelligibility. Redon's ambivalence about abstraction captures the ambiguity of the abstract line in his works, for that line is the zone between conscious and unconscious matter, between life and death. In this sense, Redon's works represent a thinking about death that emerges out of the materials themselves, that does not reflect on inanimate matter from the perspective of the living, but rather from the perspective of the dead themselves.

Balzac

In his works, Redon searched out the lowest degrees of sentience in order to imagine the experience of death as it might be perceived from the viewpoint of the dead. This he expressed in a highly controlled, biologically informed vocabulary that reflected the science of his times as interpreted through his own idiosyncratic personality. While Balzac predated Redon in chronological terms, his interest in the literary aspects of material death represented a more elaborated—one could say advanced if that did not imply a value judgment— use of its aesthetic potential, and for that reason I have waited to discuss him. With the novelist, the notion of death, as framed by an imagined medical gaze, became a figure for literary creation itself, and in particular for the fictional character. This aspect of Balzac's aesthetics is visible in one of his darkest novels, *La cousine Bette* (Cousin Bette), even though the text is ostensibly more concerned with the effects of prostitution and male sexual desire on bourgeois family structures.[78]

The novel follows the travails of the Hulot family as they attempt to manage the disorders, financial and moral, that their father's increasingly destructive sexual drives introduce among them. The narrative, as has been observed by other critics, returns regularly to the idea of an original mud from which its characters once emerged and to which they seem destined ultimately to return. The mother, the Baroness Adeline, personifies the first half of this trajectory, beginning her life as a simple peasant whose beauty caught the eye of the aspiring Hector Hulot, a dashing young figure who was laying the foundations of a brilliant career in the administration of the Napoleonic armies. "For the young peasant girl, this marriage was something like an Assumption," Balzac wrote. "The lovely Adeline passed without transition from her village mud [*boues*] to the paradise of the Imperial Court."[79] The Baron, on the other hand, figures the second, downward half of the trajectory, for as the novel follows his compulsive sexual appetites, it moves through meanders and resistances toward his final, inexorable humiliation, in which he sacrifices the noble love of his wife to marry the household scullion, a girl so repulsive that even the other servants disdain her. As wretched as its consequences may be for the social standing of the Baron and his family, the very force of his longing and his reckless self-immolation seem to have inspired a certain admiration in the narrator, who describes Hulot as a "superior man" and remarks on the "power that depravity gives."[80] And no matter how depraved the Baron's urges may be or how great the despair they inspire in those around him, they are what propels the action of the novel. In the sheer fact of writing *La cousine Bette*, Balzac acknowledged and appropriated the artistic value of this drive toward abjection.

Before descending to the scullion, whom he will make his second wife and baroness, Hulot passes through a series of mistresses and courtesans, including the singer Josépha Mirah, Valérie Marneffe, and a young girl, named Atala, whom he purchases from her parents for the sum of fifteen hundred francs. The child's beauty elicits a certain empathy even in Hulot's long-suffering wife: "The Baroness heaved a deep sigh when she saw this masterpiece of femininity sunk in the mire [*boue*] of prostitution, and she vowed to lead the girl back to Virtue."[81] The narrator's choice of words, which seem to paraphrase, in *discours indirect libre*, the feelings of Madame Hulot herself, make explicit the connection between two key themes in the novel. Prostitution was another metamorphosis of mud, that form of material abjection that returns constantly throughout the narrative as the counterpart to virtue, family, and social order. Of the prostitutes who ensnare the Hulots' *pater familias*, it is Valérie Marneffe who receives the most attention from the author and the one who functions most clearly as the antithesis to the maternal and disinterested Baroness. The rapacious mistress of three men—the Baron, his son-in-law, and his rival—Valérie is also the confident of the Baroness's cousin, Bette, and the abyss into which the family's wealth is thrown. In these multiple roles, she enjoyed a greater control over the Hulots' fortunes than her legitimate counterpart, and the force of Valérie's sexual attractiveness seems to have extended even to her own creator, over whom she exercised a certain fascination. In 1858, some twelve years after the initial publication of *La cousine Bette*, Hippolyte Taine would comment on this, writing: "Balzac is in love with his Valérie, which is why he justifies her and makes her bigger. He strives not to make her odious, but intelligible. He gives her a courtesan's education."[82] For Taine, Balzac's affection for his character was at once part of her intelligibility and somehow related to a potential odiousness.

If Valérie was not, as the critic observed, exactly hateful, she was explicitly revolting, at least in certain, crucial passages of the novel. On the one hand, she embodied a force of death—at least to one member of the Hulot family— for when Bette suggests to the Baron's daughter that her husband try to borrow money from her father's mistress, the daughter reacts with a very specific kind of fear: "Hortense gazed at [her husband] Wenceslas with the look of a condemned man climbing to the scaffold."[83] To Hortense, Valérie feels like death. This theme will be revisited and developed in the last pages of the novel, where, as the kind of fear inspired by Valérie Marneffe changes, a subtle but significant shift occurs in her relation to the idea of mortality. "Oh, Lisbeth, I sense that there is another life!" Valérie exclaims, "and I am so overwhelmed by terror that I cannot even feel the pain of my decomposing flesh! . . . To die at the very moment that I wanted to live as an honest woman, and to die an object of horror . . ."[84] Like the guillotine with which Hortense's imagination had earlier assimilated her, the courtesan originally inspired terror in those around her, but now, on her deathbed, she has become instead an object of horror. Terror, in this passage, functions as an analgesic force that dulls the pain of one's own decomposing flesh and distracts one from the revulsion it inspires. For Valérie's final days are spectacles of disgust. Even before she finally succumbs, she has been reduced to "a putrefying mass, that of the five senses retained only the power of sight."[85] Though she is still sentient and responsive to those around her, the exotic disease with which a jealous lover has infected her has left her "in a state of decomposition."[86] In its final hours, her body, which had previously functioned as a figure of the prostitute's destructive control over the social order, reveals another aspect of its powers, for it is the corpse, the living dead that now speaks through Valérie Marneffe: "Listen!" she says, "I've only a day or two left to think, for I can't say *live*. You see? I haven't got a body anymore, I'm a heap of mud [*boue*] . . . They won't let me look at myself in the mirror . . ."[87] Her deliquescent end is the representation of another form of self-consciousness, one that flows between the living and the dead, a flowing made possible by the mediation of putrefaction. And in her last hours, mud reveals another of its meanings within the novel: it is a term for an abject life in death, a force of inanimate will from which the living recoil.

Even for Balzac's contemporaries, like Hippolyte Taine, the intelligibility of Valérie Marneffe's gruesome death seems to have involved something beyond the retribution that the disfigurement of sexually active women represented for other authors, such as Laclos or Zola, since Balzac, according to Taine, felt an attachment to his character, an affection that prevented him from reducing her to an object lesson in moral odium.[88] Even her putrefying but animate body seems to have figured something else for him, something more powerful and, indeed, creative, an artistic force that only becomes apparent by teasing out the connections among a network of different figures and themes throughout the novel. Among these, two in particular need to be retained. First, Valérie Marneffe's death-bed scenes fall under the supervision of a group of medical specialists, such that this portion of the narrative is represented only through their mediation and, as it were, on their terms. The descriptions of her condition are framed by diagnostic terminology, while contact between the dying woman and those around her is carefully controlled by the doctor Bianchon—indeed, the very news of her illness is revealed only as an illustration of his medical vision of human society.[89] This use of a different, scientific kind of discourse is, however, more than a narrative device, for it is connected, through the person of the doctor, to Balzac's understanding of his own relation to his novel. In his dedication, the author described himself as a "simple doctor of social medicine, the veterinarian of incurable diseases" and compared his work to that of the naturalist Georges Buffon.[90] If Balzac saw himself as physician and pathologist, the doctors and their patients who people his novel must, conversely, represent the author, and this connection operates throughout the narrative. The deathbed scenes, which mobilize a medical personnel to construct the narrative, thus function as allegories for the relation between the author's work and his society. Valérie Marneffe does not, in other words, just die, she also reveals, in dying, something about the nature of literary creation. Second, the prostitute, as Balzac twice describes her, is a work of art: Valérie "is as fascinating as a masterpiece," while later, on seeing Atala, the Baroness "heaved a deep sigh when she saw this masterpiece of femininity sunk in the mire of prostitution."[91] Not only is the young girl a *chef-d'œuvre* but her unusual name also affiliates her with another literary character, the eponymous heroine in a wildly popular novel by Chateaubriand, and she appears, consequently, to function as a copy of a literary invention, a figure for fictional characters as such.

As off-hand as it might seem, this use of the metaphor "masterpiece" forms part of an ongoing meditation that structures the novel as a reflection on aesthetic creation. One of its central figures, the count Wenceslas Steinbock, is a sculptor, whose failures lead the author to a sustained commentary on the artistic process, "which is perhaps," writes Balzac, "explained here for the first time."[92] In a lengthy excursus on creative genius, the novelist distinguishes between two aspects necessary to the realization of an artwork. First comes the period of conception, which is marked by reverie and pleasure. This is followed by a darker, more taxing stage, that of execution, in which "the hand must be so painstakingly trained, so ready and obedient, that the sculptor can struggle soul to soul with that elusive spiritual nature he must materialize and, thereby, transfigure."[93] This is the stage that contemporaries seemed most to identify with Balzac himself.[94] It is also the stage that the young count neglects, and this repellent but necessary process of materialization is represented, at two points in the same passage, by the *glaise* or clay which a sculptor must manipulate if he is to give tangible form to his inner visions.[95] *Glaise* is a form of mud, and as such picks up on the theme of material abjection that runs through the novel, but it is also orthographically close to *glaire*, which is the mucous produced by certain membranes, and in medical terminology refers especially to that secreted by the cervix at the time of ovulation. Through a slight orthographic slippage, the mud of artistic "execution" would thus be cognate to the bodily excretions of women at the height of their reproductive cycle, a connection reinforced by the extended analogy Balzac draws between the sufferings of the artist and the travails of mothers.[96] This false cognate works only on the illegitimate level of a physical resemblance between the two, etymologically unrelated words, but the passage as a whole points to the importance of just such a material (rather than conceptual) level in art and, therefore, to the legitimacy of such a connection. The *boue* or mud of prostitution, the unspoken intimacy of the *fille*'s bodily organs, and the final decomposition of that body into a putrescent but thinking "heap of mud" can all be seen, within the logic that binds *boue* to *glaise*, as figures for the artistic process itself.

The grotesquely diseased bodies in this novel are, therefore, images of invention. As a novelistic character embedded in its own facticity and materiality, the person of Valérie Marneffe is a figure, in this respect, of the creative project itself. But since she exists in writing rather than sculpture, what she figures is not, however, caught in the materiality of *glaise*, but in the imaginary itself, in the breakdown of meaning that is represented in the fantasies of disease, disfiguration, and death themselves. If, at the end of the novel, Balzac writes that the scullion Agathe—the future second wife of Baron Hulot—is "foul in her language [*grossière dans son langage*]" that statement can be understood on a literal level as part of a larger self-reflection within the novel: her repulsiveness is a consequence of her way of being *in* language, of her status as a linguistic artifact. For her part, Valérie Marneffe, especially as she appears on her deathbed, functions as an allegory of novelistic creation as such, for the seemingly human creature that exists only in words—for that semblance of thinking that speciously, illegitimately informs the unliving characters of fiction. Her productive, putrefying body is an allegory for fictional personification, for the novelistic character as such, and the lesson of her death is that all characters are Valérie Marneffe, that they all live an allegorical death, trapped in the deceptive lifelessness of words. While Redon saw a vague sentience in the materiality of artistic creation, Balzac described a more elaborated form of this same consciousness: the fictional character who, although only apparently alive and only a product of objectified imagination, exhibits the semblance of an autonomous and identifiable subjectivity. In Balzac, this discovery was part of a meditation on the relation between literary creation and medical procedure. For Flaubert, on the other hand, the necrophilic material facticity of the novel, the assimilation between corpse and character, became the basis for a larger reflection on the process of historical memory.

Flaubert

According to the standard accounts, a reform movement swept across France in 1847, and its participants sought to raise public support for their program through a series of peaceful banquets. These were to include a gathering in Paris on February 22, 1848, which the government abruptly cancelled on the night before it was to occur. In response to the authorities' sudden obstructionism, insurgents quickly put up barricades throughout the working-class sections of Paris. The National Guard, who had been called out to suppress the disturbances, instead sided with the revolt. To prevent the situation from further degenerating, the king promised electoral reforms and removed François Guizot, his unpopular prime minister, from office. In response to these appeasements, the populace broke out into jubilation, and on the night of February 23 people took to the streets in a tumult, calling for occupants to light up their buildings in solidarity.[97] As onlookers emerged from their homes to enjoy the "spectacle" of Paris in celebration, part of the crowd forced its way into the boulevard des Capucines, apparently with the intention of demanding "illuminations" from the home of Guizot himself.[98] While the detachment of guards stationed outside the former prime minister's lodgings prepared for a confrontation, its commanding officer came forward to negotiate with the protestors. But as he attempted to defuse tensions, an anonymous shot was fired, and the guards responded by emptying their rifles on the crowd, killing sixteen people on the spot.[99] Though dead, these initial victims did not, however, abandon their revolutionary activities—in fact, it was at this point that they became most effective.[100] Once the crowd had overcome its initial panic and returned to find the street littered with corpses, they loaded the bodies into a nearby cart and brought them to the offices of the newspaper *Le National,* which described the events in its issue of the following day.[101] Garnier-Pagès, the editor, appeared at one of the newspaper's windows to harangue the crowd. The wagon then left to spread word of the "massacre" throughout the *faubourgs,* ending up at the town hall of the fourth arrondissement, where the bodies were unloaded into the central courtyard. By most accounts, it was this gruesome parade that enraged the population and catalyzed the insurgency. The king abdicated the next day, February 24, and fled to England. Under the leadership of the poet Alphonse de Lamartine, a short-lived Republic was proclaimed in the Chamber of Deputies.

The revolution of February 1848 not only set different classes and ideologies into conflict; it also threw history into opposition with literature as a means for making sense of collective human events. Contemporary observers evidenced this tension when they repeatedly disparaged the uprising's significance by comparing it to various theatrical genres. For Marx, in an often-quoted snipe, the revolution represented the degeneration of "world history" into "farce."[102] To Alexis de Tocqueville, it seemed that the protagonists were simply staging passages from *Les Girondins,* Lamartine's volume on the Revolution of 1789.[103] Maxime Du Camp wrote that he could never recall "the proclamation of the events of February 24 without thinking of an old stage farce" that he had seen as a child.[104] Literature, it would seem from this testimony, intervenes in and undermines history, reducing it to something less important, less seemly, and less adult. Flaubert's novel *L'éducation sentimentale* (Sentimental Education) and his letters from the time of the 1848 revolution show that he viewed the relation of history to literature in similar terms, but unlike his contemporaries, this relation did not discredit literature for him. Instead, he thought, the aesthetic use of language could embody a nontranscendental and meaningless but creative and emotionally charged force that the historical enterprise sought to forget and repress. He argued, obliquely but persistently, that literature underlies historiography by representing a pre-erotically charged abjection that history attempts, always unsuccessfully, to control and falsify.

The criticism that contemporaries leveled against the events of 1848 was, as I have said, harsh: the uprising was useless, meaningless, vulgar, farcical, ahistorical, and simply aesthetic. Observing that "men make their own history, but they do not make it just as they please," Marx dismissed the insurrection as a necrophilic foray into the past and argued that "to arrive at its own content, the revolution of the nineteenth century must let the dead bury the dead."[105] History, in other words, was a futural process that could only occur when the living disengaged themselves from the corpse-like remainders of the past. For his own part, Flaubert used a similar imaginary of the dead to understand the revolution. But that understanding evolved slowly, and to start with, he could scarcely contain his sheer contempt on witnessing one of the political meetings that prepared the way for the February events. He described the gathering in a letter to Louise Colet dating from the end of December 1847. "I've recently seen something beautiful, however," he wrote, "and I'm still weighed down by the impression at once grotesque and lamentable that the show [*spectacle*] has left me with.—I went to a reformist banquet! What elegance! What food! What wines! And what speeches! Nothing has so absolutely disgusted me with the idea of success than contemplating the price you have to pay for it. I sat there as cold waves of nausea passed over me."[106] Whereas other critics of the 1848 Revolution had maintained that its crucial failure derived from its aestheticism and empty artistry, for Flaubert the problem was instead the quality of that artistry. Indeed, for him, a bad performance robbed the goals themselves of meaning—history was not defined by the loftiness of its aspirations but rather by the aesthetic effectiveness of its enactment. For him, the historical was not a semantic category, but rather an aesthetic one.

Flaubert incorporated some of the events of February 1848 into his novel *L'éducation sentimentale*, structuring key passages around them.[107] The work as a whole chronicles the life of Frédéric Moreau from his arrival in Paris as a young man from a comfortable provincial family, through his aspirations and disappointments as an aspiring writer and lover, to his disillusioned return to the provinces many years later. Although they play out at the fringes of the main narrative, the evening of the cancelled reformist banquet and the subsequent insurrection in Paris mark a turning point in the action of the novel. Madame Arnoux, the inaccessible object of Frédéric's erotic longings throughout the book, has finally agreed to meet with him alone, and he has lavished money and minute attentions on preparing an apartment for what he hopes will evolve into a tryst. But she does not keep the appointment, and as Frédéric waits for her with growing despair, revolution breaks out in the adjoining streets and a female acquaintance, the Maréchale, appears. While the bodies of the massacred are piled into the cart, he leads this other woman into the apartment he has secretly rented, and as the cadavers of the fallen make their way across Paris, he finally consummates his sexual desires. "What's the matter, dearest?" the Maréchale asks him afterwards, surprised to find him crying. "I'm just too happy," he replies. "I've been wanting you for too long."[108] After months of longing, after carefully preparing the apartment and the moment, after hours spent waiting in the street, fantasy has finally been realized in the flesh of a woman.

Flaubert makes only a passing mention of the tumbrel and reduces its load from the generally reported sixteen bodies to five, but they are marked into the novel: "The previous evening," he notes on the following page, "the sight of a cart containing five of the corpses collected from the boulevard des Capucines had altered the mood of the people."[109] In the personal narrative that is mapped onto a collective one in *L'éducation sentimentale*, a sex scene covers over a heap of corpses. In confrontations with human bodies, the dispositions of both the people and Frédéric Moreau change. They set up barricades in the streets, and he weeps into his pillow. An intertext moves offstage behind these pages as the lumbering wagon leaves its visible trace in an erotic encounter. The spectacle of the corpses is thus conceived in displaced erotic terms—displaced, but not in the habitual direction, for it is not a sexual story that is being dissimulated. Instead, like an inverted neurotic symptom, a sexual act hides another narrative, and we might argue that Frédéric Moreau's encounter translates something else into erotic language.

To understand what those hidden corpses would have meant for Flaubert, it will be important to examine the texts he wrote around the events of February 1848—and by this I mean both those texts, such as the *Education sentimentale*, that discuss the insurrection and those, such as his letters, that were written at approximately the same time that it occurred. It is easiest to begin with the novel and in particular with an examination of the circumstances surrounding the erotic scene that covers over the historical narrative. Most notably, Frédéric Moreau has slept with the wrong woman. While it is Rosanette, nicknamed the Maréchale, that he has ended up seducing, his preparations were all intended for another, Madame Arnoux, who did not show up the day before and who left him, along with his carefully arranged apartment, waiting without an explanation. It is by the force of circumstances—the gunfire on the boulevard des Capucines, whose terrifying sound has left Rosanette incapable of walking, the impossibility of finding a cab in the midst of the uprising, the proximity of the apartment—and "as a refinement of hatred, in order to degrade Madame Arnoux more completely in his mind," that Frédéric Moreau leads his improvised partner to his bed.[110] The night spent with her is the displaced enactment of other intentions, of the imagined and

carefully planned seduction of Madame Arnoux that never occurred. Rosanette's body is a substitute for the desired, but only fantasmatically possessed,
body of another.

That fantasmatic other had, however, her own story, which further complicates Flaubert's version of the insurrection. The Madame Arnoux that Frédéric Moreau was supposed to meet on February 22 did not show up for her
appointment because she was concerned with the health of her feverish child,
who appeared to be dying. As Frédéric waited for her in the street, catching
glimpses of the reformist demonstration at the Madeleine that would lead,
eventually, from the fusillade on the boulevard des Capucines to the downfall
of the government and the monarchy, she was preoccupied with her son's
worsening condition. And here, Flaubert's medical attention to the bodily
details of an illness produces several curious details. The boy is having trouble breathing and he is periodically wracked by fits of coughing. When he
speaks, his words themselves are not recorded, because what is most significant about them is their sound and the physical labor that it indicates: "Convulsive movements shook his chest-muscles, and as he breathed in and out
his stomach contracted as if he were choking for breath after a race. . . . He
seemed to be puffing out his words." It is the threatening physicality of his
speech that is of importance here, the way it chokes him. "The child started
pulling away the bandages round his neck, as if he were trying to remove the
obstruction which was choking him."[111] The prolonged fit comes to an end,
and the child is declared "saved" by the doctor when at last he spits up the
blockage that was strangling him: "finally he vomited something strange that
looked like a tube of parchment. What could it be? She supposed that he had
thrown up a piece of his bowels."[112] Even the novel itself remarks on the
strangeness of this detail that seems to be part of an inner organ. While
history miscarries in the streets outside and Frédéric Moreau paces in front
of his carefully prepared apartment, the narrative dwells on this inexplicable
and foreign body whose expulsion restores a child to life. It is like parchment,
something to write on, the material support of language. The strange, the
meaningless, the physical, the unutterable excess that threatens to bring
speech to a halt is spat out and the boy's life is saved. The trauma of these
events, which take place as she was supposed to have been meeting with Frédéric, cures Madame Arnoux of her willingness to pursue an illicit sexuality,
and their two paths separate. She will stay with her child and sacrifice her

"first passion" for his sake, while her would-be lover will pursue her spectral ideal in the alienated body of another woman.

Three stories thus overlap and interact in this telling of the February insurrection: Frédéric's attempt to seduce Madame Arnoux and his subsequent tryst with the Maréchale; Madame Arnoux's alarmed reaction to her child's sudden sickness; and the fusillade in the boulevard des Capucines all coincide and interfere with each other. The first two are of Flaubert's invention, and he develops them at length, while the third derives from other, collective sources and appears only in the background or through quick references. These incidents all bear the faint traces of yet another narrative, recounted in Flaubert's correspondence from around the time of the Revolution, and it is in those intimate texts that their historical significance becomes most apparent, although in a curious and convoluted way. For the most part, the letters that survive from this period are addressed to Flaubert's former lover, Louise Colet, with whom he had recently broken. The interest he felt toward her now, he repeatedly stressed, concerned what he called "the artist" in her and led him to inquire frequently about the progress of the play, *Madeleine*, which she was currently writing, and to reflect resignedly on his own inability to write. "If my taste increases," he observed, "it only makes it all the more difficult for me to write. Sentences no longer flow, I have to tear them out and they hurt as they leave me."[113] For her part, neither the attachment Colet still felt for Flaubert nor the reproaches she directed at him for his indifference to her prevented her from discussing her marriage to Hippolyte Colet. Her husband inspired two bitter, but ostensibly altruistic remarks on Flaubert's part. In October 1847, he asked, "is the 'official one' constantly on your back and always polluting your life with his presence? There's no worse torture imaginable than to have to endure living with people you don't love."[114] Later in the month he returned to the same theme, now couching the situation in ontological terms borrowed from the philosopher Victor Cousin, another of Colet's lovers. "I'm so sorry the 'official one' is coming back!" he exclaimed. "After the dreariness of not living with the people you love, the only thing worse is to live with those you don't love. Be patient and detach yourself from the *contingent*, as the philosopher would say."[115] The situation that Flaubert describes between Colet and "l'officiel" would be echoed some twenty years later in *L'éducation sentimentale*, where the protagonist, Frédéric Moreau, finds himself caught, in quick succession, by succinct versions of Flaubert's two greatest *ennuis* or forms of suffering. On February 22, 1848, Frédéric is stood up by the woman he loves and the apartment he has rented to share with her must go unoccupied. On the following day, he leads a woman he does not love to the same apartment, where she can interpret all of its amorous appointments as having been intended for her. To put the tryst in the metaphysical terms that Flaubert himself borrowed from Cousin, Rosanette, the unintended lover, is an accident—an ontological condition that metaphysics since Aristotle has categorically distinguished from the essential and ideal. Read through Flaubert's correspondence, the unwanted lover figures the nonideal, which is to say the category of figures themselves as opposed to the unchanging but invisible essences that they represent. She not only exists in the realm of the plastic, she also signifies it, and in this respect she plays an allegorical role in relation to Flaubert's aesthetics.

The relation between the plastic and the ideal was further developed in Flaubert's letters from the months preceding the February uprising. On September 17, 1847, as he leafed through a work by Théophile Thoré sent to him by Louise Colet, the passages he read filled him with contemptuous pity. "What blabber!" he exploded. "How happy I count myself to live far away from fellows like him! What pseudoscience! What pretentious emptiness! I'm tired of everything that gets said about art, about beauty, about the idea, about Form. It's always the same refrain and what a refrain it is!"[116] Thoré, whom Flaubert does not quote, expounded a theory of sublimation through art in which the imaginable is idealized. A passage from the book Flaubert held in his hands exemplifies his approach: "The more an artist transforms external reality, the more he puts himself into his work, the higher he has raised the image toward that ideal each man carries within his heart—then the farther he has advanced into the world of poetry."[117] Art, according to Thoré, translates the objective world into an idealized subjectivity, and poetry raises the accidental—the plastic image—toward the essential. The work of art is, in this sense, an ongoing negation of the contingent. Instead of theorizations like these, Flaubert informed Colet, he spent his mornings reading Aristophanes. "It's not decent," he conceded, "it's not moral, it's not even acceptable, it's just simply sublime."[118] There follow some standard images of sublimity that could have been copied from Kant, Caspar David Friedrich, or innumerable other sources—the vast sea, threatening abysses, the world viewed from a great height—but this brief catalogue of received ideas should not distract from the originality of Flaubert's other conception of the sublime. The sublime that he evokes in reference to Aristophanes is, in his own words, inappropriate, indecent, and a- or immoral. "The Muse," he may assert, "is a virgin with a bronze maidenhead, and you've got to be a rake to . . . ," but, despite her virginity, the art that Flaubert pursues is obscene, and for all its sublimity it is not ideal.[119] Or, as Maxime Du Camp put it in a letter to Louise Colet: "above all, you know, Gustave is Mr. Plastic [*l'homme de la Plastique*]."[120]

Still, the art that Flaubert is struggling with at this time is not merely plastic, it is physical: as his sense of taste increases, he reflects, "it only makes it all the more difficult for me to write. Sentences no longer flow, I have to tear them out and they hurt as they leave me."[121] Similar to the tube of parchment-like substance that Madame Arnoux's son coughs up in agony, writing inflicts pain on the author as it emerges from him. The parchment, as an allegory of the nonallegorical in writing, of those elements that bear no meaning in themselves but support a semantic system, allegorizes as well the pain of an artistic creation whose ideal is, paradoxically, the nonideal. Rosanette, in her accidental superfluity, is the figure of this art. She is also, we should not forget, a displacement of the corpses that moved through the streets of Paris as she and Frédéric made love.

The texts around 1848 establish another opposition involving art and sexuality, for the metal genitals of art and the "impotence" of the artist contrast with Madame Arnoux's maternal fertility. The latter forgoes her illicit assignation with Frédéric to care for her desperately ill child, and when, after an anguished night spent at the border of death, he spits up the strange obstacle that had been choking him, not only is he cured of his illness, but his mother is cured of her nascent desire for her would-be lover. At the close of the sickbed scene between Madame Arnoux and her son, the vocabulary of salvation slips between the medical and the spiritual, identifying the son's physical recovery with the mother's redemption through the use of the single word *sauvé* or saved:

> Monsieur Colot arrived. According to him, the child was out of danger [*sauvé*]. . . .
> "He's out of danger [*sauvé*]! Can it be true?"
> Suddenly the thought of Frédéric entered her mind, clearly and inexorably. This was a warning from Heaven. But the Lord in his mercy had not wished to punish her completely. What dreadful punishment she would suffer later on if she persisted in this love of hers! . . . Jumping to her feet, she flung herself on the little chair; and, sending up her soul with all her strength, she offered God, as a sacrifice, her first passion, her only weakness.
> Frédéric had gone home. He sat in his armchair, without even the strength to curse her.[122]

The doctor's name, Colot, is as surprising as the tube of parchment whose ejection precipitates Madame Arnoux's renunciation of a nonprocreative sexuality, since it is separated by a single letter from Louise Colet's. Intentionally or not, it serves as an oblique reminder that in February 1848, Madame Arnoux was not the only woman from Flaubert's circle who was concerned with her own maternity.[123] In early March of the same year, Flaubert wrote to Colet in response to a letter that had apparently been sent almost directly after the brief revolution in Paris, since he makes reference in it to the disruptions the upheaval had caused in the postal service and expresses his opinions on the new government. Very quickly, however, the tone turns more personal: "And why all of your hedging before telling me the *news*?" he asks. "You could have said it right away without all the circumlocutions."[124] The news was that she had become pregnant by another man. The events in the novel and in the letters occur at almost the same time, echoing and varying each other: while Madame Arnoux sacrifices her illicit desire to her maternity, Frédéric Moreau plays through a simulacrum of the erotic encounter they were supposed to have enjoyed, and while Louise Colet brings a child to life, Gustave Flaubert struggles with the obscene ideal of art and its bronze virginity. As an object of art, Frédéric Moreau will prove, however, to be more interesting to Flaubert than Madame Arnoux, since he makes of him, not her, the protagonist of his novel. Art, it would seem, is written out of the failure of procreation.

Two other pregnancies run through the letters from this period, and the first reinforces the opposition between art and maternity. It concerns the actress Rachel, whom Flaubert has recommended for the lead in Colet's new play, *Madeleine*. In October 1847, he wrote to Colet to commiserate with her about the obstacles that the actress's condition would create: "I'm pretty upset for you about Rachel's pregnancy. What have you decided to do? If you want my advice, you should wait until she's popped the kid out before you give her yours.—I can't really think of a play with her in it that folded. If your work is a triumph without her, it'll just be even more successful with her."[125] Conflicting demands are made on the actress's person by two forms of creation, her child and her art, each of which occurs only during the suspension of the other. Even if Flaubert couches his references to Colet's play in familial terms, here as an infant and later as a daughter at her wedding, the family and the aesthetic remain incompatible.[126] Indeed, the familial terms produce an image of artistic creation as a simulacrum of biological procreation, in which the author performs a virginal and impotent copy of sexual intercourse. Once again, put in allegorical terms, art is more like Frédéric Moreau and Rosanette than it is like Madame Arnoux and her son.

The other pregnancy is far more complicated, and involves the wife of a childhood companion of Flaubert, Alfred Le Poittevin. On April 28, 1847, Flaubert announced to a mutual friend that Madame Le Poittevin would be giving birth in a few weeks. On August 10 of the same year, Flaubert informed Colet that Le Poittevin himself was dying. His demise would take months, and its approach is recorded intermittently in Flaubert's letters.[127] The overall narrative is brief and cruel: only three months after his wife gives birth, the husband is diagnosed with a terminal illness. She creates life, while he moves toward death, and on April 3, 1848, he succumbs.

Flaubert had traveled from his home in Croisset to be present at the death and funeral. "Alfred died Monday evening at midnight," he wrote to Maxime Du Camp. "I buried him yesterday and came back. I kept watch over him for two nights (all of the second), and I wrapped him up in his sheet, I gave him a farewell kiss, and I saw his coffin soldered shut. I spent two days there [. . .] two long days."[128] In the letter he describes in detail certain events from those two long days, especially the vigil of the last night and the wrapping of the corpse. "When day came, at four o'clock," he wrote, "the attendant and I got to work. I lifted him up, turned him over, and wrapped him. The feeling of his cold, stiff limbs stayed on the tips of my fingers all day long. He was horribly putrefied, it went through the sheets [*les draps étaient traversés*].—We put two shrouds on him."[129] The isolation in Flaubert's account is particularly striking, and he recounts the events of his two days as if, except for the attendant and a couple of other guests at the funeral, he had been alone with the corpse. There is, most remarkably, no reference to the wife, as if she had nothing to do with the dead man and as if the labor of caring for and burying the dead had fallen to Flaubert alone: *he* buried him, watched over him, wrapped him in his shroud, kissed him farewell, and stood by as he was sealed in his coffin, all in the first person singular. If the child was her business, the corpse was his.

When Maxime Du Camp wrote his *Souvenirs littéraires* for the year 1848, he devoted several pages to Le Poittevin's death in a chapter titled "En révolution [*In Revolt*]," including a slightly edited version of the long letter Flaubert had written him to describe their friend's burial. Although Du Camp's transcription is largely unaltered, it does contain one significant—and unmarked—elision: the words "it went through the sheets," which in the original letter follow Flaubert's remark that Le Poittevin's body "was horribly putrefied."[130] The leakage from the corpse that Flaubert had remarked is wiped clean in Du Camp's version: what had oozed out from the body and marked the sheets is erased, and then the erasure itself is erased, since there is nothing in Du Camp's text to indicate the omission. The seeping of the cadaver, the signs that it leaves on the blank sheet, are apparently inadmissible, even in a text that acknowledges that the body was "horribly putrefied," and Le Poittevin's corpse is censored in a quick act of literary hygiene. But the elided detail recalls another moment in Flaubert's correspondence that argues for its significance. In a letter to Louise Colet on April 13, 1847, he had written: "recently you did all you could to hide your pain from me, but it showed through all the same. Like the form of a dead body under its white sheet, no matter how clean it is, how perfumed."[131] Even before he had encountered it in the flesh, the scene of Le Poittevin's corpse was present as a metaphor in Flaubert's imagination, where it spoke of pain in a mute language that was able to cross the sheets, washings, and perfumes that were intended to disguise it. Just as surely as one will try to clean the corpse away, the image contends, it will resist. The oozing cadaver thus becomes the figure for something that cannot be successfully repressed, and in its seepage it speaks an obscene, insistent language that hygiene unsuccessfully combats.

The meaning of the corpse is unstated and unclear, but Flaubert makes a gesture toward explaining it in the strange last words of his letter to Du Camp: "Farewell, my poor dear old fellow," he wrote after his lengthy description of the two days spent with their friend's cadaver. "A thousand tender thoughts. I send you a kiss and I want to see you in the worst way, for I need to tell you incomprehensible things [*dire des choses incompréhensibles*]."[132] For Flaubert, the two days ended with the pressing need to tell things that cannot be written, that make no sense, and that can only be spoken in an other's presence. It is an odd language that he evokes here, an idiom of powerful emotions without meanings, whose foreignness is so profound that it cannot be comprehended or translated into signification, a tongue that will always be strange. It is also a language of desire, the language that Flaubert wants and needs, as he puts it, since it is not the message that he longs for (there is none), but the words themselves. Word things: *dire des choses*. If they were writing, they would stain the sheets of paper in undecipherable shapes that only looked like signs. Is it really Le Poittevin's corpse that inspires this longing? That can never be said for sure, but what *is* sure is that for Flaubert what inspires his desire can *only* be said and never understood. It is *not* a hidden meaning but a type of language without signification. It is something that adds no meaning to a communication and whose omission will not interrupt its intelligibility, indeed will improve it. It is something that can be edited out without sacrifice of meaning and that, for this reason, would be in excess if it remained. It is a leftover, like the words, "it went through the sheets." Nobody among these pages, whether writer or readers, it seems likely, knows what the corpse is saying, only that it is saying something and that this is the language Flaubert longs for.

There is one final observation to make about Le Poittevin. In Du Camp's opinion, the young man would have become a historian. "The cast of his mind, which was inclined toward speculative deductions, would doubtless have drawn him for some time to metaphysics, which he enjoyed . . . ; but he had a sense of precision and a need for clarity that would have led him to historical criticism, at which he would have excelled."[133] While living, his clarity, precision, and critical sense would have led him to write history. Dead, he speaks another, very different language. A language utterly foreign to history. A language that goes on speaking after the clarity, precision, and critical acumen of history die.

The author's version of February 1848 is structured around a missed rendezvous that marks the divergence between two narratives, one involving motherhood and salvation, the other sexual expediency and frustration. These two narratives also encapsulate conflicts that emerge in Flaubert's correspondence from the period during and around the 1848 insurrection: the plastic and meaningless in opposition to the ideal and conceptual, the nonsemantic in opposition to the semantic, Le Poittevin's dead body in opposition to his wife's childbearing body. I would like to argue that the personal experiences recorded in Flaubert's correspondence inflected his memory and perception of 1848 and that this series of oppositions can be understood as the intellectual apparatus through which he constructed, many years later, his interpretation of the February uprising in *L'éducation sentimentale*. Art, in the form of the novel itself, is juxtaposed with a (necessarily) absent other to which it repeatedly refers. That other would be the events of 1848 as they entered the historical record, beginning with Tocqueville, Lamartine, Garnier-Pagès, and Marx and following through to writers such as Crémieux, Seignobos, and Bernstein. In this sense, with his novel, Flaubert entered into a contemporary discussion about the historical significance of 1848, arguing, against all the others, that literature is the best way to represent the pre-erotic, affectively charged plasticity that both resists and underlies historiography. If, as Marx contended, the revolution was not historical, that was, by Flaubert's reading, because it concerned something more fundamental and important, something whose force could only be brought out through the sterile and unintelligible emotions of art.

With its metaphorical richness and historical significance, the corpse plays a role in making this argument. According to Flaubert's letters, it pokes through the sheets that would disguise it, seeping through the shrouds and pretty allegories that, like Rosanette, would cover but cannot contain it. It disfigures the intelligible figure with the substance of figuration, a substance that chokes off words like a tube of indigestible and meaningless parchment, the materiality of a communication that has become incomprehensible. The dead are thus the trope for figuration itself and for the aesthetic as the end of intelligibility. As the figurative, as the incomprehensibly plastic, they are an obscenity more indecent than sex. They are a dirtiness against which a program of conceptual hygiene will necessarily but unsuccessfully be deployed. They represent a nonprocreative creation, a world of artists and men, where friends bury friends in the absence of their childbearing wives, the image of a dark, indistinct, oozing language of desire. They represent art as the death of history. This, I have been proposing, is what Flaubert longed for in his letter to Du Camp. His longing, when taken in the larger context of his novel and letters, is an expression of the limits and the function of history. It is an argument that the putatively meaningful analysis of collective human time could be a sheet thrown over a horrible but fascinating abjection. But to conceptualize his longing in such propositional terms is, of course, to falsify what is most important in it: an unutterable desire for a humiliating remnant of the human.

The Written Dead

"Consider," wrote Louis-François de Borsbeek to denounce the closing of urban graveyards, "how cemeteries were pushed aside and hidden away from sight and memory."[134] But if corpses could be forgotten, it was because they represented memories. They were elements from the past, and as such had a special temporality, even a peculiar ontological status, for they neither were nor were not, but lingered, instead, between the two, in a state of no longer being, a persistence, in the present, of what is not but once was. Perhaps this is part of their uncanniness: they are not what they are; they are what is no longer, or the dead. They resemble what they were but now are not. They are, in this sense, reduced to remnants and signs. And tellingly, for Hegel, the symbol of the sign itself was a tomb.[135] For language indicates what is missing: the past writes or disappears, remaining, if at all, in marks that tremble between existence and nonexistence, in a state of protracted and determinate nonbeing. The relation between the dead and literary creation that Balzac and Flaubert allegorized and, in their own ways, analyzed, was based on this other, more primordial connection, which linked the dead and language itself. And this aspect of the dead was significant, in a strict sense, because it associated them with the processes not only of memory but also of meaning.

One does not have to look to such a powerful and original thinker as Hegel, however, to find a nineteenth-century awareness of language's curious ontological status. The former peer of France and *conseiller d'Etat*, Auguste-Hilarion Kératry voiced similar opinions in more common and impassioned terms. He argued that human beings, no matter how simple, inherently recognize the enduring power of language against mortality. "In vain will the death knell sound," he wrote, "we refuse to give up our hold on life. And to lend it some sort of perpetuity, we seek the aid of books, posthumous memoirs, medals, testaments, and even the tomb itself, which we burden with an epitaph."[136] Even the simple and barely literate farmhand betrays his conviction in the strange force of language, according to Kératry, when he scratches his name in the stone parapet of the local steeple. Words endure, perpetuating the absent and eternally lost, and even when we speak, we can scarcely keep ourselves from signifying, in the same gesture, both our death and our ability to exceed it, for Kératry observed that every individual constantly uses words that negate his finitude:

> That symbol of eternity, the word *forever*, will accompany his vows of faithfulness. If he writes a letter, that expression, laden with years, will flow from his pen; if he presses a beloved hand to his heart, it will pass from his lips. That other, opposite figure of eternity, the word *never*, will consecrate his thanks or arm his hatred. Never will he forget the services or indignities that he has received. Feeble creature that lasts but an instant, his frail organs will fall with the first breath of autumn, and yet he shrinks from thinking of it, and the language of the immortals is in his mouth![137]

Human beings frequent and internalize absolutes that infinitely exceed their capacities of experience. Kératry used these observations in an attempt to prove that all people have a sense of, and indeed a conviction in the immortality of their soul, but the arguments themselves undercut his conclusions. If concepts such as eternity demonstrate the ability of human beings to speak a language whose significance infinitely surpasses us, they also reveal, as a result, that we do not need to derive such concepts from extralinguistic sources. The knowledge of the soul's immortality cannot come from experience, since that experience is never finished, but rather from an *a priori* intuition—and yet that intuition is itself the negation of experience, the sign of what can never be experienced, the sublime, as Kant describes it in the *Critique of Judgment*. It is, in fact, curious that Kératry, who published a study on Kant's aesthetics of the sublime and beautiful, should not see the problems they represented for his own reasoning and at least attempt to address them, but he did not.[138] It is in signs that we exist as nonbeings, constantly uttering a language of immortality from whose perspective we are already consigned to the past and dead. In language, we mingle with the past and its former inhabitants, moving among their polymorphous remains, entering into an existence of nonbeing, the indications of something that infinitely escapes us. And what infinitely escapes us is not our immortality, for we have assumed that in our speaking if not in our experience. Instead, what we have lost is our finite, living self. We have become corpses of our own experience.

In a strange, oblique way, Kératry seems to have indicated that he was aware of this other, proleptically posthumous kind of existence, this corpse being that is opened to us in language. He was not a prolific author, but alongside his philosophical publications he did find time to write at least one novel, the four-volume *Les derniers des Beaumanoirs, ou la tour d'Helvin* (The Last of the Beaumanoirs, or the Tower of Helvin). The work was repeatedly cited in nineteenth-century studies on sexual deviance, because it centered on a scene of necrophilia with the dead body of a young virgin.[139] Along with his belief in the immortality of the soul, Kératry thus betrayed an interest in the persistence and activity of the corpse, its autonomy in relation to the person it once incarnated, and its ability to interfere—in peculiarly human ways—with the living. For the crime, as represented in the novel, is an outrage not merely against the morality of the perpetrator, but also against the deceased; and the latter, in turn, reveals an ability to perform uniquely human acts of sexual intimacy. In being deflowered, the corpse in Kératry's novel goes on to participate in behaviors that change the status of the person who no longer is, thereby revealing a strange connection to the nonexistence of the past. The corpse, somehow, is still in the past, but it is also left over from it, vulnerable and misplaced in the present. That Kératry himself did, or ever could have, articulated a parallel between his observations on the afterlife of language and that of the corpse is highly doubtful, but others among his contemporaries did make the connection.

Language was, from this perspective, not only a form of objectified memory and, as such, a connection to the past, it was also a charnel house of the dead. In few places does the imaginary of the corpse seem at once so florid and so integral to a massive and canonical intellectual enterprise, and while the confusion between language and death is probably one of the great conceptual characteristics of the nineteenth century, the role of the corpse in it is probably one of its strangest and least appreciated aspects. For the pamphleteer Jacques Fernand, cemeteries enclosed the "touching archives of our hearts."[140] Conversely, for Jules Michelet, archives were a sort of cemetery.[141] The preeminent historian in nineteenth-century France, Michelet was acutely aware of the strangeness of the past, its "mysterious" ontological status. To express this alienation, he regularly figured his work as an encounter not merely with the deceased, but with their earthly remains. The description of how he discovered his vocation is, for instance, marked both by an unusually affectionate necrophilia and by an attention to precise physical details of the dead. "What these mysteries concealed," he wrote, "I couldn't guess when I was a child. As a young man I sought it out with studiousness and good will, compassionate as I am towards all the dead. I met a lot of them, I studied their sarcophagi, I pulled aside their wrappings: I found their remains and the cold ashes from which their spirit had escaped."[142] Studying history was strangely material for him, and repositories of documents frequently took the form, in his imagination, of tombs. The encounter with the living past, the reanimation of its fugitive and living spirit seems, however, to have always escaped Michelet, despite his Herculean efforts and partial victories. Even when he describes his successes, the scenes are remarkable for their ghoulishness. The deceased do not return in them as they once were, but, rather, changed, marked by the deformities of death. "And as I breathed upon their ashes," he wrote, "I could see them rising up. They dragged from the tomb here a hand, there a head, like in Michelangelo's Last Judgment or the Dance of the Dead. They circled about me in a galvanic round, and that is what I have tried to capture in this book."[143] The dead, it had been found, could ape life, jerking and convulsing when electrical current was applied to their muscles. But this induced animation was the life of the dead, not of the living. And this, according to Michelet, was history. Elsewhere, he recognized still more clearly the darker aspect of this metaphorics, describing his historiographical method as a confrontation with the material horrors of death: "The broken-down gods and rotted kings appeared without their veils. Bland, conventional history, that shame-faced prude who once satisfied us, had disappeared. From the Médicis to Louis XIV a grim autopsy exposed this government of corpses."[144] History is autopsy, and the past a putrefying mess, normally guarded by reactions of shame. It is not the nakedness of their living humanity, their pettiness, passionate excesses, or pusillanimity that creates unease here, but rather their pastness itself, their deadness, written all over their bodies in the signs of decomposition. This is their mystery, their condition, their status, their form of being. And their pastness was legible, in this metahistorical figure, through the semiotics that Bouchut had systemized in his *Traité des signes de la mort*.[145] They rot. Their rotting is the expression of their ontological condition. It is history confronted in the nakedness of its paradoxical existence.

This rotting, this independent activity of the past in the present, is part of the imaginary of the corpse, and it is linked, for Michelet, to the notion of language. "To hear them tell it, said a certain gravedigger at a battlefield, not a single one of them was dead."[146] So goes a passage from the 1833 draft of the preface to his *Histoire de France*. The joke about the gravedigger relies on the relation between living and speaking, on the unstated propositions that one cannot speak without being alive and that the form and content of an argument would consequently be comically irrelevant for someone trying to demonstrate that he or she is not dead, since the sheer fact of being able to express an argument—any argument—would in itself be sufficient proof. But documents complicate this situation, since in them the dead do continue to talk. It is the separability of language from its referential context as well as its ability to exceed—indeed to exceed infinitely—the experience and imagination of its user, as Kératry observed, that allow it to persist as the negation of the life that spawned it. In this respect, Michelet's anecdote about the gravedigger is both a joke and the negation of the joke, for the dead in it demonstrate, through their eloquent materiality, that the presuppositions that would make one laugh are false: the dead do talk. Language, as Maurice Blanchot would later argue, is a thing, physical, sensuous, and subject to material laws.[147] It signifies life without being alive, pursuing, in this way, an experience of death. Blanchot argued that the object of language, the ever vanishing point of its longing, was the corpse, the corpse in its foul-smelling putrefaction, the Lazarus on whom death had left its indelible and unmistakable signs. But language is already a corpse, as Michelet and Kératry reveal. The conceptual model of the dead, the fantasmatic program for understanding cemeteries and their contents, was in the mouths of the living, in the very words they spoke. It was this link that allowed the dead to become allegories of literature and history themselves, but allegories in the De Manian sense of a figure that produces, rather than simply expresses a meaning.[148] And this figuration, in turn, represented the extension of a medical imagination of death, an intentional and sustained interpretation of contemporary science by artists and novelists.

Building on his understanding of biology and evolution, Redon revealed the creative possibilities inherent in the ambiguity and mystery of matter itself and sought, in his works, to make the unconscious forces of nature visible, intelligible, and sentient. As idiosyncratic as it may have seemed, his visual language was intended to be a universal idiom that could express the hidden sensitivities of the inanimate world and the intelligence that lurked in the darkest corners of creation. In his images, it was, consequently, matter itself rather than abstract concepts that spoke, and although he may not have been fully aware of it, his vision of the dead was consistent with theorizations of death by contemporary physiologists, such as Claude Bernard. Through the medicalized figure of the corpse, Balzac and Flaubert reflected on how this sentient materiality exists in language itself, lending it the plasticity necessary for artistic creation. For Balzac, the corpse represented the apparent animation of a fictional character, impressed, like an artist's clay, with the abstractions of thought. For Flaubert, the corpse figured an object of unspeakable longing that organized the historical discourses that at once expressed and attempted to disguise it. In both cases, the dead body functioned as the remnant of an archaic and buried world that allegorized how language both relies on physical events—spoken and written words—and embodies the persistence of the past into the present. In the next chapter, I will theorize the structures of that relation to the past and their effects on meaning. I will do this through an analysis of the concept of the city and the persistent myths about its origins, myths that seek to explain the relation between reason and desire, between subject and abject.

SEVEN

Abstracting Desire

The rise of the modern, hygienic city, as I have argued, is based in significant part on irrational or imaginary motivations that coalesced around the indeterminacy of death. In what follows, I will attempt to understand those forces through recourse to the psychoanalytic principle of the *fantasm*.[1] And since this principle cannot be dissociated, in the relevant literature, from stories about origins, I will look at such stories, concentrating on those that imagine the city as a space devoted to and protected by reason. To this end, I will take the fantasm in a broad sense, understanding it both as a factor within reason itself and as a driving force within what I have earlier described as the medicalization of society, especially as that medicalization manifested itself in urban space. And if the city emerges from this discussion as a place devoted to and protected by reason, the fantasms of its origin reach back to an inexhaustible scene of desire, a scene that explains the existence of the city by framing it as an unbearable, and incomprehensible question. That question, I will argue, took plastic form in works by the popular novelists Victor Hugo and Eugene Sue, who consequently represented not only an aesthetic analysis of medical fantasms about abjection but also the penetration of those ideas into what one might term the public imagination, bearing in mind that such a concept is itself probably an imaginary construction.

Intimations of Another Reason

The energy behind the movement to expel the dead from Paris can be gauged in part by the resistance that it had to overcome, for it encountered a steady and determined opposition, from whose perspective the deceased constituted a legitimate segment of society—sometimes compared to an age group by later commentators—that continued to play a vital role in the community and required, in turn, certain unique accommodations.[2] These reactionary forces were led by the Church and its representatives, who fought a vigorous and unrelenting rearguard battle to preserve the integrity of their funerary practices. From the earliest years of the movement, these parties had made their voices heard, and even before a single law had been enacted or a corpse moved, the fictional priest of Porée's 1745 *Lettres sur la sépulture dans les églises* (Letters on Sepulchers inside Churches) defended the inhumation of bodies inside places of worship by arguing, on the one hand, that the custom was a form of recognition owed to those who had served the faith with particular distinction and, on the other, that its suppression would unfairly bankrupt the *fabriques*, which enjoyed a monopoly on funerary services.[3] Some twenty years later, in response to the edicts of 1763 and 1765 that had ordered the removal of cemeteries from urban centers, the *curés* or parish priests of Paris issued a memorandum repeating the themes of Porée's cleric while adding a new twist—they now contended that the stipulated removals would in fact pose more of a threat to public health than the procedures they were meant to replace.[4] But while they seemed, in this way, to accept the basic principles espoused by the hygienists, the *curés* also mocked beliefs, widespread among the scientific community, that a subterranean evil lurked in the urban soil and could be attributed to the decomposition of corpses. Noting that in many large cities, the custom of burying the dead *intra-muros* had never before led to objections, they argued that "one would have to say either that the problem had labored [incubated?] over the course of centuries without anyone ever having noticed it, or that although they were aware of it, they spent several centuries without thinking to complain and solve it."[5] The handwriting is difficult, at points, to decipher, and it is unclear whether the churchmen meant to say that the disease had labored (*œuvré*) during this period or had incubated (*couvé*), but in either case, there is the sense of a hidden pestilence awaiting its moment to emerge. More significantly, however, the *curés* add something subtly, but fundamentally new to these scenarios of hidden disease: they offered the possibility that the latency occurred not in the ground but in the imaginations of scientists, *philosophes*, and the people they frightened. Perhaps, according to the authors, it was simply that no one previously thought to be disturbed. Seen from this perspective, the subterranean world of infection was an act of thought, a psychological rather than a physiological state.

In 1824, after the hygienists' arguments had been broadly accepted and the transfer of remains was largely complete, a certain Louis François de Paule-Marie-Joseph de Robiano de Borsbeek reopened the old debate with a pamphlet entitled *De la violation des cimetières* (On the Violation of the Cemeteries). Like his predecessors, he emphasized the long-standing tradition that was being violently and—according to him—senselessly disrupted by the new injunctions. The "violations" of his title refer to the removal of dead bodies that had been taking place over the previous several decades, the legally mandated displacements of human remains to burial grounds outside the city, and de Borsbeek, for one, was not convinced by the hygienic arguments for these transfers, viewing them as so many tricks to rend the fabric of Christian life. "Whenever there was a contagious outbreak, these philanthropists would not fail to attribute it to the neighboring cemetery," he wrote of the hygienists.

> It was the insalubrity and the danger of such proximity that was and still is the heart of their argument. But how were they able to spread this terror in cities whose population so flourished and grew, in villages as populous as cities? I could go on to cite a great number of cities where the population was five times higher in the period when the dead were buried within their walls than it is today.[6]

As far as de Borsbeek was concerned, hygienic science was an instrument of other concerns, wielded within the context of a bitter struggle for cultural domination. The main problem with his approach was not so much that he based it on the premise that scientific truths might be epiphenomena of a hostile ideological system. Its principal weakness was rather that it attempted to replace that ideology with an older and increasing discredited one: Christian doctrine.

But de Borsbeek was not the only contemporary observer to feel that hygienic arguments about the dead might be so many illusions created to hide deeper and more troubling interests. The methods used by researchers themselves rarely approached later standards of rigor and objectivity, and they were often shrouded in a vague methodological unease, even by the investigators themselves. With rare exceptions such as Lavoisier, late-eighteenth-century scientific arguments concerning public health were, as Owen and Caroline Hannaway have observed, based more on individual anecdotes than on precise measurements or statistical comparisons, which were not conceptually available at the time. In short, hygienic reasoning was most often shaped by the choice of examples that were focused on, and this choice was itself oriented by unexamined motivations.[7] Even in the work of chemists such as Cadet-De-Vaux, one can see the subordination of clinical procedures to a preexisting certitude about what those procedures would reveal. This predisposition is betrayed in phrases like "such a pile of corpses could not but spread infection through such a narrow enclosure."[8] Here, the author reveals an incapacity to imagine other scenarios than the one he subscribes to. "I shall not enter here into the details of my experiments," he wrote elsewhere, or again: "but I little insisted on these physical details."[9] More tellingly, Cadet-De-Vaux repeatedly undermined his value as a clinician by interrupting experiments before they could yield results. As a consequence, he frequently did not actually see what he nonetheless seemed to believe he was witnessing. "It will be understood that I was little concerned with physical experiments there," he wrote of his attempts to comprehend and combat an outbreak of disease in a street adjoining the Saints-Innocents cemetery.

> The first one nearly cost the man who tried it his life. Besides, almost always called upon in circumstances where men's life is concerned, I do not wish to have on my conscience the instants I devoted to any other object. In such cases, the selfish pleasure of discovery must yield to humanity, and the happiest result that one can obtain is this: I have saved the life of a citizen.[10]

The author recognized that he did not comprehend the phenomena he observed and that, despite his original intentions, his actions had done nothing to advance such an understanding. In order to excuse himself, he described a conflict between two opposing interests: on the one hand a human life and on the other scientific knowledge. Nor was this mortal incompatibility an isolated or aberrant situation; it seemed instead to have been his normal working condition as a chemist, for, as he put it, he is "almost always called upon in circumstances where men's lives are concerned." By the very nature of his vocation, the applied scientist, and especially the hygienist, thus found himself operating under a contradictory imperative in which he must systematically sacrifice comprehension to action. As a consequence, he must consistently interrupt his experiments to save his associates from a danger that only the experiments themselves could prove to exist. He saved them, in short, from his fear itself. Scientific knowledge, in such a context, must have a very special meaning: structurally, it was more closely related to speculation than to experimentation.

On the face of it, it is difficult to understand why Cadet-De-Vaux's reasoning would seem more convincing than de Borsbeek's, say, and how it could have prevailed, leading to such massive upheavals in the treatment of the dead and the organization of the city. It was certainly difficult for the historian Jules Michelet to understand, for he remarked that hygienic fears about the corpses of those guillotined under the Terror were demonstrably spurious and manifestly served to displace other sorts of anxieties: "The living took fright," he wrote. "What they did not dare say in the name of humanity, they said in the name of hygiene and salubrity."[11] To demonstrate his point he observed that:

> if one considers the great massacres that occurred at different periods under the monarchy, without Paris having felt the same fears, it is astonishing [*on s'étonnera*] that twelve hundred criminals executed over the course of two months should have raised concerns about the public health.
>
> The faubourg Sainte-Antoine, which, for some two hundred and fifty years, buried its dead and those of the adjacent neighborhoods in the Sainte-Marguerite cemetery (thousands of dead per year) without suffering from its proximity, declared that it could no longer bear the added influx of the guillotined, even though it was minimal in comparison.[12]

Still far from a statistical analysis, Michelet's observations nonetheless represent an attempt to expose and give numerical value to the contradictions in hygienic concerns. For Michelet, there is something "astonishing" in the fear of the dead, in the belief that they will affect public health, and his choice of vocabulary indicates that for him the underlying fears that the language of medicine expressed lay, in reality, beyond the realm of the rational. By quantifying the inconsistencies in an argument, one exposes its marvelousness and its wonder, which leads to the question: If the hygienic arguments were invalid, how, as de Borsbeek asked, does one explain the terror that was felt? What were the origins of the very real fear that seems to have seized some of the most intelligent, most driven and—ostensibly—least credulous members of society over a period spanning several generations? What was the "humanity" in whose name, according to Michelet, the population of Paris took fright?[13]

Ghost Machines

There was, in the last years of the eighteenth century, an individual named Etienne-Gaspard Robertson, who attempted to create a scientific device for understanding and curing just such irrational fears.[14] He called his apparatus a *fantasmagorie* or "ghost machine [*machine à fantômes*]," as he put it, and according to contemporary reports it met with extraordinary success across all levels of society, even attracting Joséphine Bonaparte to one of its sessions.[15] Spectators would enter into a darkened room, where, through a series of projections and other optical illusions, the operator sought to terrify and entertain them, with the ultimate intention—or so, at least, he claimed—of disabusing the public of its fears. It little matters whether Robertson genuinely believed in the curative powers of his invention or whether they were simply a pretext; to be useful, the argument had to have the value of plausibility, and as such it must have answered contemporary aspirations and corresponded to beliefs about how they could be realized.[16] But simply fabricating *ersatz* "ghosts" does not mean that real ones do not exist. It therefore seems more reasonable to understand Robertson's idea of a "cure" to mean that the ability to produce frightening images allowed some sense of mastery over the processes of fear themselves. If this was true, the theater of the *fantasmagorie* was designed to stage psychological conditions, to function, in other words, as a partial recreation of the psyche itself. With this prosthesis, then, the inventor sought to recreate the "fantasms" of the mind and to demystify the irrational by literally bringing it to light.

What is particularly remarkable in Robertson's apparatus, however, is that the register of the irrational was limited in it almost entirely to ghosts, as if the potentially limitless category of the fantasmatic had been reduced to visions of the living dead. Articles reporting on the *fantasmagorie* exhorted their readers to "come breathe the air of the tomb," and to enter "into the fictional regions of the dead."[17] "Seated in a funeral vault," according to one account, the spectator was confronted by "a succession of the most hideous fantoms, in all the illusion of reality. . . . A trumpet's dreadful blast heralds the arrival of death, and death suddenly reveals itself in all its horror."[18] And the success of Robertson's invention seems to have transformed Paris itself, as imitators sprang up throughout the capital. By *pluviôse* of the year VII (January–February 1799), "the fantasmagorie had become a very common thing," according to its inventor, "and operated by fantasmagorists of all classes, they made Paris seem like the Elysian Fields for the sheer number of shadows that inhabited it, and it took but a slightly metaphoric imagination to transform the Seine into the river Lethe."[19] Not only did the projections offered by Robertson and his imitators clearly respond to some deep desire among Parisians of all walks, but they also illustrated another kind of distinction operating in urban space, for as the inventor describes it here, the line separating the Paris of the living from the Paris of the dead was nothing but a bit of metaphor. The difference between science and fantasm was, in this sense, no more than the difference between the literal and the figural, and the latter was the world of the irrational, the realm of illusion projected in the images of the *fantasmagorie*.[20] Robertson treated fantasms as misconceptions that eventually yielded to rational investigation, but by indirectly attributing the origins of these misconceptions to figurative discourse and by effectively restricting the entire category to representations of the dead, he made of the latter allegories for metaphor. Indeed, by this sort of conflation, metaphor itself became another word for the realm of the deceased. An equivalence was thus established between figurative language, irrational fear, and revenants; and, as the funerary décor of Robertson's stagings made clear, these three manifestations of a single principle were associated with a specific place: the graveyard. From this perspective, the walls going up around cemeteries during this period can be understood as apotropaic barriers against something more complicated and elusive than hygienic concerns: on the one hand they represented concrete embodiments of the divide between the literal and the metaphoric, and on the other safeguards against the fantasmatic projections that the dead represented.[21]

Robertson's *fantasmagorie* was not merely a "ghost machine"; it was also a mechanism for freeing the public from the illusions of discourse, and he conceived of that liberating process as a journey to the underworld, a journey in which the nonexistence of the dead, their futility and nullity, were to be revealed. But Robertson's spectacles exceeded these intentions, for the difference between forgetting that nullity and exploring the illusions created by it was itself sometimes forgotten, so that the treatment seems at times to have replaced the cure as the object of desire. In the wake of the Enlightenment and French Revolution, something about nineteenth-century Paris found itself caught between these two tendencies. On the one hand, there was a need to hide the dead away, to exclude them entirely from the city, and to create a hermetic seal between them and the living: to transform Paris entirely into a city of the living, to make it coterminous with life by arguing that death is nothing, or an eternal sleep, or something legally, even constitutionally outside the city. On the other hand, the dead had been freed to circulate among the living in ways never before possible. Under the watchful gaze of the Church, they had previously been held in check, their role in the community of the living assured but rigidly controlled. With the transfer of the cemeteries and with the Revolution, however, they began to walk again, disturbed and perhaps vengeful.[22] And through a horrible paradox, even in their demystification they seemed to become all the more interesting, attracting even the future empress to their haunts, taking over the city, turning the Seine into the Lethe, the river of forgetting, now transformed into a forgetting of the river for an illusion, a living in metaphorical fantasms that the ghost machine was supposed to exorcise and that the partisans of scientific method were relentlessly trying to debunk. The dead, in other words, were restless. The very attempt to dispel beliefs in their powers only increased them. And despite a public discourse of scientific rationalism, there seems to have been an awareness that concerns about the deceased represented something different, less defined, and more exciting than pragmatic questions about public health. This was what Robertson, somewhat unconsciously, identified in his fantasmagoria, lending not only a powerful new instrument to the investigation of the irrational but also a label that would play an increasingly crucial role in the theorization of the human psyche.[23] For with the advent of psychoanalysis, as I will argue, a language emerged that was capable of analyzing the otherness of fantasms—their alternate logic and their strange, erotic potency—in terms that sought not only to represent and dispel, but also to understand them. Insofar as the dead were a fantasmatic property, they fell, therefore, under that other logic that psychoanalysis has attempted to decipher.

Anal Erotics

Medical arguments acquired an unprecedented authority in early nineteenth-century France, they were able to reshape Paris physically and ideologically, but they were, at the same time, informed by a significant irrational element that expressed itself in more or less conscious fantasms of abjection and desire. The force of the hygienic movement, for instance, did not derive from pragmatic concerns about longevity and vigorous good health alone, for the latter entailed a horror of filth that seems to have exceeded mere concerns about physical well-being. This horror, as I have shown in my discussions of Bichat and Claude Bernard, expressed itself as indecision about the limits of consciousness. Certainly, there had been other historical periods when life and death had been confused and other figures for that confusion besides the corpse, the oyster, and putrefaction. Earlier centuries had been haunted by ghosts, or imagined the bodies of their dead to lie in wait of glorification while their spirits suffered in the intermediary space of purgatory. But the fantasies of indeterminacy that characterized the eighteenth and nineteenth centuries were different. On the one hand, their notions of indeterminacy appear to have derived naturally and necessarily from recent discoveries in chemistry, physiology, and pathology, and as such to be legitimated by some of the most authoritative and avant-garde voices in contemporary society. The ambiguity of death could not, in other words, be attributed to folkloric beliefs but evolved, instead, of out some of the most advanced, codified, and accredited thinking of the day. On the other hand, this was not the idea of an afterlife in the sense of an immaterial exaltation of consciousness, but instead the suspicion that death might, conversely, be the degeneration of consciousness into a material state—not a progression from the animate to the purely intelligible, but instead a regression to the inanimate and sentient. And whereas the idea of death as transcendence strengthened the division between it and life, the idea of death as putrescence weakened the distinctiveness of animation. What had to be expelled from Paris in the course of its hygienic reforms was not so much the danger of an abrupt and definitive end to life, therefore, as an inanimate continuation of it, the prospect of a dead and materialized subjectivity. But just as important as this idea of a sentient death itself was the fact that it was never clinically demonstrated. For although speculation on the question had been literally galvanized by experiments in which electrical currents provoked muscular reactions in corpses, no one ever proved that the dead could feel or that death itself might exist and be inhabited by some dim awareness. Powerful as these ideas may have been, they were, in short, imaginary constructs, and even contemporaries recognized a strong irrational component behind the hygienic handling of the dead. But if these fears were imaginary, the question of their motivation arises. Why, in other words, would anyone *want* to be horrified by death?

Despite his forthrightness in speaking of his crimes, Sergeant Bertrand never attempted to explain *why* he was so attracted to the dead. Nor did Zola account for the mixture of revulsion and sexual excitement that the morgue provoked in his characters. In fact, despite the fascination with representing necrophilia during this period, there was very little attempt to understand it: one could almost say that it existed entirely on the level of experience without ever being mastered by comprehension, as if there were something peculiarly nonconceptual about the dead. Even the doctors who studied Bertrand's case made no attempt to explain why he might be interested in corpses or what the dead might signify within a pathological (let alone nonpathological) sexuality. It is true that Gautier justified his characters' necrophilia by imagining it to express an aspiration toward the transcendental, but his approach is of little service in understanding an erotics of the abject, such as one finds in Bertrand, Baudelaire, Zola, or even Gautier himself. With their insistence on putrefaction and material corruption, these latter expressions of desire related more closely to forms of sexual deviance such as coprophilia than to the quasireligious transports of Gautier. And in the medical and popular imaginations of the late eighteenth and the nineteenth centuries, the dead, as I have shown, were in fact regularly assimilated with feces. From this particular perspective, one does, however, find a rich explanatory literature, especially in psychoanalytic studies on anal eroticism. The relation to corpses, the erotics of the abject dead and the putrefying wastes of life, might, in other words, be understood as a form of anal libidinization, and it is from this perspective that I will try to sketch out an initial understanding of the unacknowledged desire that manifested itself in the medical, and especially hygienic, imagination.

For the most important early writers on the subject, such as Freud and Karl Abraham, the tremendous physical pleasure that children derive from defecating is linked to more abstract feelings of narcissistic power, which are both sadistic and creative in nature. Abraham, for instance, saw a close connection between anal stimulation and "infantile impulses of love," a connection that led certain children, as they developed and learned to control their bowel movements, to express converse feelings of hostility through their excretory functions.[24] This hostile expression, which Freud also remarked, seemed to be a consequence of the creative aspects of defecation, for with their feces, children are able to produce something that previously did not exist, a wondrous achievement that is translated, according to Abraham, by such divergent forms as Biblical creation myths—where human beings are shaped out of "earth or clay, *i.e.* from a substance similar to excrement"—and an inclination toward artistic production, especially if it involves "painting, modeling, and similar activities."[25] As Abraham understood it, however, this creative ability had a negative corollary, in that it engendered the fantasy of an immense power over existence and nonexistence, which the child believed he could turn against others in moments of rage.[26] Infinitely fungible, more-over, feces were connected to gifts and money, and linked people in a tactile and peculiarly potent way both to a lost period of presocialized existence and to the determining experience of toilet training, during which they learned to subordinate the narcissistic immediacy of bodily pleasures to the more abstract and ethically significant desires of others.

What positive traits the early psychoanalysts detected in the anal complex were almost all explained as reaction formations or defenses against the tre-mendous power of the fecal world. The obsessiveness that characterizes this sort of personality indicates, for its part, the persistent proximity of that world, the way that it presses, at all moments, against the psychic structures erected to protect social conduct. Insofar as it represents a constant and minute vigilance, that obsessiveness suggests as well the dangerousness of the fecal, as if in the briefest lapse or the smallest displacement something overwhelming and horrible, worth sacrificing one's life to defend against, threatens to erupt. Ernest Jones could admire the "extraordinary and quite exquisite tenderness" that such people are capable of, their dedication to orderliness and lucidity of thought, but both were, in his estimation, protec-tions against the more basic feelings of hatred and destruction that torment the anal character.[27] Similarly, according to Jones, "such people are always pleased at discovering or hearing of new processes for converting waste prod-ucts into useful material, in sewage farms, coal-tar manufactories, and the like," but this apparent positivity actually had more tortuous origins, deriving from the anal personality's retentiveness and its horror of dirt, for as refuse is made valuable, it loses its status as refuse.[28] The English word *waste* nicely embodies the dual tendency that Jones alluded to in his explanation of the enthusiasm for recycling projects, for it contracts the notion of futile expen-diture into that of a useless and potentially noxious residue. Filth is excess. Applying this insight to a larger frame of reference, one could say that filth is anything that cannot be assimilated into the social order, the people, ideas, discourse, and stuff that resist integration. And indeed, the abject has been explained in similar terms.

Picking up on the proposition that dirt is "matter in the wrong place," which was extensively mined by early psychoanalysts such as Jones, the structuralist anthropologist Mary Douglas determined that "our pollution behavior is the reaction which condemns any object or idea likely to confuse or contradict cherished classifications."[29] Her reading of the abomination laws in Leviticus, for example, understood the unclean to be that which defies categorization according to the taxonomies in force at the time of Moses. Thus animals that "swarm" (Hebrew *shérec*) were characterized by "an indeterminate form of movement" and were therefore deemed to be polluted.[30] It would be hard to lend credence to Douglas's argument on the basis of such an abbreviated description, and her contention that a reaction as powerful and physically spontaneous as revulsion could be elicited by stimuli as arcane and intellectual as an inability to make precise taxonomic determinations might seem ridiculous. But her point was that such indeterminability places the very structures of society in jeopardy by confusing the conceptual frameworks that give it order and allow the impression of meaning; the disgust that such ambiguities provoke would, from this perspective, resemble the nauseous reaction caused by sudden disorientation, the spinning and lurching of a world abruptly deprived of its reference points. When such structures of determination are lost, or when they are shown to be frail or arbitrary, it is meaning itself that is threatened, and the world teeters on the brink of absurdity. The significance of filth, and the horror it evokes, would thus result from the danger it represents to the very possibility of making sense.

As the first attempt to interpret, in a sustained and coherent manner, the fantasmatic signification of these substances and behaviors, the psychoanalytic work on fecality represented a historical turning point in the study of abjection and an unprecedented act of creativity in its own right, but as rich and important as these theories were, they tended to reduce questions of coprophilia to an analysis of the anal character, which was painted in grim terms such as parsimony, automatism, compulsiveness, anger, and sadism. Lost in this all were the image, briefly evoked by Abraham, of the artistic creator and the notion that there is a tremendous, loving pleasure at the basis of the other, more negative expressions. One can even track the disappearance of these traits in his writing, the way that the ideas of love and creativity appear, like Eurydice, only long enough to vanish, subsumed almost immediately into the vision of a darker world ruled by hatred, destructiveness, and avarice. For before turning away to concentrate on somberer, more destructive drives, Abraham also alluded to the intimate ties that bind "infantile impulses of love"[31] to the pleasures of defecation. One might wonder what those quickly occluded positivities are and how they bear on an understanding, or at least a fantasmatics, of the abject world, since they suggest a conversion and perhaps, to borrow Leroux's utopian approach, a redemption. To understand such a fantasmatics of abjection, however, one would have to have some definition for the term *fantasm*.

Fantasms of the Abject

Although Freud made only passing references to the fantasm, and those were mostly in his early writings, the concept has subsequently played a crucial role in psychoanalytic theory. Indeed, some would argue that its importance cannot be overstated: for Laplanche and Pontalis it is "the psychoanalytic object *par excellence*," while Jean-Paul Valabrega called it the "*alpha* of psychoanalysis."[32] And if the fantasm is so fundamental to psychoanalysis, that is not, according to these theorists, simply a disciplinary idiosyncrasy, but rather a reflection of its function in the most basic psychological and epistemological structures organizing human experience as a whole. As René Kaës argues, the fantasm organizes all human thought and activity. For Lacan, it is the unjustifiable and originary axiom of truth itself.[33] So theories of the fantasm represent an attempt to formulate a crucial and generalizable structure of thought, valid for human beings in general, rather than simply for an individual pathology.[34] It is in this larger sense that Lacan speaks of a "logic" of the fantasm, since the latter constitutes, according to his theory, a crucial element in the production of meaning, with the rigor, necessity, and universality of logical propositions.[35] And if, in what follows, I have chosen to focus on Lacan and some relevant commentaries on him, it is because of the complexity and sophistication of his approach, because of its broad-reaching implications, and—perhaps more than anything else—because of its sheer audacity. In this sense, he has provided the most important means to account for the role and significance of the fantasm in human experience, both normal and deviant.

At least in his earliest moves, Lacan organizes his explanation around an analysis of Descartes's *cogito*, or the proposition "I think therefore I am." As an initial step in that analysis, he draws on linguists' distinction between the subject of enunciation and the subject of the statement to distinguish the subject that thinks or speaks from the subject who is. He then turns to the nineteenth-century logician Augustus de Morgan's formula "not (a *and* b) = not-a *or* not-b," and recasts the linguistic difference between subject of enunciation and subject of the statement on its basis. With this, he creates his own version of Descartes's *cogito*, which he summarizes in the proposition that the subject either is *or* speaks.[36] It is one or the other, but not both. The disjunction between speaking and being produces, in turn, a logic of sexual difference in relation to *jouissance* or pleasure: one *is jouissance* (and therefore "unbarred" in Lacan's terminology) or one *says jouissance* (and is "barred" or, in other words, a signifier to other signifiers).[37]

Casting the *cogito* in terms of a relation to *jouissance* and sexual difference may seem arbitrary, but this shift of perspective is not gratuitous, if one takes it within the larger terms of Lacan's psychoanalytic theory. For Lacan, sexual difference enters the equation because in experiential terms, the *cogito*'s seemingly abstract structure expresses itself through the relation to the phallus as *having* or *being* it, so that the questions of castration and the Œdipus complex, both of which are central to his notion of subjectivity, can be understood as the difference between logic (or being) and grammar (or speaking), while the fantasm can be understood as an attempt to reconcile them. In other words, the fantasm attempts to resolve this disjunction in the relation to *jouissance*, which consequently becomes the basis for the fantasm's logical legitimacy— and therefore universality.[38]

Now, psychoanalytic theories of the fantasm are often contradictory, at times on crucial points, but they have enough in common that certain salient features consistently reemerge, two of which are particularly important for a discussion of abject desire. First, there is general agreement that the classic or paradigmatic fantasm centers on a scene of incest. This is not particularly astonishing, given the central importance of the Oedipal complex to Freudian and post-Freudian thought. Still, under closer scrutiny, this *Urphantasie* reveals a little surprise, a structurally necessary remnant that functions like— and often *is*—bodily remains, a leftover that provides a material support for the subject's displaced desires.[39] Second, the fantasm entails a breakdown of the category of the other. To a certain extent, this is intuitive: a conscious fantasy is a substitute for the partner in an erotic encounter, a stand-in produced by an individual's imagination, often in order to accompany masturbation.[40] The situation becomes more complicated, however, when one recognizes that fantasms can function unconsciously and that they can intervene even in the presence of an erotic partner, thereby altering the latter's role both in sexual acts and more generally. Because he understands sexual difference as two incompatible relations to the phallus, this situation is not, for Lacan, an occasional event, but rather the nature of sexual relations as such, leading him to declare, infamously, that there is no such thing as a sexual act—since sexual acts and relations "exist" only in the impossible ontology between being and saying.[41] To put the case somewhat brutally, the self *is* or it *signifies* in relation to another. And the status of that other changes accordingly.

Juan David Nasio's reading of Lacan is especially useful at this point because it helps explain the functioning of the fantasm within this impossible ontology of sexual difference. It is important to remember that although Nasio speaks specifically of neurotics in this passage, the structures of the fantasm that he describes should be understood universally, since the neurotic is recognized by Lacan—and Nasio himself—as the paradigm for all fantasmatic productions. "The fantasm," Nasio writes, "takes shape when one is confronted by a danger. It is a solution, a solution in face of the danger inherent to the speaking being, which is to find oneself completely effaced in the signifying chain. Now the neurotic's relation to that repetitive, serial chain of signifiers is not a relation of metaphysical alienation but rather a confrontation with *jouissance*."[42] He goes on to explain the origins of this menace: "Now under exactly what circumstances does this risk of *jouissance* arise?" he asks. "It is when we are faced with a bit of speech, with the fact of having been surprised by some bit of our speech, and are immediately led to wonder what the Other wants."[43] The danger against which the fantasm protects is, in short, the desire of the other, and the fantasm protects against this desire by replacing it with some alternative object. That object is subsequently invested with the subject's own desire, which it serves to materialize and thereby immobilize. This produces an oscillating movement between the two roles that each element in an intersubjective relation can play. If, on the one hand, the subject denies the desire of the other, the latter is reduced to a fantasmatic object constructed in the imagination of the subject. On the other hand, if the subject recognizes the desire of the other, the subject itself is reduced to the role of a fantasmatic object for that other. Nasio describes Lacan's formulations of these two situations in the following terms:

> Let us then consider one of the two principal equations of the fantasm, the one that leads Jacques Lacan to write $\mathcal{S} \lozenge a$ or, in other words, that the subject is made an object by the intervention of the partial image insofar as it is a signifying sign and the envelope of the real. . . . The second equation specific to the fantasmatic structure is given by the decline [*chute*] of the Other into an object, the degradation

of the A into *little a*. One caveat: when we say "Other," we must translate it, in terms of the fantasm, as "desire of the Other" and not, as is usually the case, as "the symbolic Other."[44]

The problem is, accordingly, the impossibility of the subject's simultaneously recognizing both its own and the other's desire, rather than the impossibility of its relating to the other within a linguistic order, or what Lacan calls the symbolic register. Desire, according to this paradigm, breaks down the possibility of an intersubjective relation, thereby reducing the self or its other to a fantasmatically constructed, generally unconscious image.

The fantasm, then, materializes and supports a crucial intersubjective relation, or rather, the attempt to negotiate the impossibility of that relation. It is the attempt to mediate between two noncompossible forms of desire. And, as we have already observed, Lacan understands these forms as two different relations to the phallus. The qualities of this latter term consequently inflect the fantasmatic relation that derives from it, leading Lacan to argue that the impossibility of the sexual act can be located in specific characteristics of the phallus itself. "What separates us from the sexual act," he writes, "is the relation between the body and something that is separated from it after having been part of it."[45] This means that the crucial element alienating the subject from the sexual act as an act between two desiring subjects is its relation to a detachable element of the body. In part, Lacan describes the phallus as detachable because of its role in the Oedipus and castration complexes. But in his writing on the fantasm, he emphasizes another reason, which is the fact that the phallus can become detumescent, thereby indicating the end or limits of *jouissance* while simultaneously revealing the male organ to be a bodily part that can disappear or become detached.[46] Significantly, for Lacan, the phallus functions in this role as a signifier for other detachable elements of the body, or, as he puts it: "the phallus, insofar as it represents the exemplary possibility of the lack of an object, is nothing but the sign of those absences of *jouissance* that are the breast, excrements, the gaze, and the voice."[47] For his part, Nasio uses the generic term *déchets* or detritus to describe these cognates and sees their loss as a necessary corollary of *jouissance*.[48] The phallus, then, is a sign, and as such it signifies other removable parts of the body, which Nasio calls *déchets*.

In short, the phallus means something else within the logic of the fantasm, and what it means is a removable remnant of the body, something like an excrement. And this remnant marks the disappearance of the other as desiring subject. The fantasm is, therefore, the human remains that both instantiate and signify the end of the other's subjectivity, its reduction to object. The language for describing this excremental remnant of the subject's disappearance suggests, however, that among the various cognates that the phallus can signify, one plays the role better than the others. So one should listen carefully to that language. Nasio writes: "when, in the fantasm, the desiring other is exposed to violence, it remains, either by contempt or caress, a lifeless being, an inert and dead object. That death is very close to the real one and sometimes, in fact, the two converge."[49] Or as he puts it a few pages later: "To summarize, the fantasm consists in the *mise-en-scène* through which the Other is annihilated [*anéanti*], reduced to a pure object at the mercy of the subject, abolished as a speaking being and negated as a desiring one. In short, the fantasmatic apparatus stages the putting to death of the Other."[50] The transposition of the other into other-object (or *objet petit a*, in Lacanian mathemes) constitutes, in Nasio's violent but very astute reading, the death of the other.

Why is it so astute of Nasio to speak of death, when Lacan himself only refers to reducing the desire of the other to a nonlinguistic object, the *objet petit a*? Because Lacan *should* talk about death here but does not. He speaks about death elsewhere, in his writings on Sophocles's *Antigone*, for instance, where he calls it the intervention of language, of the symbolic, in human life.[51] Death is, accordingly, subjectification, the integration of the self into the symbolic register. But Lacan also speaks of Antigone as being caught between two deaths, and that other death, the death that is *not* subjectification, he leaves unstated and unexplained. In his reading of *Antigone*, the other death would, presumably, be the death that desubjectifies, that reduces the heroine, in the play's last lines, to a corpse. And in the logic of the fantasm, the desubjectification of the other, his or her reduction to *objet petit a*, should also be a form of death, a reduction to a corpse. Nasio, in short, adds the word that Lacan, for some reason, does not want to utter here.

Still, Nasio's description of that putting-to-death is slightly, and significantly, inconsistent in its choice of terms. He writes that the other is annihilated and, as such, reduced to a *pure* object. According to the logic of the scene he describes, however, that cannot be the case. First, the other is not annihilated, since that means reduced to nothing and, in fact, neither death nor the fantasm reduces the other to nothing. There is a body or bodily part left over, and it is, precisely, this excess that constitutes the material support for the fantasm. Second, this object is not pure, since it is not clearly and absolutely an object: it is, as I have argued, variously the objectification of the subject and of the other, and as such constitutes an object not entirely—that is, not purely—distinct from the subject or, in other words, an object not purely an object. Following Julia Kristeva, one can call that particular, impure status between subject and object abjection.[52]

In the fantasmatic resolution of the impossible relation between desiring subjects, the *objet petit a* thus emerges as the remnant of a death, or, in other words, as a cadaver. And it is in just such terms that Nasio describes the detachable bodily part or "the decrepitude of the body: a lost entity, the rotting or missing piece that returns to the status of a pulsional object."[53] What this means, in the end, is that the cadaver—more even than the phallus, which only signifies it—represents the fantasm as such. It is the replacement of the other's desire with the erotically charged, bodily residue of that desire. So, we substitute the cadaver for the phallus, not only in the notion of the fantasm, but more importantly, in the conceptions of desire and intersubjectivity that Lacan organizes around it. Unlike the phallus, however, whose particularities Lacan discusses at some length, the characteristics of the corpse go unexamined.

From all of this, then, one makes the somewhat surprising discovery that the fantasm cannot explain the affective force and meaning of the corpse. There are two principal reasons for this failure. First, because the fantasm derives from the corpse. Second, because the concept of the corpse is never mentioned, let alone analyzed, by Lacan within this particular context. This does not mean that his theory of the fantasm is without importance for an understanding of dead human bodies, for it does, ultimately, attribute to them a key role in the production of truth. More important, his model situates them within a rigorous nexus of terms, notably language, desire, intersubjectivity, and abjection. The fantasm, in other words, does not explain the corpse, but it helps us to position it in ways that can allow us to understand its meaning within other, nonpsychoanalytic contexts.

To help move toward those other contexts, one should recognize that there is another crucial aspect to the fantasm: it is always in some way about an origin. According to Piera Aulagnier, for instance, the fantasm explains the advent of the "I" and resolves, through the notions of the parents' love for each other and their desire for a child, the difference between experience and language.[54] In a similar vein, Valabrega describes the fantasm as a myth and argues that "all myths are accounts of the beginning."[55] For Laplanche and Pontalis, too, the concept of the fantasm is inseparable from this question of origination, as is evidenced in the very title of their principal essay on the subject. And for Lacan, the fantasm is an axiom, the inexplicable starting point that grounds logic in truth rather than knowledge, in being rather than saying.[56] His description of the fantasm's axiomatic nature recalls, moreover, Valabrega's ideas about the rhetorical nature of beginnings. "Problems about origins never end in an answer," Valabrega writes. "Instead, they always open onto a question, a quest, a hesitation. Because every origin *poses a question* [*fait question*], every origin *is* a question."[57] His originary myth may be formulated in language, but it does not *say* anything in a propositional sense. In that respect, it can be understood to open the fantasmatic place that, for Lacan, links grammar and logic. For the incomprehensible origin, according to Lacan, is not a proposition but, rather, a place—a place that depends conceptually and structurally on the corpse. That place, one could also say, is the city itself, the city as an instrument for excluding abjection and rationalizing desire. Valabrega himself, in fact, uses the term in this very way.[58] And so, in order to understand the hygienic imagination and the role of abject fantasmatics in it, one would have to look at what might be called the origin myths of the modern city. To do that, I will need to go back in time to ancient Athens, the city, as Gillian Rose argues, that stands as the mythical beginning of western rationalism.[59] The fantasm instructs us that this is the place that will allow us to situate the corpse in terms of meaning.

The City as a Space of Reason

While still young and untried, less a philosopher than an aspirant, Socrates described a brush with meaninglessness that had once shaken him. He recalled the incident while outlining his theory of forms and just after describing how every object imperfectly mirrors a perfect and transcendental type. He was speaking with Parmenides, a leading sophist and, as such, a master of the *dissoi logoi*, or the ability to argue opposite propositions with equivalent force. The young man was thus confronting someone who championed an absolute relativity of reason and order and who therefore represented a threat to the discursive bases of democracy, for the latter was grounded on the possibility that the best ideas would prevail in discussion, whereas the sophists contended that *any* idea could be made to prevail. So although Socrates was apparently discussing abstract principles, it was the state itself that was in the balance. The older philosopher asked:

Are you also puzzled, Socrates, about cases that might be thought absurd [*geloia*], such as hair or mud [*pēlos*] or dirt [*rhupos*] or any other trivial [*atimotaton*] and undignified [*phaulotaton*] objects? Are you doubtful whether or not to assert that each of these has a separate form distinct from things like those we handle?

Not at all, said Socrates. In these cases, the things are just the things we see; it would surely be too absurd [*atopon*] to suppose that they have a form. All the same, I have sometimes been troubled by a doubt whether what is true in one case may not be true in all. Then, when I am standing at that point [*epeita hotan tautēi sto*], I am driven to retreat, fearing [*deisas*] lest I tumble into some pit of nonsense [*eis tina buthon phluarias*] and be utterly destroyed [*diaphtharo*]. Anyhow, I get back to the things which we were just now speaking of as having forms, and occupy my time with thinking about them.[60]

The concept of nonsense that Socrates sketches out here is complex and somewhat mysterious. On the one hand the idea that mud or hair might have a transcendental form is *geloia*, or "laughable," which suggests a social condition—a feeling of disgrace that attaches itself to philosophical missteps. What would seem to hold the young man back from certain investigations is thus the fear of being reduced to a laughingstock and humiliated in the eyes of his peers. A little later on, Parmenides picks up on this idea of shame, assuring his interlocutor that when he finally ceases to care about the opinions of others he will turn to such apparently trivial questions and, in so doing, attain to philosophical maturity.[61] According to him, the accession to thought thus requires a certain shamelessness, an ability to reject the opinions—or *doxas*—of others. At that moment, apparently, Socrates will be able to engage those things that are *atimotata*, entering into a world without *timē*: the notion of honor, value, and price, of social standing, that was one of the great, guiding concepts of ancient Greek culture. The one who deals with abject or *atimotata* things will himself, it seems, become abject. But what Parmenides describes as a form of embarrassment, Socrates feels as an overwhelmingly powerful and terrifying force. It is a place—or absence of place—into which one drops. There is no footing here: one goes from standing to falling with one small step. It is a vertiginous moment, when the body plunges nauseously, but also a moment of absolute destruction. Embarrassment is not just unpleasant, it disorients, revolts, and ultimately annihilates. This, apparently, is what it feels like to violate the *doxa* and transgress the social order. Or so it seemed to the young Socrates. But Parmenides had entered that world. To hear him tell it, this place, so carefully guarded by

fear and shame, is a mystery of adulthood awaiting certain privileged thinkers. And from the point of view of the young, uninitiated Socrates, in this,
other, heterodox world beyond the boundaries of social convention and intelligibility, things must be only as they seem to be—individual, unhaunted by
a higher meaning or a vocation to resemblance. They are sheer matter in its
endless, swarming profusion—formless.

What lies beyond the *doxa* and conventions of collective intelligibility—or
collectivity *as* intelligibility—is thus bounded by fear, revulsion, and the possibility of annihilation. Now this threat of death was sometimes seen by
Plato's contemporaries to be a natural consequence of social transgression
and at others appeared to require human enforcement, such that the avoid-
ance of the abject blended with definitions of the state as a legislative entity.
One finds this connection between revulsion and legislation in another dialogue, where a sophist named Protagoras explains the origins of mankind by
recounting the fable of Prometheus. Despite their god-like skill with fire and
their wisdom stolen from Athena herself, according to this account, the earliest human beings were constantly falling prey to wild beasts because they
lacked "the art of politics" and consequently could not band together for
mutual protection. "They sought therefore to save themselves by coming
together and founding fortified cities," Protagoras explains, "but when they
gathered in communities they injured one another for want of political skill
[*tēn politikēn technēn*], and so scattered again and continued to be devoured."[62]
It is in the unintended order of things that those who cannot come together
in civic union should be destroyed by something that lies constitutionally
outside the city, and this latter is the irrational or *aloga* forces embodied by
the beasts.[63] The boundaries that are constantly being transgressed in this
preurban world are those, therefore, between words and wordlessness,
between thought and appetite, between the human and the inhuman. To preserve mankind, Zeus therefore found himself obliged to send down political
skill—the skill of the city or polis—and this in turn comprised two qualities:
"a sense of shame and a sense of justice [*aido te kai dikēn*]."[64] The latter were
evenly apportioned among human beings, such that they became the barrier
between them and the animal world. But apparently there were some individuals who did not willingly accept this gift, some human beings who preferred
to continue frequenting the state of bestial irrationality, and so Zeus proclaimed a law to counteract this tendency—but it was not just *a* law, it was
the *first* law of the city, the law that legislated the possibility of legislation,
the one that separated between those capable of accepting justice and those

incapable, that condemned the latter to death and created the polis as a place of legality. "[Y]ou must lay it down as my law [*nomon*]," Zeus tells his messenger, "that if anyone is incapable of his share of these two virtues he shall be put to death as a plague to the city [*hos noson poleos*]."[65] The founding of the cities, their condition of possibility, comes in this act of violence, this enforced distinction between the rational as that which will submit to justice and the irrational or *alogon* as that which will not. And the latter is seen to be like a sickness, so that the originary act of justice is also an act of hygiene, a separation between *nomos* and *nosos*, in which the nonpolitical is construed as a form of disease.

The Protagoran vision of the relation between abjection and the state, or some vague and persistent memory of that vision, seems to have reasserted itself in Enlightenment political ideology, especially in the latter's call for a systematic exclusion of irrational forces from civic life. Protagoras echoed, for example, throughout Diderot's article on *droit naturel*, or natural law, in the *Encyclopédie*, which attempted to demonstrate that the laws of nature laid the universal and immutable bases of human justice. For despite Newton's discoveries that physical behaviors could be understood as expressions of consistent underlying forces and that those forces and their interactions could be formulated in mathematical absolutes, the late eighteenth century was still uncertain about how to understand the relation between those absolutes and human behavior.[66] The first of Diderot's nine points in his article on *droit naturel* thus established the specificity of mankind in respect to other animals, and it did so through the difference between appetite and reason. Men, Diderot contended, are not free so long as their actions spring from material causes alone, and insofar as they do, "there will be no rational goodness or evil, although there might be goodness and evil of an animal kind."[67] Unlike human beings', beasts' judgments are determined not by the free exercise of reason, but through the dictates of their physical conditions and are, in this way, a living expression of speechless drives both animate and inanimate. As dimly conscious bits of matter, subhuman species are, so to speak, unwitting prisoners of their unwittingness. Consequently, "the animals are separated from us by invariable and eternal barriers."[68] To be human, from this perspective, is to rise above matter through the force of reasoned thought. To be free is to be rational and immaterial. Such is the vocation of mankind, its defining characteristic, and whoever declines, therefore, to submit his will to the force of reason and to seek the truth is dehumanized and "denatured": a beast, a madman, or evil in a profound and immutable sense.[69]

One must, consequently, choose to be human and choose to be natural, which one does by subordinating individual desire to the will of the group. "Individual wills are always suspect," Diderot wrote. "They can be good or evil, but the general will is always good. . . . It is to the general will that the individual must turn, when he wants to know the extent to which he must be a man, a citizen, a subject, a father, or a child, and when he should live or die."[70] In all his relations with others—and even in his relations with himself—the individual must thus submit to the determinations of an abstract universal, which is embodied in the collective state insofar it negates the particular will. For this is what the general will is: the negation of the particular. To be *a* human is always to be *the* human, and anything else is a form of madness or bestiality or evil. And anything else is not just *other* to the state: it is a hostile agent. "The man who listens only to his individual will," Diderot wrote, "is the enemy of the human race," and he expected that any such individual would quickly and necessarily be snuffed out or *étouffé* by his more enlightened fellows.[71] As in Protagoras's fable, Diderot saw the fundamental act of legislation to be an enforceable separation between the rational and the irrational, the human and the animal. But Diderot took the point further by understanding animality to include a sort of sentient materiality, the forces of lifeless matter that speak through the drives and appetites of beasts. For him, irrational individuals fall not merely outside of the human, thereby sacrificing their right to the state, they fall, as well, outside of the natural, and consequently lose their very right to exist. As a certain legibility became the defining characteristic of the natural and reason the key to deciphering it, the illegible and meaningless were cast out not merely from the city, but also from the universe. The proscription that Zeus laid on mankind now extended to the world at large. As an embodiment of a rational order, the state, paradoxically, became the guarantor and protector of the natural. Since the category of the natural could be violated, it too must be enforced, and this on pain of death.

Although not in any overt way, capital punishment was thus foreseen in Diderot's project for the state, and its role was foundational, since it preceded the possibility of justice and legislation themselves.[72] This role did not remain purely theoretical for long. After Louis XVI was arrested in his attempt to flee France, arguments derived from Diderot and Rousseau's political theories led to his execution as an enemy of the nation.[73] The first to make this case was the young Saint-Just—Michelet's "archangel of death," the "living sword" of Taine—who addressed the Convention on November 13, 1792.

Already, in positioning himself as a speaker before his fellow legislators, Saint-Just explicitly adopted the point of view of the general will and described it as the negation of his own, individual will. "You will never see me place my personal will against the will of all," he told the assembly. "I shall want what the French people, or the majority of its representatives, wants. But since my personal will is a portion of the law that has yet to be made, I shall openly explain what I mean."[74] The law of the state was not yet established, for in fleeing and denouncing the Revolution, the king had effectively abrogated the constitution. On December 3, Robespierre would step to the tribunal to expand on his colleague's observation and to draw out the consequences of this strange, stateless moment. "It is a blatant contradiction to suppose that the constitution could preside over this new order of things," he argued. "That would amount to saying that it could outlive itself. What laws replace it? The laws of nature and that law that forms the very basis of society: the welfare of the people [*le salut du peuple*]. . . . But the people! What law are they to follow if not justice and reason, seconded by their almighty force?"[75] It is the will of nature as expressed through reason and the people that guides the legislators in this state that is not yet one, that is striving for itself, listening carefully to the symptoms of its own future being in an attempt to translate them into intelligible signs of a justice to come.

What those signs indicated is that in dissolving the constitution, the king had violated the social contract; but his crime laid bare, for Saint-Just at least, a more fundamental violence against the general will. To be a king was in itself a refusal of the social contract. "What relation of justice is there between humanity and kings?" he asked the Convention.[76] Because he lived outside the social contract, Louis could not, according to his prosecutors, even be judged, since the law only applied to citizens. In a powerful, but still groping attempt to subordinate the foundations of the state to the order of reason, Saint-Just laid out two arguments for why Louis could not be considered a member of the social pact. On the one hand, the king, by *being* who he was, by his status as king, fell outside the general will. "The pact is a contract between citizens," Saint-Just observed, "and not with the government. Without obligations, one has no part in a contract. Consequently, Louis, who had no obligations, cannot be tried in civil court."[77] On the other hand, the king excluded himself from the social contract by *doing* what he had done. At this point in the argument, however, the logic grows more tortuous and troubling. "Louis is a foreigner among us," Saint-Just continued. "He was not a citizen before his crime. . . . He is even less one since it. And by what miscarriage of justice would you make him a citizen in order to condemn him? As soon as a man is guilty, he leaves the city."[78] Or as Robespierre put it: "[T]ribunals and judicial procedures are created only for the members of the city."[79] The problem is that the reasoning seems to be circular here: once a person has committed a crime he exits society and cannot be judged, but in order to know if he has committed a crime must he not be judged? Apparently not. Because of his crime, Louis, according to Saint-Just, could not be tried for his crime. The tribunals of the Terror, under which hundreds of individuals were sentenced to death on the slimmest evidence and with virtually no hearing, have been dismissed as mockeries of justice, but their peremptory decisions did conform to the notion of law laid out here by Saint-Just. According to his reasoning, there really should be no courts at all, since those who would be brought before the law were systematically excluded from access to it.[80] Indeed, the Law of Suspects, passed on September 17,1793, brought these arguments to their necessary conclusion, for it mandated that citizens could be executed not only for what they did but for what they were suspected of having done.[81]

Saint-Just's complicated logic cannot be dismissed as merely a momentary lapse in the rigor of his thinking. It represents a different and a more radical notion of justice, but one that was already present among the Enlightenment theorists. Rousseau had advanced a similar argument in the *Contrat Social*.[82] Diderot had prefaced his exposition of the system of natural law by observing that "it is necessary to start from the top, and to accept nothing unless it is evident, at least to the degree that moral questions can be and that satisfies any man of sense [*homme sensé*]."[83] The standard of evidence in natural law is thus that a proposition satisfy any reasonable man. Any citizen is by definition reasonable, and so, in a moment such as the Terror, when the state is under the laws of nature, any man is judge and need only appeal to his innate sense of right.[84]

It must have been an extraordinary feeling to live in such a moment, when those of good faith—and perhaps those of bad faith too—saw the world illuminated and transcendent with their own deaths, and when they seemed, joining into the higher will of the state, to survive themselves. To those who believed in it, the Terror must have looked like a secular and rationalized version of the beatific vision. But that transcendence could only be bought with death. Robespierre summed up the situation with brutal economy: "The Republic! And Louis is still alive!"[85] At the beginning of his tenure in the Constituent Assembly he had argued against capital punishment, but now he embraced it. On December 3, he attempted to explain this apparent contradiction to the Convention:

> Yes, the death penalty is generally a crime, for the sole reason that the indestructible principles of nature authorize it only when the safety of individuals or of the social body demand it. Now, public safety never exacts capital punishment for ordinary crimes, because society can always prevent them by other means and thereby protect itself from further harm. But a deposed king at the heart of a revolution so utterly unsecured by law, a king whose very name brings down the scourge of war on a roiling nation? Neither prison nor exile can make his existence a matter of indifference for the public happiness. And this cruel exception to the ordinary laws endorsed by justice can only be imputed to the nature of his crimes.[86]

Such were the first steps toward the Terror. The king had to be killed because his sheer existence represented a constant threat to the security of the state. This was the condition of being for the city; it was also the precondition for its laws, since in this period when they did not yet exist, a death must be imposed without judgment. And while for the moment Robespierre considered this execution to be an exception, soon the same threat would be seen everywhere, tribunals would proliferate, and under the direction of the *Comité de salut public* (Committee for Public Safety), led by Robespierre and Saint-Just, the guillotine would devour the suspected enemies of the state, who now seemed, by sheer force of numbers, to represent as great a threat to the nascent republic as the king once had. "As for Louis," Robespierre called out a few moments after explaining his apparent change of heart on capital punishment, "I demand that the National Convention *immediately declare him a traitor to the French nation and a criminal toward humanity*."[87] There was a limit to the state, an infinitely narrow line between inside and out, where judgments were preemptory and death immediate. It was the thin edge of the guillotine's blade, which cleaved the individual from his idea, the living from the dead, the criminal from the city. It was, if one recalls the logic that led up to the Terror and came to be institutionalized in it, the difference that separated the human from the inhuman, reason from matter, and the intelligible from the abject. The terror of death had made possible a clean break with the unnatural crimes of the past.

The Reign of Terror against the Anarchy of Horror

The division between the city and its other was thus a privileged expression of the difference between law and nonsense. It was privileged in the sense that law—even natural law as it applied to human beings—might depend on the city to define, maintain, and enforce its legitimacy. Simultaneously, this same difference manifested itself more immediately in the distinction between two different types of fear, which thus functioned as analogues to state and statelessness, thereby translating an underlying political structure into affective terms. Although it remained untheorized, this division emerged during the Revolution as a crucial and ongoing theme. Robespierre, for instance, played on it when he demanded not only that the king be put to death, but that the memory of his execution sustain the nation across the future. "I ask," he told the Convention, "that this memorable event be hallowed by a monument destined to nourish in the hearts of all peoples the feeling of their rights and the horror of tyrants; and in the soul of tyrants, a salutary terror toward the justice of the people."[88] In his terse description of the two different publics targeted by the same monument, Robespierre imagined two, complementary emotional responses to the same event. Terror, on the one hand, is the fear inspired by the force of transcendent reason as it annihilates the individual, the feeling of the tyrant as he succumbs to the common will. Horror, on the other, is the reaction of the just state to its excluded, to the bestial forces of individualism that the king embodied. For individualism was not, within the political writings of the Enlightenment figures that Robespierre is echoing here, a heroic transcendence of the common lot, but rather a perverse attachment to appetite over reason and a consequent abnegation of one's inherent vocation to humanness. As a rejection of the commonality through which reason, the *lingua franca* of intelligibility, expressed itself, this egotism also represented a rejection of the very possibility of communication. The horror felt by the just was, in this regard, a fear not only of the unnatural and the unclean but also their repugnance toward an idiolect so personal as to be meaningless. Reason was the shared language of the group. Horror was the reaction to any threat to that language.

This distinction was also expressed in other, crucial ways. Theories of the sublime, for instance, represented one of the defining innovations of this period, and according to their most important formulations one could literally get over death—or rather, death itself was a getting over. For the sublime, at least as described by Kant in the *Critique of Judgement*, represented the accession to a higher law, the identification of the individual with the principles of reason and so with the power of abstract thought that synthesizes an otherwise inchoate and limitless world into precisely delimited concepts. But that accession to reason, to a higher freedom and a higher law, necessarily entailed, for Kant, the annihilation of the individual as individual and, concomitantly, the negation of the imaginable world. And for that reason, the awesomely destructive force of freedom was met with intense fear—which Kant calls *Schreck*, or terror—both by the individual and by everything in him or her that was still attached to the world of the senses, to the world of images and concrete specificities.[89] In this respect, reason is the death of the individual in his or her individuality. This particular death was, moreover, functionally equivalent to the state that the citizen, in Rousseau's sense, inhabited, for the citizen attained to that status by a negation of his or her particular will. And so, if the apolitical was a realm of horror, the enlightened republic was, by definition, a state of terror.

Never explicitly theorized, this fundamental distinction between two fears hovered nonetheless at the edges of consciousness during the late eighteenth and early nineteenth centuries, marking its traces surreptitiously but deeply in the imagination and across conceptual structures as different as hygiene and aesthetics. Terror was sublime, sudden, and bracing, the emotion that marked a transcendental encounter with death. Horror, on the other hand, welled up whenever the absoluteness of death seemed to be in doubt. It was slow and nauseating and attached itself not to the clear abstractions of mortality but to the deliquescent world of putrefaction. For death and the dead belonged to different ontological categories. The former was a fundamental political operator, a principle that allowed the organization of individuals into a rationalized social collective capable of making sense and of vindicating the laws of nature. But death seemed to get mired in the dead themselves, to linger excessively in their flesh, to materialize away its transcendental force, and to reveal its temporality in the slow degenerative march across the body that Bichat and others had observed.[90] One finds images of this physical entrapment throughout the literature of the nineteenth century, and despite their disparate genres and origins, they all represent attempts to think through a category essential to politics, but which could not be theorized politically since it was, precisely, the apolitical. Never entirely eradicable, the horrifying lurked like a persistent memory beneath the city that rose up in negation of it. One catches glimpses of it not only in images of the dead themselves, but in other instances, where it often betrays itself only through the reactions it provokes.

A passage from Victor Hugo's 1862 novel *Les misérables*, for instance, meticulously traces the devolution of terror into something more hideous and abject, conjuring up, as it does so, the impression of a persistent dreadfulness that informs matter itself. The scene is worth analyzing in some depth, since it shows the plasticity of horror and the way it works on aesthetic structures as basic to intelligibility as time itself. The scene takes place in the sewers of Paris, which the novel's hero, Jean Valjean, has entered in order to escape from a group of soldiers intent on killing him. One danger, however, yields to another, for in the darkness Hugo's character finds himself faced by new threats, infinitely more frightening than the ones he had avoided. The language of the sublime, such as the thunder of battle, give way to the horrifying coils of abjection. "After the blazing whirlwind of battle," Hugo wrote, "the cave of miasmas and treachery. After chaos, the cloaca."[91]

In the imagination of the city's inhabitants, the sewer, according to Hugo, is a realm of death, a place where it is paradoxically born and lives, for "it was with an almost holy dread that the masses viewed these beds of stagnation, these monstrous cradles of Death."[92] This is, therefore, an unclear, ontologically ambiguous sort of death, one that lives and that swarms with the indistinct bodies of vermin, as if its existence expressed itself in their masses: "this network of caverns has always had its immemorial population of rodents, which pullulate more than ever."[93] And although it reaches back into time immemorial, the sewer is a place of memory, a reservoir that holds the lost consciousness of the city and that remembers, in a material, degraded, but somehow more authentic form, the ancient turmoil of those above.[94] For among the relics that linger in its bowels, Hugo remarks in particular a single scrap of cloth that bears the enigmatic inscription LAVBESP. "They realized that what they held before their eyes was a piece of Marat's shroud," Hugo imagines. "In his youth, Marat had had affairs. . . . From his affair, historically attested, with a great lady, he had kept this bed sheet: wreckage or reminder."[95] Among the detritus of memory preserved beneath the streets is this frail text dating from the upheaval of the Revolution, from the originary moment of the Republic and the death of Louis XVI. But this object recalls not only the Marat of the Terror; it reaches back to an earlier period and to a glimpse of sexual intimacy, a primal scene in which the origin of the state is physically confused with the young man's loves and coitus. It is the sheet itself that binds these moments together in its material persistence, and the letters inscribed on it point to the wordless signification of their physical substrate. The sewer is not merely a place of swarming and abjection, of memory and the mysteries of origin, it is also a place where text yields to materiality, the symbolic to the semiotic.

Among the dangers of this noisome, fascinating realm, Hugo reserves one until the end, creating from it a climax of wretchedness that he had been carefully preparing through a series of staggered descriptions. In the first of these, he imagines a solitary man making his way across a vast and lonely northern beach until he gradually notices something amiss in the sand on which he has been walking. At last, the imperceptible changes progress to the point where he can no longer ignore them:

> Clearly he is not on the right path. He stops to get his bearings. All of a sudden, he looks to his feet. His feet have disappeared. The sand is covering them. He pulls his feet from the sand, he wants to retrace his steps, he turns back; he sinks more deeply. The sand rises to his ankle. He drags himself out and lunges to the left. The sand reaches to his calves. He lunges to the right and the sand reaches his knees. Then, with an unspeakable terror, he realizes that he is caught in quicksand and that he has beneath him that dreadful medium in which a man can no more walk than a fish can swim.[96]

The whole of the description builds over several pages, and in its very length, its graduated progression, and the repetition of words like *feet* it shares some of the slow temporality of the moving sands themselves. Part of their experience is imbedded in the inexorable time of the description itself, so that one cannot skip its details and repetitions without losing an understanding of their object. Like Marat's shroud, the writing turns here to its own materiality, its duration and resistance in the act of reading, its refusal to release its meaning in the synthetic timelessness of a concept or proposition. The traveler, in contrast, reacts with terror to the initial moment of recognition, when he captures his situation not as an impenetrable mystery but in a sudden realization. His terror comes simultaneously with his ability to name and conceptualize his problem as "quicksand." As the meaning of the description is attached to the slowness it imposes, the victim's terror is, conversely, linked to the instantaneity of his understanding, its clarity and intelligibility. But this initial response gives way to another fear, already suggested in the "dreadful medium" on which he finds himself. "He is condemned," Hugo writes some lines later, "to that frightful burial [*enterrement*], long, infallible, implacable, impossible to slow or hasten, that lasts hours, that does not end . . . that forces a man slowly back into the earth. Such a burial is a tomb that rises like a tide from the bottom of the earth toward a living being. Every minute is an inexorable grave-digger."[97] As it does in the description, time itself becomes palpable in the sand. It is not just that the process is slow and long, but that time changes in it: hours become endless, and the minutes themselves are transformed; they are not merely expressed in the sinking ground—like light nearing a black hole, they react as if they were trapped by the moist soil and shaped by its peculiar properties, slowing, stretching, burying. Rather than the *a priori* axis of a transcendental aesthetic grid on which experience is plotted, as in Kant's *Critique of Pure Reason*, time has become imminent here, involved in, indeed determined by the substances it is logically supposed to precede.[98] The behavior of this materialized time, even its very materialization itself, is driven by a force that rises from the lowest depths of the earth, from its most intimate and remote recesses. And those who are caught by the materialization of time are dragged down living into the heart of that earth. *Enterrés*, they are not merely buried, they also *become* earth, the hostile, minerality against which they have struggled all their lives; and what the earth hides where it is farthest from the light and the living, where it is most extremely earth, is the sepulcher and the realm of the dead. The English term *quicksand* inherently resists Hugo's efforts at depicting a viscous temporality here, since it evokes ideas of liveliness and speed, but the connection between life and quickness that the term incorporates is useful, since the peculiar movement of the sand suggests a certain animation, as if it were controlled by life itself. Only the life they embody is the life of the dead, of the blind and inexorable earth, the grim and purposeless purposiveness of the tomb.

"This funereal accident, still possible here and there along the ocean's coast," Hugo continues, "was also possible, thirty years ago, in the Parisian sewer."[99] For the description of the traveler dying on the seaside is itself only a preparation for the real description, that of the *fontis* that Jean Valjean will have to cross in the depths of the sewer. And it is here that the devolution of the original moment of conceptualizing terror reaches its nadir.

> What inexpressible horror to die in such a way! Death sometimes redeems its atrocity through a certain terrible dignity. On a pyre or in a shipwreck one can rise to greatness; among the flames or spindrift, a gesture of defiance is possible, and one is transfigured in being engulfed. But not here. Death is dirty. It is humiliating. The last, fleeting sights are abject. Mud is a synonym for shame. It is small,

ugly, vile. . . . To struggle in it is hideous; one wallows to death. . . . The dying man does not know if he will end up as a ghost [*spectre*] or a toad.[100]

Hugo now distinguishes explicitly between the two forms of death we have been discussing: on the one hand the dignity and terror of the sublime, in which the infinite abyss transfigures its victim. On the other, horror, humiliation, filth, and abjection, death as disfiguring, the death of the dead. The *fontis* is a patch of quicksand in the sewer, a culmination of misery, in which tomb seals tomb, earth and waste conjoin, and the horror of death expresses itself in a complex, physical system under the city. The one who perishes there is caught between two deaths, unsure whether he will be released from the earthly coils that squeeze around him or surrendered to them for all eternity. He hangs between the specter—pure light and Enlightenment, the clarity of thought freed of matter—and the toad, who exists in the darkness of its material sentience, thinking but unreflecting, unknowing and animal like the oyster. The *fontis* is not, in an important sense, part of the action of the novel, since the event it threatens never actually happens in the plot; instead, the story of the dying traveler is subsumed into the service of a description. Transformed in this way, it loses its apparent narrative function to become instead an instrument for revealing the nature of the sewer. The tiny story is not, in short, about its putative protagonist, but rather about the sand that devours him, not about narrative time, but about descriptive time. The abject, in this sense, seems to have a capacity for shaping texts through its peculiar affinity to description, and perhaps description should be understood in this light: a fascination with materiality, a dwelling in it, a partial submission to its slowness and blind imperiousness. This is the world of the sewer, a nightmare of living death that devours subjectivities, deforms time, and gnaws endlessly, stupidly, at the foundations of the city. And in his description of this world, Hugo offers an aesthetic analysis of a key element in the fantasmatics of contemporary hygienic programs.

A contemporary and literary rival of Hugo, Eugène Sue, elaborated similar fantasies of the abject in two passages from his wildly successful novel *Les mystères de Paris* (The Mysteries of Paris), but unlike Hugo, he conceived them in terms that derived more from contemporary discoveries in medicine and physiology than from notions of the historical past. In this sense, Sue testifies more clearly than Hugo to the effects of clinical practices on the broader public imagination, especially as they bore on ideas of abjection and death. The first of these passages appears as part of a dream, in which the sleeper has been forced to revisit his most gruesome crimes. The scene in question represents a drowning, and although its location prefigures the sewers in *Les misérables*, the dreamer's psychological state lends to his vision a hallucinatory symbolism that will be absent from Hugo's text.

> At first, one can see that the bottom of the canal is covered with a thick mud made up of innumerable reptiles normally invisible to the naked eye, but which, now enlarged as if under a microscope, take on monstrous shapes and enormous proportions relative to their actual size.
>
> It is no longer mud, it is a swarming compact mass, an inextricable, living confusion that throngs and pullulates, so densely, so tightly packed that its dull and imperceptible undulation barely raises the level of the sludge or, rather, the layer of those foul animals. [*Ce n'est plus de la bourbe, c'est une masse compacte vivante, grouillante, un enchevêtrement inextricable qui fourmille et pullule, si pressé, si serré, qu'une sourde et imperceptible ondulation soulève à peine le niveau de cette vase ou plutôt de ce banc d'animaux impurs.*]
>
> Above it, there slowly, slowly flows a turbid water, thick and dead, carrying along in its sluggish current the refuse that the sewers of a great city constantly belch up, detritus of all sorts, animal cadavers [. . .] . . .
>
> Through a crowd of bubbles that rise to the surface, he sees a woman sinking rapidly into the canal as she struggles [. . .] struggles [. . .] . . .
>
> Scarcely has the drowned woman let out her final breath, already she is covered by a myriad of microscopic reptiles, the horrible and voracious vermin of the mud [. . .]
>
> The corpse floats for a moment, still rocking slightly, then it slowly sinks, horizontally, the feet lower than the head, and starts to follow the current between two waters.
>
> From time to time, the corpse circles around with its face toward the School Master. Then the specter stares up at him with its two glaucous, glassy, and opaque eyes [. . .] its purple lips start to move [. . .][101]

The insistence on the time and materiality of the text itself that had marked Hugo's description of the *fontis* returns in this passage, where Sue slows down his description by repeating certain phrases and expanding others through a series of synonyms (for example, "*grouillante . . . qui fourmille et pullule, si pressé, si serré*"). The precision of language is at the same time undercut by this technique, which gestures toward a referent that neither *fourmille* nor *pullule* but moves in a manner lying somewhere between the nuanced differences separating these words. Even the syntax is open-ended, with sentences left unclosed by ellipses, as if the clauses did not stop but rather faded off into the unspeakable. This style is brought to bear on the description of a filthy death, and the filth itself is given an intense scrutiny in these lines. On closer examination, the mud reveals its true nature, and it does so in a way normally made possible only through scientific instruments, such as the microscope. This is, therefore, the otherwise invisible world that science has revealed to human observation—or, rather, a novelistic fantasy of the scientific gaze.[102] And what that gaze uncovers is that filth is a writhing, animate thing, a swarming mass of vermin. The cluttered canal and especially the mud that chokes it operate as a symbolic extension of the crime itself, so that, somewhat like the physiologist's microscope and scalpel, they make visible what the victim experienced as she died. Most remarkably, at the moment of death, her body succumbs to the creatures that constitute the filth surrounding her. Their appearance on her is exactly contemporaneous with her demise and as such seems to function as a manifestation of her death itself—or, more precisely, it seems to function as an image of her putrefaction, which was recognized medically at the time of Sue's writing to be the sole physical sign that reliably and invariably marked death. The seething life of filth that Sue depicts here would thus be a fantasm of rotting. More significantly—and this is the turn in the text that makes it a genuine revelation about the state of death at this historical moment—the abject creatures, as allegories of putrefaction, objectify death into something that can actually exist in itself.

This reification, which objectifies the woman's death into her surroundings and thereby establishes the two as consubstantial, reveals itself through certain details of the passage. First, Sue insists on the unusual movement of the woman's corpse in the immediate aftermath of her death, and the key elements in his description indicate some form of indirection. She moves slowly, which emphasizes the process rather than the result of her disappearance, its status as an event caught in time and material circumstances. She also sinks not vertically but horizontally, as if there were something noteworthy and repugnant in oblique motion. And she is caught between two waters. She occupies, in other words, an intermediary state, like the movements of the filth itself, which cannot be decisively described by any single word, or like the syntax, which shades off into the unspoken. Second, this ambient emphasis on indeterminacy then focuses on the figure of the corpse itself. The transparency of its eyes has failed, so that the organ that had, in a literal sense, allowed enlightenment is blocked by its own materiality. Perception, awareness, and, by figurative extension, thought are all entrapped when physical properties reassert themselves in the body. This figure of the dead nonetheless turns to speak, its lips move, and so it serves as an image of life in death, or rather, of the life of the dead. Sunk into the materiality of its own person, it has become part of its swarming but unthinking environment. In its moving lips, in its unseeing eyes, the corpse blends with its surroundings and reveals the whole passage to be the description of a place between life and death, a shadowy realm of filth where the two ontological categories cannot be distinguished. It is a depiction of the dead as putrefaction, as a liminal sentience embedded in matter itself.

This notion of a subanimate sentience is developed under a different guise much later in the novel. This second scene takes place in the psychiatric hospital of Bicêtre, a location that had become famous at the time of Sue's writing as the institution where Pinel had revolutionized the treatment and understanding of the mad. After encountering various types of monomaniacs, one of Sue's characters enters a courtyard populated by idiots, who are said by the narrator to represent the lowest state of mental incapacity into which the human mind can sink. Their infirmity deprives these creatures, according to the text, not only of their humanity but even of their animality—and yet they are alive.

> The complete absence of verbal or intelligent communication is one of the most sinister features distinguishing a group of idiots. Despite the incoherence of their words and thoughts, lunatics at least speak to each other, recognize each other, and seek each other out, but among idiots there reigns a dull indifference, an isolation that shrinks from company. One never hears them utter an articulate word, only, from time to time, some wild laughter or groans and cries that have nothing human about them. Scarcely a handful among them even recognize their keepers. And yet, let us repeat with admiration, out of respect for God's creatures, these wretches, who, by the complete annihilation of their intellectual faculties, seem no longer to be members of our species—or even to be animal—these incurably afflicted beings who seem closer to the mollusk than to an animate being and who pass in this same state through all the stages of a long life, are surrounded by solicitous attentions and a well-being they are not even aware of.[103]

The mollusk, it would seem, incarnates a sentience that is neither human, nor animal, nor even alive. A creature from the muddy ocean depths, it somehow embodies a lifeless life. Its existence is characterized by the absence of language, the inability even to make articulate noises, and the absolute isolation that results from an incapacity to recognize other beings. In this description, the idiots are seen as inhabiting the same fantasmatic zone as the invertebrate and, by extension, as putrefaction, for the mollusk is analogous to that inanimate life that had appeared in the depiction of the canal. Their consciousness, in other words, is essentially that of the drowned woman in the earlier passage—and, ultimately, of the dead as a whole. A continuum of abject sentience is thus established among idiots, corpses, rotting, and mollusks. They are all the embodiments of another, horrifying world toward which recent clinical discoveries intimated.

Some of the broader significance of this becomes apparent when one considers that Sue stood at the juncture between two types of perception. On the one hand, he was an educated and affluent member of society. In his youth, he served for six years as a military surgeon, although with a sketchy formal training and perhaps even less distinction.[104] His father, Jean-Joseph, was a prominent surgeon who descended from a long line of distinguished doctors and authored an influential study on the guillotine as well as a monograph documenting his experiments on the physiological aspects of vitality.[105] The elder Sue was particularly concerned with issues of postmortem sentience, which he framed in terms of the materiality of death, writing at the end of his "Opinion sur le supplice de la guillotine [Opinion on the Guillotine]" that "everything is alive in nature, and death, in the eyes of the naturalist philosopher, is only a state of material being."[106] In short, although he chose not to follow in the footsteps of his father, Eugène Sue grew up in a medical milieu that stretched back for generations. He was intimately aware of the issues that were currently under discussion by anatomists and pathologists, especially insofar as they concerned questions of life, death, and material sentience, and he integrated them into his novel. *Les mystères de Paris* had other connections to the higher intellectual life of the nineteenth century as well. It became, for instance, a reference point for certain philosophical circles, with Marx and Engels using analyses of the novel as the basis for an extended critique of Hegel in *The Holy Family*.[107] On the other hand, however, Sue was writing for a wide audience, and his success across different classes testified to his ability to resonate in, if not shape, the public imagination. His perception of the idiot's consciousness can thus be understood to represent a popular medical fantasy, and it is in this sense that one can take it as a historical document. As such, it represents not only an aesthetic analysis of contemporary medical thought, but also the penetration of more specialized scientific discourses into a broader social milieu. In this respect, Sue was able to represent the fantasms of horror and abjection that haunted both

the hygienic and the popular imaginations. Most importantly, in his depictions of the drowned woman and the idiot, Sue offered an image of the city's
opposite. This was the abject other from which political thinking—from Socrates and Protagoras to Rousseau, Diderot, Saint-Just, and Robespierre—
recoiled, but which it was unable to describe in any sustained detail. It is here,
in a descriptive passage from a literary text, that that other takes shape. The
drowned woman and the idiots thus offer medically informed images of the
opponent to reason and its city. They are pages from the repressed fantasm
that underlay the state.

The city, then, represented a fantasmatic construction of reason that was
defined by its distinction not so much from an other as from an abjection—a mobile and fluid category that demanded a constant vigilance. And
although the word itself was rarely used in such contexts, that abjection was
elaborated in medical terms that were then, in turn, reconsidered through
aesthetic approaches. By identifying the medical—and especially hygienic
—representations of the city as fantasmatic, we have moved those representations from the category of utility (for instance, the protection from disease) to the category of desire and, by following the "logic" of the fantasm,
to the category of meaning. The final chapter of this study will accordingly
attempt to recast the fantasmatic forces underlying the hygienic reform of
Paris more explicitly in such terms. But to do so, I will need to move away
from the historical period in question, for the problem of meaning is not
limited to, or best approached by, the documents and debates of the nineteenth century.

EIGHT

What Abjection Means

> When you feel yourself borne along by a pure and white idea, you can cross
> through the mire without getting soiled, like the swan that cleaves the water
> without dampening its feathers.
>
> —ALPHONSE ESQUIROS[1]

Death changed in early nineteenth-century Paris, and Paris, as a result, did
too. I have documented those changes as a way to establish the role of irrational, desiring forces in them and to describe the fantasmatic logics that organized that desire. The mythical city of the fantasm was, I argued, a place of
reason and indeed of truth, an axiomatic space that attempted to resolve primary ontological and epistemological problems, to give them form and some
sort of resolution, as temporary or illusory as it may be. In this respect, the
city was an instrument—in the scientific and artistic senses of the word—for
representing, grasping, and potentially resolving questions about time, memory, death, meaning, and interpersonal difference. For various reasons, however, including anxieties and the search for means to express them, these
questions were often dissimulated in other issues, which tended to frame matters of desire in terms of utility. I will now, in ending, analyze the role of
meaning in that fantasmatic structure of desire, refining my description of
the imaginary power of material death by framing it in terms of language
and subjectivity. For the question of the "meaning of meaning," to borrow

Emmanuel Levinas's disturbing formulation, seems to depend on the relation between experience and language, in which the latter term necessarily introduces the category of intersubjectivity. The abject is a breakdown of otherness and of sense. Consequently, the city, insofar as it is an instrument to control abjection, is the place—or means—by which experience is organized into something communicable and meaningful. This way of understanding the connection between abjection and the city represents a synthesis of observations I presented at the end of chapter 6, where I discussed the affinities between corpses and language, and the fantasmatic intersubjective structures that I described in chapter 7. But to develop this last part of my analysis, I will have to take some distance from the documents I have discussed so far, moving to more strictly philosophical texts and beyond the chronological limits of the eighteenth and nineteenth centuries.

The Language of Abjection

In 1964, Louis-Ferdinand Céline fulminated: "Men don't have to be drunk to ravage heaven and earth! They've *got carnage in their bones!* . . . It's a wonder they've survived, after all the time they've spent trying to reduce themselves to nothing. All they think about is nothingness, the nasty business, the little delinquents. They see red everywhere. Can't dwell on it, that would be the end of poetry."[2] For Céline, this fury to annihilate was not the personal quirk of a sociopath like Sergeant Bertrand, it was the pathology of the human itself. To be human was, for him, to think of nothing but nothing while attempting to put that nothing into practice through carnage and ravaging. Although the point is perhaps obscured by his convulsive enthusiasm, Céline is essentially reiterating what several of the most prominent philosophers of his time had already formulated in a more dispassionate way—a theory of human thought as annihilation. It was an idea that dated back at least to *The Phenomenology of Spirit*, where Hegel had described abstract language as both the truth and the negation of its sensuous referents. Using the word *now* as an example of indexing material presence, Hegel argued that simple thought experiments can demonstrate that the *now* is, in its linguistic invariability, the negation of every particular but impermanent predicate that can be applied to it (e.g. night or day), and that it is, in other words, "a *negative* in general." "[S]uch a thing," he concluded, "we call a *universal*. So it is in fact the universal that is the true [content] of sense-certainty." And it is this universal, this negating truth of sensuous existence, that we pronounce when we speak:

> It is as a universal too that we *utter* what the sensuous [content] is. . . . Of course we do not *envisage* the universal This or Being in general, but we *utter* the universal; in other words, we do not strictly say what in this sense-certainty we *mean* to say. But language, as we see, is the more truthful; in it, we ourselves directly refute what we mean to say.[3]

To those who consider it, language reveals that the material world is a nothing in the making. This is an insight that has haunted philosophy since its earliest manifestations, and even beasts, according to Hegel, are aware, on some level, of this truth, for it can be put into practice:

> Even the animals are not shut out from this wisdom but, on the contrary, show themselves to be most profoundly initiated into it; for they do not just stand idly in front of sensuous things as if these possessed intrinsic being, but, despairing of their reality, and completely assured of their nothingness, they fall to without ceremony and eat them up. And all Nature, like the animals, celebrates these open Mysteries which teach the truth about sensuous things.[4]

Like people, animals philosophize with their mouths, but instead of uttering they devour, and in so doing they reveal not just that the material world is a nullity, but also that in its relation to the world language is like eating.[5] We consume the sensuous with our words, phenomenalizing its inherent nothingness. But there is a paradox here: if the world of our senses has no being, how can we annihilate it? This passage is troubled by an elusive something that neither is nor is not, that cannot be said to exist and yet awaits destruction. For all of its vacuity, there must be something to speak about, to eat. This is a something that never entirely disappeared from the legacy Hegel left and that continued to trouble reappropriations of his work.

The return of Hegel in the mid-twentieth century was accompanied by an increased acceptance of his notion that thought is a form of negative abstraction. As Alexandre Kojève argued in his epoch-making seminars on the *Phenomenology*: "Hegel's method is an *eidetic abstraction* (Husserl). He considers a concrete man or a concrete epoch, but in order to discover in it the possibility (i.e. the 'essence,' the 'concept,' the 'idea,' etc.) that is realized in it."[6] Hegel's approach, according to Kojève, is to consider a concept at the expense of a concrete reality, and in this his method is itself only a particular—if particularly perfected—example of human spirit in general. Like Hegel's system, intellect by its very nature essentializes its object. It intervenes in the world not only as will and creative force, changing what was before it into a human artifact—i.e. not merely by physically shaping it—but, more importantly, by the sheer event of thinking itself, which occurs as the negative sign of the world it designates.[7] In essentializing its object, thought abolishes the object's difference from thought, negates the object as something other than itself, and consequently annihilates it as a concrete reality. Intellect is, in Sartre's word, "nihilating."[8]

As an annihilation, thought does not merely eat, it also kills; or as Kojève phrased it, "a human being . . . is death living a human life."[9] From this proposition, he deduced that human beings need war to ground themselves morally and epistemologically. "So it is really murderous war that assures the historical liberty and the free historicity of Man," he wrote. "Man is historic only to the extent that he actively participates in the life of the State, and that participation culminates in the voluntary risk of life in a purely political war. So it is that man is only truly historical to the extent that he is a warrior, at least potentially."[10] It should be clear that Kojève is not speaking about the necessity of war in terms of contingent, historically specific threats that only a military intervention could defend against, since in his terms, history is not a prerequisite for battle; it is, rather, the other way around, with history being an effect of war. Only by exercising its essential negativity on itself through armed conflict can the human achieve the condition of humanity. Like Céline, Kojève contends that man has war in his fibers, but if war is, in its historical and human significance, an essentialization—a transformation of matter into thought—then any essentialization should be able to fulfill the same human historical function. This was, in fact, an idea that gained currency in the aftermath of World War II.[11] Maurice Blanchot, one of Kojève's students, clearly articulated this more subtle way of understanding the relation between human thought and destructive essentialization when, in 1949, he wrote: "A word gives me what it signifies, but by first suppressing it. For me to be able to say 'this woman,' I have to somehow take her flesh-and-blood [*chair et os*] reality away from her, making it absent and annihilating it." To name is to kill, and from this he concludes: "So it is precisely accurate to say that when I speak, death speaks in me."[12] For Blanchot, speaking is already a "hecatomb."[13] But if thought itself is annihilation, why go to the trouble of actually engaging in combat, dirtying and disemboweling oneself on a field of battle or in the muddy trenches of the front? Why do anything but think? Why this excessive killing in the flesh, when flesh and blood—*chair et os*, as Blanchot puts it—are already banished in the words that designate them? The answers to these questions come only obliquely, if at all, and force a consideration of the flesh that is left over from the putative sublimity of war and that war, despite its putative sublimity, requires.[14] They demand an investigation of that nothing that is not quite nothing and that haunts the Hegelian annihilation.

For war to be necessary, there would have to be some negation that language could not accomplish, something left over from what Blanchot calls the "hecatomb" of naming, a remnant that would put the carnage into man's fibers. Blanchot himself identified such a linguistic excess, a surplus that naming could not reach: "Negation can only be effected on the basis of the reality of what it negates. Language draws its value and pride from being the accomplishment of that negation; but to start with, what has it lost? The torment of language is what it lacks [*manque*] by having to be its lack [*manque*]. It cannot even name it."[15] In order to exercise its essential function as negation, language—the human—demands something to negate, a positivity without which there would be no language and no human; but language, precisely because it is a lack (*manque*), misses (*manque*) what it is structured to negate, and this "missing" has the double sense of a perceived absence and the inability to attain a goal. Language cannot reach what it aims for because it is structured as the absence (or negation) of that goal, and by its very structure language is therefore inherently *manqué*, or a failure. Since to name is to negate, that something that words by their very essence cannot abolish is unnamable. The reality of discourse, Blanchot states, depends on the reality of this unspeakable leftover, while the value and pride of language depend on the impossible annihilation of that same remnant. Beyond the reach of words there is, then, a reality that supports the negative reality we speak, and this unspeakable, primordial existence torments language with its tantalizing nearness and absolute absence. For its archaic age, this absent something is astonishingly nimble—as in a nightmare, every time we get it in our sights and fire a name at it, we find we've missed. But what would happen if we hit? Since the reality of discourse depends on the reality of that other, the negation of our target would logically entail our own negation as speakers and as human beings.

Still, language exists as the endlessly frustrated attempt to name that unnamable. The terms and structure of Blanchot's argument recall the way Lacan formulated the relation between language and desire, where the latter exists as the ineradicable difference between a need and its expression.[16] Like Hegel, who argued that "it is just not possible for us ever to say, or express in words, a sensuous being that we *mean*," Lacan saw speech as inevitably missing what we want to convey. Since it is by nature alienating, language invariably estranges needs from the needy, expresses them always as the wants of an other, and thereby creates a discrepancy between the preverbal and the verbalized need. In the case of Lacan, as in the case of Blanchot, language by its very essence engenders an inexpressible excess as a byproduct of its attempts to articulate something. That excess, that postlinguistic remainder of frustrated need that Lacan calls desire, is what Blanchot names "torment." This suffering is what literature, according to Blanchot, attempts to assuage, and to calm the frustrations of an impotent utterance it tries to reach that intractable remnant that language, by its very nature, cannot attain. And when literature tries to grasp what other forms of discourse cannot, it finds itself, like the young Socrates, confronted by an abyss in the dirt. It is a grave that opens:

> The language of literature is the search for the moment that precedes it. Generally, it names that moment existence; it wants the cat as it exists, the pebble in its commitment to being a thing [*le galet dans son parti pris de chose*], not man, but this one here, and in this one here what man rejects to say him, which is the basis of language and which language excludes in order to speak: the abyss, the Lazarus of the grave and not the Lazarus come back to the daylight, the one who already smells bad, who is bad, the lost Lazarus and not the saved and resuscitated Lazarus.[17]

What language misses and literature tries to supply, the desire and torment of the human condition—of Kojève's "death living a human life"—is a corpse. The poetics of Francis Ponge, alluded to in the expression "*parti pris de chose*," the nausea with existence that the "*galet*," or pebble initiates in Sartre's *Nausea*, literature, the Hegelian formulation of language as the annihilating essence of the sensuous world that Blanchot is addressing in these passages, Lacanian desire, the Kojévian construction of the human—all are, in Blanchot's terms, necrophilic. Not in the sense of loving death, but of loving the dead. They long not for the sublimated essences that slough off earthly existence, since they cannot help but produce such essences anyway, since it is their very nature to sublimate in this way; they want instead the body moldering at the bottom of the pit, its "dark, cadaverous reality."[18] This is no longer the purity of a structural differential, like Lacan's notion of desire. This is desire as a precise but complex figure, rich in associations, pungent. Hegel, in his *Aesthetics*, dismissed the Romantic movement as a chasing after empty tombs; Blanchot, conversely, argued that literature and philosophy are by their very nature an excavation of occupied ones.[19] The endlessly frustrating object of their desire, he asserts, is a corpse. It is, moreover, a corpse that is already beginning to smell bad. This is no embalmed effigy that he is describing here, no theatrically preserved Madame Necker, nor are these the mummified remains that the sign entombs, according to Hegel's semiotics.[20] Instead, language is structured for Blanchot as the craving for something far more troubling, something that, despite all the endless, unrequitable desire it engenders, fills its beholder with a profound uneasiness. The corpse is malodorous and repellent and yet we long for it with every word we speak.

At certain moments, however, the excavation succeeds, at least partially, and the subterranean world breaks through, even within the works of writers whom Kojève had taught, like Georges Bataille and Maurice Blanchot himself. The latter imagined, for instance, something left over from the linguistic negation of the sensuous world, something that returns within the very language that denies it. That remnant is the materiality of words themselves. Even within my utterances, the object of my naming does not simply and purely disappear. "The word *cat*," Blanchot observed, "is not merely the nonexistence of the cat, but that nonexistence made *word*, which is to say a perfectly determinate and objective reality."[21] In this sense, the corpse, what language excludes, reappears in a discourse that at once longs for and repulses it, a discourse that the dead body fills with insatiable desire and unfinishing disgust. Blanchot elaborates on this return:

> Then what hope is there for me to reach what I push away? In the materiality of language, in the fact that words are also things, a kind of nature, something that is given me and that gives me more than I can understand. Just a moment ago, the reality of words was an obstacle. Now, it is my only hope. The name stops being the ephemeral passage of nonexistence to become a solid ball, a block of existence; language, abandoning the meaning that it wanted only to be, tries to make itself meaningless. All that is physical moves to the forefront: rhythm, weight, mass, figure, and then the paper on which one writes, the trace of ink, the book. Yes, fortunately [*par bonheur*], language is a thing: it is a written thing, a scrap of bark, a piece of a clothing, a clay fragment in which the reality of the earth subsists.[22]

Language itself is not all meaning. Its negative, semantic force depends on words, which have, themselves, a sensuous determinacy, a feel and heft. Utterance and writing exist beyond their essence, since words are spoken in a time and place, under certain accents and conditions; since they are inscribed on substances that, when unfamiliar, shock us with their clumsy materiality: a napkin, a shirtsleeve, the back of a hand, a clay tablet that the archeologist surprises in its shroud of dirt. Language is a thing that includes its own unnamable nonsense, its gurgling and rhythm that have no meaning, its Lewis Carroll and Antonin Artaud.[23]

The corpse is poetry, the interruption of signification by the music of words. It is the rhythm, the weight and feel of syllables, their physicality—literature, in Blanchot's sense—and the feel of language in an infant's mouth as it crows with pleasure at the very possibility of creating sounds.[24] But at times its materiality interrupts my speech more completely, surprising me with its forgotten physicality, not just in those moments when it seduces me, as when I am delighted by the accents and timbre of a certain voice or the rhythms of a poem. It is also, less pleasingly, the words that stick in my throat, that gag me like a "solid ball," as Blanchot puts it, and that threaten to smother me. It is the "something strange that looked like a tube of parchment" and that asphyxiated Eugène Arnoux the night before a tumbrel filled with bodies set off across the Paris of Flaubert's *Education sentimentale*.[25] "He seemed to be puffing out his words" the novelist wrote.[26] That "something strange" and unnamable, like a substance on which words are inscribed, returns to steal words away, to silence the speaker, and take his life. A short while before the cadavers of history bring history to a standstill, a little boy chokes on the dead body of language. He cannot breathe. He cannot speak. This too is the corpse: the moment when words stifle and murder their speaker. Poetry brings a weight and a rhythm to utterance. It can fill the throat and mouth with a materiality that always threatens me and towards which all my language is aimed.[27]

Certain authors from the period around Kojève, such as Artaud or Céline, offered a more commonplace vision of the cadaverous and subterranean force that is at work in language. It is in this respect that Julia Kristeva's *Pouvoirs de l'horreur* [Powers of Horror] presented Céline as the exemplary modern writer of the abject, arguing that his entire literary output was oriented towards death and massacre, which were, in turn, most fully realized in the figure of the corpse. "It is the human cadaver," she wrote, "that provides the place where abjection and fascination reach their most intense concentration. All of Céline's stories converge towards a site of massacre or death."[28] But if the corpse gives direction to Céline's writing, making his work testify to the torment of language and the allure of its unnamable object, it is not primarily through a thematics that it does so. Rather, the corpse, in the sense that Blanchot means it, is most present in the text at precisely those moments when its thematics are disrupted, when another aspect of language overwhelms its semantic function. Some of this eruption is visible in Céline's description of the human drive to war.

> They've *got carnage in their bones!* . . . All they think about is nothingness, the nasty business, the little delinquents. They see red everywhere. Can't dwell on it, that would be the end of poetry.

> *Ils* ont le carnage dans les fibres*!* . . . *Ils pensent qu'au néant, méchants clients, graines à crime! Il voient rouge partout! Faut pas insister, ça serait la fin des poèmes.*[29]

The text is marked by a superficial incoherence in the grammar and syntax that is offset by a more palpable rhythm and affective expressiveness. The passage is structured around a series of ejaculations, punctuated by exclamation points, that disrupt grammatical structures (the missing *ne*, in *"ils pensent qu'au néant,"* for instance, or the absent *Il* of *"Faut pas . . ."*) and proliferate metaphors (*"méchants clients, graines à crime"*). While Kojève, say, can rise to a memorable formulation ("a human being . . . is death living a human life," for example), his description of war maintains a tone of studied detachment, in which the horrifying fatality of his propositions is untroubled syntactically or grammatically by any apparent effect those pronouncements might have on the author's ability to communicate them.[30] By contrast, there is something else, destructive in its own right, that intervenes in Céline's text: a violence disrupts it that does not appear in Kojève—or rather, in Kojève's writing, that violence exists primarily on the semantic level of the signified, whereas in Céline it intervenes powerfully on the level of the signifier. The lifeless body of language forces its way into the foreground of discourse at moments like these, occluding the possibility of meaning and obstructing the abstractive power of signification.

The corpse, as I mentioned, is a precise but complex figure, rich in associations and pungent. Artaud tried to capture that pungency in his own writing. "*I don't like poems or superficial styles of language* that breath of happy leisure and intellectual success," he stated.[31] Instead he was drawn to what Blanchot called the other Lazarus, "the one who already smells bad, who is bad," to the literary stench of decay, and for this reason he criticized Lewis Carroll's style of nonsense as an effete toying with the genuinely disturbing powers of language:[32]

You can invent your own language and make pure language speak with a meaning that goes beyond grammar, but it has to be valid in itself, which is to say that it comes from anguish [*affre* (*sic*)] . . . When you dig down into the caca of being and of its language, the poem has to smell bad, and [Carroll's] Jabberwocky is a poem that the author has been very careful to keep away from the uterine being of suffering, that place where every great poet has bathed and where, in giving birth, he smells bad. There are passages of fecality in Jabberwocky, but it's the fecality of an English snob, who likes his fecality in ringlets, as if he curled it with a curling iron . . . It's the work of a man who ate well, and you can smell it in his writing.[33]

According to Artaud, the problem with Carroll is that his excrements smell too good. A class consciousness inhibits him from fully delving into the abject depths of existence and incorporating them into a poetic language that they would irreparably disfigure. A social fastidiousness translates itself into his writing, maintaining a sense of decorum even within its excesses, and for that reason his poetry falls short of greatness.

Still, unlike the plastic aspects of language that Blanchot described, the stench of poetry that interests Artaud can only be taken metaphorically. Words have a physicality, but they do not smell. They sound, they seize you by the throat, or they take up space, inscribed somewhere, on something concrete—to be words they must; they cannot do their work of semantic negation without sounding, without rasping in the throat, without filling a written surface. But they do not need to smell in order to function. They may, but it is not inevitable that they will. And while the music and tangibility of language will always recompense the annihilating force of its meaning, its odor, on the other hand, comes and goes. The smells of breath or leather cannot be written down or captured in the syntax of a phrase, will not always accompany and belie the words that negate them. The sounds and rhythms of discourse can be fixed in poetry, their shapes in calligrams, but their scent escapes. Blanchot himself wrote, "I call passionately for . . . that scent crossing through me and that I cannot breathe": he can conjure only an absent smell, its mere idea, but this, again, is just the annihilation of that smell.[34] The cadaver, on the other hand, reeks. Once it rots, it lets out a stench, and, conversely, as the miasma theorists argued, all that decays and stinks is cadaverous. The corpse is defined by its relation to a certain odor. The pungency of decomposing flesh that fills the tomb and the battle field, or that rises from my body on a summer's day, this is the index of that other Lazarus, "the bad one," towards whose subterranean existence intelligible language futilely tends. It is the smell of the dead that marks to me the opening of another realm, the elsewhere of fulfilled desires but also, perhaps, the place where "I" melts away into something formless and unspeakable. It is not Carroll's fault that his language does not stink. His failing is instead that he was not sufficiently troubled by the impossibility of language to capture that sensuous plenitude, that he was complacent about its ability to physically betray its own semantic import. This is the "anguish" of which Artaud writes, the "torment" that Blanchot describes: the refusal to accept language's incapacity to smell. The great poet is the one who suffers as long as possible the odorlessness of words, who forces language against itself in the delirious and futile attempt to make them stink. And not just to smell, but to smell bad, like excrement or corpses, because the cadaver is the figure of linguistic desire.

Death is clean and annihilating; it converts concrete reality into concepts and has no odor, since it is the absence of sensation.[35] The dead, in contrast, are filthy and foul-smelling leftovers. Death elicits terror, the affect of sublimity that accompanies, for theorists like Kant and Burke and Schiller, the translation of apprehension into comprehension, of the sensuous and imaginable into the conceptual and intelligible. The dead, on the other hand, fill us with horror, a queasy mix of disgust and fear, the anxiety that the corruptible material world could penetrate through our senses to infect our insubstantial being. This distinction between the clean and the foul informs the very words we speak at their most basic level; it is the primordial difference of language itself, its relation to all that it is not. Or, as Blanchot formulates it, the difference between death and the dead, between sublimation and corpse, is the difference between language and the reality on which it depends. Every time we open our mouths to speak we are making this distinction, separating between death and the dead with the thin and tenuous line of words. The torment of language is that the line holds, and we forever miss what we want to say. Its *bonheur*, or happiness, on the other hand, is that it does not hold altogether, and that the physical sensuousness of that absent object of desire can return in the materiality of words themselves. What Blanchot did was try to round out the picture of Hegel's philosophical animals. In the *Phenomenology*, they were only mouths, and philosophy itself a disillusioned devouring that revealed the nullity of the sensuous world. Hegel wrote as if animals did not defecate, but they do, and their other end reveals, for its part, a certain insistence of the material, a cloaca of discourse where the feces of an entire human existence is its corpse, that indigestible something that remains after having been spiritually masticated for a lifetime. Hegel's metaphor, when we turn it around, depicts philosophy as coprophagy and sarcophagus, the unending attempt to consume its own final leftovers.

Hegel's conflation of uttering and eating disguises a potential disorder in the very language of philosophy, a disorder that is evidenced and celebrated in literature—in the works of Carroll and Artaud for instance. In analyzing their poetry, Gilles Deleuze argued that language is divided between transcendence and materiality and that this divide is meaning itself. "Things and statements stand less in a radical duality than on both sides of a border represented by meaning. That border does not mix them or join them (it is not more a case of monism than of dualism), it is more like the articulation of their difference: body/language."[36] And since the things and bodies that are excluded from propositional discourse can all be considered "consumable" objects, he adds: "from this stems the alternative that runs through all of Lewis Carroll's works: eat or speak."[37] Whereas for Hegel uttering and devouring are equivalent philosophical operations, for Deleuze they would represent two opposite aspects of language. The work of philosophy, of intelligibility, would, as a result, be the labor to maintain the line that separates those two aspects:

> It is this new world, of incorporeal or surface effects, that makes language possible. For, as we shall see, it is what draws sounds out of their simple state as bodily actions and passions; it is what distinguishes language, what prevents it from getting confused with the noises of the body, what abstracts it from their oral-anal determinations. . . . It is the expressed, in its autonomy, that grounds language or expression, which is to say, the metaphysical property that sounds acquire and that lets them have a meaning and, secondarily, to signify, manifest, designate, instead of belonging to bodies like physical qualities. . . . Language is made possible by the border that separates it from things, from bodies, not least of which are the bodies of those who speak.[38]

The body is the end of language, wracked by the partial objects that Melanie Klein observed in the fantasmatic worlds of children:

> Orality, the mouth, and the breast are at first bottomless depths. . . . The introjection of partial objects into the infant's body is accompanied by a projection of aggressivity toward internal objects and a reprojection of these objects into the maternal body. In this way, the introjected elements are also like venomous and persecutory substances, explosive and toxic, that threaten the child's body from inside while ceaselessly reconstituting themselves in the mother's body. This makes a perpetual re-introjection necessary. . . . And orality naturally extends into forms of cannibalism and anality in which the partial objects are excrements

capable of blowing up the bodies of both the mother and the child. . . . Bodies explode and make others explode in this system of the mouth-anus, or of the food-excrement, this universal cloaca.[39]

If language is understood in these terms, philosophy is not merely the frenetic and unending attempt to devour its own feces, it is the attempt to eat them before they can, for their part, destroy philosophical—i.e. propositional—discourse. The two aspects of language are not laid inertly one next to the other; they are, instead, mutually antagonistic, such that the vertigo of the body, like the abyss that the young Socrates glimpsed, threatens to overwhelm meaning and convert the intelligible into the physical, the organic, and the bodily. The opposition is therefore not so much eat or speak as it is speak or rot. Although language cannot reach the cadaver, cannot capture its smell in words, the cadaver, for its part, constantly threatens to contaminate language. Language, as Deleuze describes it, is thus caught in an endless bind along the border separating its coprophilic physicality from its conceptual transcendence. That border does not have a meaning, according to him—it *is* meaning. This is the place where language signifies. Meaning is produced in the contact of statement and corpse, in the reluctant desire for its smell, in the ambivalence of revulsion and delight. This is the meaning of meaning, the logic of sense.

Corpse and Subject

Robespierre put his fellow legislators on guard against what he called "the abjection of the individual 'I' [*l'abjection du moi personnel*]."[40] The mouthpiece of the Terror promulgated an impersonal "I," an agency of no one in particular, purified from the filth of individuality. Reason, the general will, a proto-Habermasian community of rationalized communication would supplant the tyrannies of capricious individual taste that had dominated the *ancien régime*. I am dead, and only so do I attain the right to speak and legislate: as the negation of my particularity, of my abjection.[41] True to his word, the "incorruptible," as he was known to his fellow revolutionaries, met his death at the guillotine, that most insubstantial of executions known at the time, an imperceptible intervention of the abstract into the commerce of the city, so sudden it could not, according to contemporaries, be either felt or seen.[42] The citizen-subject that Robespierre personified enacted its own sublimation by converting itself into the language of a purified and general thought. "The individual consciousness . . .," Hegel wrote of the Terror, "has put aside its limitation; its purpose is the general purpose, its language universal law, its work the universal work."[43] The citizen is an abstraction of its own individuality. It is its own death as a person and resurrection as an impersonal. The guillotine is infallible, regardless of whose head should fall, for the executed is always either a revolutionary or a counter-revolutionary. In the second case, the punishment was just and necessary to preserve the Republic, and in the first harmed no one, since all that was touched was the individuality of the victim, which had already been willingly sacrificed when he or she assumed free and impersonal citizenship. The citizen had attained, as Kojève put it, "the political right to death."[44] And then, writing in the long shadow of the French Revolution, Hegel, according to Kojève, uttered a truth that no philosopher had yet even glimpsed: human existence, all human existence, is "death living a human life."[45]

Since the time of the French Revolution, the history of the subject has been the protracted conceptualization of a human agency that dominates the material world through thought, especially an annihilating thought. It is a history that can be traced from theories of the sublime in Kant and Schiller and Burke through Hegel to Heidegger and to Kojève and then to all those whom Kojève's readings of Hegel influenced, such as Blanchot and Georges Bataille and Jacques Lacan.[46] Like an amplified version of Hegel's proposition, "Now is the night," my self-sameness, my immaterial constancy to myself as a subject over time refutes every temporal experience or condition that can be predicated of me, indeed, every experiential particularity. I am death: my own death. But the figure of the corpse traces a counter-history, or rather, the a-history of a nonsubjective existence. It is a thinking imbedded in what the subject excludes, in the impurities and filth and materiality of the inhuman world. Corpses are still not perceived as utterly dead, and for that reason we are obliged to them, treat them with care or deference, and fear their unsolicited return in moments of personal crisis or historical upheaval. In them, death is not an absolute or an epistemological premise on which anything can be grounded with certainty: too bad for abstract individuality, for subjects, and for the modern, democratic polis that they permit. The dead have faces and eye-sockets that seem to stare. They look as if they were able to return our gaze, although we know they cannot, and with their resemblance to people, it is difficult not to imagine that cadavers retain some sort of consciousness as they rot into the dirt, offering the image of a thinking that defies both death and the limits of the subject.

The corpse oozes: it must have been a familiar experience during a period when vigils were held at home and the body washed by members of the family. There would have been an intimacy with the dead, with how they leak and fall apart and yet retain the name and semblance of a friend, with how they write their nonsense across the blank sheets in which the living wrap them. And yet, for all its impenetrable mystery, theirs still seems to be a language. It is scrawled on the shroud by a subject beyond meaning: that subject without subjectivity that can be glimpsed in the fantasmatics of the corpse, that flows like the gases and fluids seeping from its body, that collects like a miasma. When the dead return our gaze, they do so with a consciousness based on the imagery of a decomposing body, speaking a language that fills us with an endlessly strange and unintelligible longing, like Flaubert at Poittevin's deathbed. The "I" that is projected onto the dead, as Robespierre said, is abject. It is embedded in their corrupted bodies. It comes not with the cleanness of terror but with a filthy and lingering horror, a *dé-terreur*. The language of the Revolution and its citizen-subject, Hegel wrote, is the universal language. The language of the corpse is the specificity of a certain stain or smear. When the guillotine severs a head, no one dies, but when we look at a corpse, someone unspeakably particular looks back.

In *Pouvoirs de l'horreur*, Julia Kristeva presented the cadaver as not only the *déchet*, or leftover, par excellence, but also as the final degree of revulsion, the summum of the abject. She described the effects of this abjection on our concept and experience of subjectivity:

> No, like a theater of the real, without make-up or mask, detritus and the cadaver *indicate* to me what I permanently push aside in order to live. These humors, this filth, this shit are what life tolerates only barely and on pain of death. Here, I am at the limits of my status as living being. From these limits, my body emerges as living. These bits of detritus [*déchets*] drop off in order for me to live, until, loss by loss, there is nothing left for me, and my body falls entirely beyond the limit, *cadere*, cadaver. If filth means the other side of the limit where I am not and which allows me to be, the cadaver, the most sickening of detritus, is a limit that has invaded everything.[47]

Like the miasmas of digestion that threatened the Enlightenment imagination with fantasies of a mortal putrefaction cohabiting our bodies, the corpse that Kristeva describes already dwells in me and disrupts my sense of subjective definition, threatening me in my very self. With their ripe putrescence, the dead, as Kristeva observes, never cease menacing the limits of the "I" and threatening to dissolve the finitude that gives to amorphous living the form, meaning, and communicability of subjective experience. The corpse, smelling now of excrement and rot, pushes ever nearer, smearing with its messy touch the lines that make of me a someone and not a something. The swollen body of the dead does not wait patiently elsewhere for me to die. It is not another. It is I, since the corpse is always already here, none other than this body that is mine, this body that will survive me, that I think of as subordinate but that will remain after I last close my eyes. It is the remnant that comes from before, that persists after, and on which I inscribe myself, like words in a book.[48] Only through a constant vigilance do I keep it at bay, expulsing it with a verbal stream and by the careful elaboration of an "I." The abyss that Socrates had seen opening in the dirt has moved infinitely close with Kristeva, but already Parmenides had foreseen this intimacy, since he spoke not just of mud and dirt, but also hair. It seems strange to include this last term in the list of formless things, since hairs touch close to the limit of the immaterial and their fine linearity seems more closely related to a pen stroke, to the subtle *trait*, or feature that gives contour and identity, than it is to the blotchy mass of moist earth that defies form.[49] But the sloughed whisker remains as a trace of the body, and thence of the body itself as trace and residue. The hair, like fingernails, pushes up with its own autonomous activity inside my body, and I cannot help suspecting that it will continue after I am gone. Nor am I the only one who has suspected as much, since the legends abound of graves dug up that yielded coffins filled with hair and where the decomposed bodies were ringed around with fingernails that would not stop growing after death.[50] In French *ça pousse*—it grows. But also, *ça pousse* means it pushes. The body, as it grows and follows its own history from conception to decay, presses against "I," threatening to force me out, to exclude me, as Kristeva writes. The corpse is already here, in short, menacing not only my language, but also my existence as a finite subject. Anything that cannot be put into words lingers like an odor—but not like any odor; it is the smell of the dead, the frightening, amorphous autonomy of my own body that words cannot annihilate.

That smell carries with it the threat of becoming like a corpse, of yielding a Kantian, rational and categorically structured consciousness to a corpse-consciousness, a consciousness that exists not as the Hegelian negation of the physical, natural world, but on the model of that world. The dead are thought in a mess, figured as the decaying body, and to the extent that the cadaver and hygiene are both metaphors of consciousness, the cemetery objectifies an internal subjective limit, the limit of subjectivity itself. This corpse-being, this corpse-thinking frightens with its transgressivity and its easy availability at all moments. It beckons with its very facility: come to me, embrace me, risk the peril of being me. It is breathtakingly close: in one's feces, one's belly, in the very structures of one's thought. And a horrible fear attends its seductions, a fear whose origins and motivation cannot be explained, until one can account for the desirability of being a subject in the first place. At most it is possible, for the moment, to speculate that in a world unmoored from the absoluteness of death and in which individual experience can no longer be organized through mortal subjectivity, the category of the individual begins to fail, taking with it all that is familiar, and then the "I" itself. All whom we know die there, including the one who knows them. All the bonds of love are falsified and what remains is dreadfully alone, a vagrant consciousness that collects meaninglessly here and there, like miasmas in the cellar.

This fear dates back at least to the Enlightenment. Rather than founding or confirming the integrity of human individuality, as it does in Hegel, Kojève, or Heidegger, death as it was viewed by the Encyclopedists was a vaguely limited condition that tended instead to decompose that individuality, for if death itself is indeterminate, if it is not itself a clean break, it cannot ground absolute distinctions, whether they be the difference between thought and matter or the limits of the individual subject. Once the fantasmatics of the cadaver have blurred the lines of demarcation, personhood can be established neither through bodily integrity nor through mortality. The limits of the individual living entity are open not merely because death itself is a vague limit, but also because it is communicable among such entities. The barriers of the body, like those of the tomb, will never be perfectly sealed; the dead will always, eventually, spread their condition to the living; no one resists forever. Fecal matter, that concentrated slough of cadaverousness from which we must try to distance ourselves daily, is, as Mathieu Géraud wrote in 1786, "heterogeneous to our individuality."[51] Heterogeneous, but not heterogeneous enough, for it threatens to slip the boundaries between that individual and its surroundings.

By its very nature, then, the cadaver is a menace, and for Kristeva it indicates with its crude nakedness what "I" must permanently hold off, or *écarter*, in order to live, as if the corpse were always reaching at me, always trying to get hold of my person and reduce me to its level. It is, in her estimation, the most nauseating of detritus not only because it signals to me the other side of a limit that I must maintain in order to persist as "I," but also because it constantly tends, in its mindlessly unintentional way, to ooze over its borders and to expel the "I" from the determinacy that makes of it a finite, singular "I," this "I." "The cadaver," she writes, "considered without God and out-side of science, is the pinnacle of abjection. It is death infesting life. Abject. It is refuse that one cannot get rid of, that one cannot protect against, the way you can with an object. An imaginary strangeness and a real threat, it calls to us and ends up by swallowing us."[52] The dead, in Kristeva's theory of abjection, are far from inert, for they appeal to us, reach for us, act on us, and insinuate themselves into our being. Restlessly they call and press, like insis-tent offspring refusing to be abandoned, or like intractable remnants that stick to us after we thought we had finished with them. For Enlightenment theorists, the hygienic issues raised by the corpse were only more intense versions of those already associated with fecal matter. More generally, the dead body is that which is excreted and left over from the person as a whole. It is the slough of his or her living existence, and, conversely, when we defe-cate, we see ourselves mirrored as cadavers. It is the erotized substance of a consciousness following our existence, of a living subsequent to our subjectiv-ity, that is reflected in the fecal world. Freedom from the terrifying and abstract subject is figured in a homunculus of our inadvertent creation, for in the verticality of the fecal stick we see the image of our own bilateral symme-try.[53] It is a puppet form that functions, as Freud argued, equivalently to a baby in the infantile imagination; and babies in turn are thought, by way of analogy, to originate in the anus.[54] The puppet child returns to us an image of ourselves, and that image implies a consciousness, at once too disturbing to be tolerated and too fascinating not to become a potent social and subjective operator.

Discourse, for Hegel, consumes sensuous existence, but the devoured returns in feces and corpses. The "I," as discursive entity, must constantly, vigilantly defend itself against the reappearance of an indestructible and non-discursive materiality, the excremental accumulations of its thought, the miasmas left over from its annihilating relation to the world. The subject is haunted by the fear of this remnant. So it is that at the same historical moment when subjectivity is most sharply brought into focus as a social, political, and epistemological category, the issue of hygiene simultaneously attains its most intense currency in social discourse and behavior. The rise of death-based subjectivity in the nineteenth century is attended by the unprec-edented appearance of modern hygiene as a generalized social program.[55] The filthy threat to the subject takes shape in the imaginary form of a rotting person, a character that embodies the fantasm of a linguistic but unintelligible consciousness. This figure, in turn, provokes powerful but contradictory affects in its creator: revulsion and unspeakable longing. Inscribed in the very materiality of language, the cadaver intimates a consciousness beyond language, a thinking that is alien and frightful, but that also beckons us—in perhaps its only recognizable gesture—to join it.

The Other Ends

For Kristeva, then, abjection does not just create an ambiguity between life and death, it also threatens subjectivity. At the same time that it confuses the distinction between thought and matter, it blurs the line separating "I" from what is not "I." In its affectively charged materiality, it forces the question: "How can I be without a limit?"[56] The fear seems to be that without limits I would cease to exist. In one sense, this is true. The subject is a product of its limits and is able to give meaning to its experiences through that determinacy. But the fear of the abject—even if it is associated with death—is not that it will kill me, since the fear of death confirms the limitations of the subject and reinforces it as a structuring principle. Indeed, a dominant post-Enlightenment current of thought has, as I have observed, understood the subject to result from the permanent threat of an inevitable and absolute end of consciousness. But if one accepts such a concept of subjectivity, then the converse must be true as well, and this is the problem that Kristeva attaches to the abject. Once the end of consciousness is uncertain or vague, the subject falls apart. That falling apart is not dying, at least not in the terrifying sense of an absolute vanishing. Instead, it is a decomposition of identity in which the subject's consciousness continues, but outside of itself. The subject, consequently, can therefore be understood as a withholding of consciousness from material things, a refusal to be determined by them. Insofar as that materiality can have its own sentience, subjectivity is also a will to establish limits to what thinking is me and what thinking is not.

The materiality of the abject can take subtle forms, such as language. One thinks of Blanchot, Lewis Carroll, Artaud, and Céline and their fascination with the physical properties of linguistic expression, its dangers and attractions. But the objective aspect of language that they refer to supports another, ghostlier form of materiality, what one might call a quasi-materiality. This is the impersonal objectivity of words, the way in which they continue to move before, among, and after the individuals that use them. Ideas themselves are passed around without anyone being able to identify where they came from, or they acquire their apparent validity through their sheer, anonymous circulation. This is the *Gerede*, or idle chatter that Heidegger censured so severely in *Being and Time*.[57] These are also the received ideas that filled Flaubert with contempt and that he tried to master by organizing them into a dictionary.[58] Indeed, the past itself, insofar as it impinges insidiously on the present, is part of that thinking that is both "I" and not "I," and for that reason is revolting. The received ideas, the work of previous generations that is handed down and lingers in the present to disturb the originality and self-definition of the subject, open its borders to the past and the dead. To become a subject is, therefore, to determine the difference between this preexisting material and one's own self. Hegel described this process in the preface to the *Phenomenology of Spirit*: "This past existence is the already acquired property of universal Spirit which constitutes the Substance of the individual, and hence appears externally to him as his inorganic nature. In this respect formative education, regarded from the side of the individual, consists in his acquiring what lies at hand, devouring [*in sich zehre*] his inorganic nature, and taking possession of it for himself."[59] This past information is a human residue, substantial and inorganic, corpse-like in short, and the work of subjectification is to eat it— conceptually, at least. Through that process, the individual makes the past his. Without that process, however, the deceased inhabit the individual in an uncontrolled and unassimilated way. His motivations, agency, and borders are all consequently unclear, and he remains caught in the indeterminate zone between the living and the dead, between the organic and the inorganic, between substance and thought.

All human artifacts look at us with the eyes of the dead or of the dead who will be, since they, as artifacts, have separated themselves from their makers. Any nineteenth-century painting stares at us with the gaze of the deceased. We can turn our backs on paintings, but language is different. With it, our mouths and minds are full of the residue of past thinking, for words are not entirely transcendental, not just because of their sounds and written traces, but because of the history they bear, what Hegel called their inorganic substance. We feel this quasi-materiality particularly strongly, I think, in words without general concepts, like proper nouns. Their referents do not change (unless one accepts that a certain generation is filled with people more Stanley-ish, say, than another), but the value of the names does. A Gladys or Waldo or Adolf can sound remarkably strange in the wrong context or time, and this is not a reflexive judgment, since the strangeness is an involuntary reaction. The word *spangled* is inflected by associations with the American flag, a connection created by a national anthem and deriving, in turn, from one individual's experience of a naval battle and his choice of words. Or the pronoun *I*, which is not just the negation of the person it intends to indicate, but also, now, the memorialization of the originality of Hegel's insight, and it bears, in this way, that history. It bears the stamp of a past thinking the way that *being* bears the stamp of Heidegger. Words are inflected, or infected, by the specificities of their history, their embeddedness in other people's thinking, and probably never more so than when someone, like Heidegger, tries to reject that history.

Following Kristeva, I have framed the notion of abjection as a loss of the subject, but how does one reconcile that with Robespierre's contention that the "individual 'I'" is abject? One could argue that the two are describing different notions of abjection, but it seems more likely that they are describing different notions of the "I." The "I" of Robespierre is one that cares only for itself at the expense of others, but his idea of others was the abstraction of the state itself, the purity of its impersonality. Kristeva, on the other hand, is referring to the specificity of an individual consciousness, but that individuality is a permanent fending-off of the inorganic world and everything that is not "I." And that "I" is not the same as the self. A consciousness continues after the collapse of the subject and in the moments, such as idle chatter or drunken conversation, when it oozes out into an indeterminately interpersonal place of thinking. This, following Hegel, one might call *inorganic substance*. It is figured also in the swarming of vermin or the pullulating of life under the microscope. This, I have argued, is the world the nineteenth-century medical imagination glimpsed in the idiot, the mollusk, and the dead and that was reappropriated by artists and writers and probably by much of the population at large.

What Kristeva's insight about abjection reveals is that this world, with its abiding sentience, represents, on the one hand, the destruction of the subject and, on the other, the limitless expansion of the self, its uncontrolled hypertrophy. But as the consciousness of the self extends, something else disappears in the dim and swarming world of putrefaction: the *other*, for there is no difference here between matter and thought, between me and my world. As the subject loses its ability to recognize itself, it also loses its ability to recognize what is not itself—most importantly other consciousnesses. The quasi-materiality of language, for example, does not threaten my sentience, but it can kill my ability to see that something or someone is not me. The characteristically human capacity to see what is not, to think and speak in negatives, need not be thought of as an ontological issue manifested in the nonbeing of death, as it is for Hegel and Heidegger, but as an ethical relation manifested in the mystery of other people, as it is for Levinas. Ethics, in this sense, is life. And what horrifies in the corpse is therefore not the loss of one's own identity, but rather the overbearing plenitude of the self.

The abjection of the other—the Lacanian and Kristevan abject that is not another subject—is, as I have argued, a fantasm, a projection of our own desire. It functions, in that sense, as an image of our loneliness in the annihilation of that other. That abject loneliness finds common and indeed prosaic expressions. It permeates our relations to the deceased and their memories, insofar as those relations manifest our ability to continue to attribute to human remains the impression of the life that has left them, of the person who is gone. It takes the form of artistic creation, which always entails, as a result of its fantasmatic nature, a certain element of horror or uncanniness, for the artistic creation is only a semblance of the living. And the horror of the abject is a function of the latter's relation to desire. In the desire for the abject—in abject desire—one finds embedded the longing for a lost and mythical world of plenitude, a plenitude of sentience and self. But the limit of that plenitude is the other in their subjective alterity, the possibility of their difference. And so abject desire is an annihilation of that difference. The queasiness that such desire produces seems, in turn, to be related to that annihilation, for it is the desire for a world we can no longer imagine without marking, in that very imagining, the death of the other. Every time we evoke a plenitude of the self, a sentience without limits, without subjectivity even, a trace of that missing other surfaces, the fantasmatic remainder of their death in the very structure of plenitude, the indigestible corpse of the lost. We feel the impossibility of ever returning to an *otherless* world without some vague memory, some leftover, some remnant of the lost other, without an indigestible corpse. Revulsion would be the attempt, both psychic and physical, to expel the remnant that blocks our appropriation—and digestion—of the material world. That obstruction, I would argue, is the other, who invariably surfaces as a corpse in the fantasmatic structures of desire themselves.

Conclusion

"Natural history, in the Classical period," Michel Foucault wrote, "cannot be established as a biology. Up to the end of the eighteenth century, in fact, life does not exist: only living beings."[60] Until the end of the eighteenth century: in the writings of Xavier Bichat and all those grouped around him, his contemporaries and his later followers, I have shown how profoundly things changed at the turn of the nineteenth century. Death changed. It became a scientific problem. One could almost say that modern medicine was born out of the desire to understand death and to separate it conceptually and clinically from life. But as the two questions—What is life? What is death?—increasingly organized the field of medical research, as death and life *became* questions, their meaning opened to new forms of doubt. These new doubts, in turn, raised new anxieties, a new imaginary, and new desires. And while generations of researchers failed to isolate and conceptualize the two states, certain factors emerged clearly enough. Life resisted death. Death, for its part, was material, horrifying, and abject, part of a noxious continuum that could be broadly grouped under the category of putrefaction. These were the imaginings that arose around the new death. And those imaginings, in turn, guided the way that medical researchers thought of death. It was not that they were reading Balzac or Zola or Flaubert, or that they were studying the depths of Odilon Redon's *noirs*. It was just that artists were expressing the operative fantasms in ways that were not accessible to the medical corps itself.

A new Paris rose up in the image of those fantasms. The hygienic city was not only a place or even an ideal, it was also an instrument by which the abject could be removed from contact with the human. As such, it represented a new interpretation of a long-standing idea, the polis as a place of reason. And this was an idea that was formulated in classical Athens and taken up with passionate intensity during the French Revolution. The story of death in the nineteenth century is also, therefore, the story of Paris. The Paris of smells that no longer exist, that have vanished more completely, perhaps, than any other aspect of the period. A Paris that I have tried to resuscitate, briefly, in the darkest, unloveliest corners of nineteenth-century art and literature, in the readings of Walter Benjamin, in the very fabric of language from the time, as if it still clung to the materiality of those words, to the communality of their ideas, like an odor in an unwashed shirt.

But the force of abjection came not merely from abjection itself. What made it dangerous, what let it slip back into the city that was built to exclude it, was the fact that it was as desirable as it was revolting. Its danger was, in fact, its attractiveness. The figure of the prostitute taught us that. And in that desire, one sees traces and indicators that point toward the meaning of abjection. It is the breakdown of alterity, the murder of the other, the expansion of the self beyond all limits, including death. It is desirable because it represents a plenitude of the self. It is revolting because that plenitude is at once infinite and sensuous, like the vertigo that takes us over, like the attraction of an open chasm before we are saved by intimations of the sublime. It is revolting, too, because in the image of that plenitude a figure returns inescapably. It is the reminder of our crime, of our loneliness and guilt. It returns with the nauseating intractability of a body that cannot be buried, that will not be sublimated.

Perhaps this return to the past will help us reconsider contemporary and future issues of public utility in other terms—as translations of more pressing, but less speakable, desires and needs.

INTRODUCTION: THE TOXIC IMAGINATION

1. Jean-Joseph Sue, *Recherches physiologiques et expériences sur la vitalité. Lues à l'Institut national de France, le 11 Messidor, an V de la république. Suivies d'une nouvelle edition de son Opinion sur le supplice de la guillotine ou sur la douleur qui survit à la décolation* (Paris: chez l'auteur, an VI [1797]), iii–iv.

2. "All known precautions and all the usual aids against the insalubrity of the air must be brought together and applied with the greatest care" to exhume and transfer the remains (Jacques-Guillaume Thouret, *Rapport sur les exhumations du cimetière et de l'église des Saints-Innocents; Lu dans la séance de la Société Royale de Médecine, tenue au Louvre le 3 mars 1789* [Paris: Ph.-Denys Pierres, 1789], 9).

3. Thouret, 11–12.

4. Those who resisted the removal of the dead from cities and churches frequently cited these long-standing traditions. See, for example, Louis François de Paule-Marie-Joseph de Robiano de Borsbeek, who defended *intra-muros* burials partially on the grounds that the earliest Christians had gathered in cemeteries, "where so many martyrs lay buried," and that later, under the emperor Constantine, "cemetery and church were one and the same place" (*De la violation des cimetières* [Louvain: Vanlinthout et Vandenzanden, 1824], 21–22).

5. In his *Topographie médicale de Paris ou Examen général des causes qui peuvent avoir une influence marquée sur la santé des habitans de cette ville, le caractère de leurs maladies, et le choix des précautions hygiéniques qui leur sont applicables* (Paris: J.-B. Baillière, 1822), Claude Lachaise remarked on the singularity of this history: "Convinced that the proximity of the dead could only be deleterious to the living, the ancients took care to remove dead bodies from their cities and to bury them in places consecrated by religion. All peoples practiced inhumation and were in agreement about it. The Roman laws, the decrees and councils of the various churches, the statutes of our kings expressly ordered it. In the first centuries after its founding, Paris did not depart from such a wise and generally observed law, but ceased to obey it when, having been made a capital city, it saw its inhabitants reach beyond the natural boundaries of the Seine and spread their dwellings to

its northern side, where, at the time, the terrains were larger and more commodi-ous. The Saints-Innocents cemetery was at that point enclosed within the limits of the city, and this abuse continued for more than ten centuries, although at different periods certain unbiased philanthropists, magistrates, and doctors raised their voices against its dangerous effects" (140–41).

6. See Antoine-Alexis Cadet-De-Vaux, *Mémoire historique et physique sur le cimetière des innocents par M. Cadet de Vaux, Inspecteur Général des Objets de Salu-brité, de plusieurs académies, Censur Royal, &c. &c.; lu à l'Académie Royale des Sciences en 1781. Extrait du Journal de Physique 1783* (N.p.: n.p., n.d.), 1–2, and Thouret, 2–3.

7. The history of the transfer of the dead from Paris has been broadly docu-mented. Many of the relevant ordinances and decrees can be found in Vicq d'Azyr's "Discours préliminaire" to Scipione Piattoli's *Essai sur les lieux et les dangers des sépultures*, trans. Félix Vicq d'Azyr (Paris: P. Fr. Didot, Libraire de la Société Royale de Médecine, 1778), xli–cxvii, and in Félix Gannal, *Les cimetières depuis la fondation de la monarchie française jusqu'à nos jours. Histoire et législation* (Paris: Muzard et fils, 1884), 1–274 of the appendix entitled "Pièces justifica-tives." Documents related to the question have been gathered in Bibliothèque Nationale, Fonds Joly de Fleury, 1207, including the "Arrest de la cour de parle-ment extrait des registres du parlement du 21 Mai 1765" (fos. 50–55). For good overviews of the process, see M. Pinard, *Le cimetière du sud (Montparnasse)* (Paris: Retaux Frères, 1866), 4, and more recently: Robert Vovelle, *La mort et l'Occident de 1300 à nos jours. Précédé de: La mort, état des lieux* (1983; repr., Paris: Gallimard, 2000), 461–67; Armando Petrucci, *Writing the Dead: Death and Writing Strategies in the Western Tradition*, trans. Michael Sullivan (Stanford, Calif.: Stanford Uni-versity Press, 1998), 104; Thomas Kselman, *Death and the Afterlife in Modern France* (Princeton: Princeton University Press, 1993), 167–80; and Richard A. Etlin, *The Architecture of Death: The Transformation of the Cemetery in Eighteenth-Century Paris* (Cambridge, Mass.: MIT Press, 1984), 22, 32, 295, 299–300.

8. Still, nearly a third of incorporated areas in the regions of Calvados and Normandy had isolated their cemeteries in 1804. Kselman, 176–78. See also Vovelle, 564–69.

9. Ibid., 201.

10. For Mercier, see "Rotting Waste" in chapter 5.

11. Jacques Léonard dates the liberalization of the medical profession to the passage of the loi Le Chapelier on August 4, 1789 and the decree of August 18, 1792 (*La France médicale: Médecins et malades au XIXe siècle* [Paris: Gallimard, 1978], 69).

12. On Auguste Comte, see "Death Becomes a Medical Condition" in chap-ter 3.

13. Foucault described how in the nineteenth century medical authority spread beyond its "traditional" limits of illness and the ill so that at the time of his writing there was, as he put it, no "outside" to medicine (*Dits et écrits 1954–1988*, vol. 3, ed. Daniel Defert, François Ewald, and Jacques Lagrange [Paris:

Gallimard, 1994], 48–53). According to Foucault, this rise of authority derived in large part from a shift in the object of medical knowledge from the individual to the body politic, or "population," and as such represented a political activity, a noso-, or medico-, or bio-politics or a "somocracy." Foucault was less concerned with the specific relations between various institutions of power, such as the Church, the courts, and the doctors, than with the larger control of a collective entity—for example, the population, the (ab)normal, the pathology—that exceeded the individual (see, however, "L'évolution de la notion d'«individu dangereux» dans la psychiatrie légale du XIXe siècle," in *Dits et écrits*, 3:443–64, on the "pathologisation of crime"). *The Birth of the Clinic: An Archaeology of Medical Perception*, trans. A. M. Sheridan Smith (New York: Random House, 1973) describes the epistemic shift that, according to Foucault, occurred in medicine around the turn of the nineteenth century and details some of the political implications of this change (see esp. 22–53). A clearer sense of the overall argument he is making however, can often be found in his shorter writings. See "La politique de la santé au XVIIIe siècle" (*Dits et écrits*, 3:13–28), "Crise de la médecine ou crise de l'antimédecine?" (ibid., 40–48), "La naissance de la médecine sociale" (ibid., 207–28), "La politique de la santé aux XVIIIe siècle (725–42, and somewhat different in its first pages from the earlier version of this article). While *Naissance de la bio-politique: cours au Collège de France (1978–1979)*, ed. François Ewald, Alessandro Fontana, and Michel Senellart (Paris: Gallimard, 2004) represents a first step towards examining the bio-politics of the rise of medicine, it concentrates almost entirely on the epistemological preconditions for that event, focusing especially on the advent of economic liberalism. We should note that Foucault's argument that there is no outside to medicine is somewhat disingenuous, since he contrasts medicine to antimedicine rather than nonmedicine, thus creating a dialectical impasse for thinking beyond its terms.

14. See Michel Foucault, *Madness and Civilization: A History of Insanity in the Age of Reason*, trans. Richard Howard (1965; repr., New York: Random House, 1973), 287–88. Foucault's understanding of the relation between madness and discourse has not gone uncontested, however. See, notably, Marcel Gauchet and Gladys Swain, *Madness and Democracy: The Modern Psychiatric Universe*, trans. Catherine Porter (Princeton: Princeton University Press, 1999).

15. See in particular Gaston Bachelard, *The Formation of the Scientific Mind: A Contribution to a Psychoanalysis of Objective Knowledge*, trans. Mary McAllester Jones (Manchester: Clinamen, 2002), 136–53, 185–210.

16. It is worth noting, in this respect, that Jean Joseph Sue was father to the novelist Eugène Sue, who, as I argue in chapter 7, performed his own literary analysis of medical theories.

1. MEDICINE AND AUTHORITY

1. Ambroise Tardieu, *Etude médico-légale sur les attentats aux mœurs* (Paris: J.-B. Baillière et Fils, 1878), 117. There is a significant body of literature on Sergeant Bertrand, but it is quite dispersed. Aside from the materials cited below, one

should add Michel Foucault, *Abnormal: Lectures at the Collège de France*, ed. Valerio Marchetti and Antonella Salomoni, trans. Graham Burchell (New York: Picador, 2003), 283–87, which provided much of the bibliographic orientation for what follows; Dr. [Charles?] Pajot, "A Monsieur le rédacteur en chef," *Gazette hébdomadaire de médecine* 4, no. 8 (February 20, 1857): 200, which describes the wounds inflicted on some of the corpses that Bertrand mutilated; Jean Raimond, "Feuilleton," *L'union médicale: Journal des intérêts scientifiques et pratiques, moraux et professionnels du corps médical* 3, no. 92 (August 2, 1849): 365–66; "Le Sergent Bertrand," *Le siècle* 14, no. 181 (July 11, 1849): 4–5; and Cesare Lombroso, *L'homme criminel, criminel-né, fou moral, épileptique: Etude anthropologique et médico-légale*, vol. 2, trans. Regnier and Bournet (Paris: Félix Alcan, 1887), 189, which diagnoses Bertrand as an epileptic.

2. Henri de Castelnau, "Pathologie mentale et médecine légale. Exemple remarquable de monomanie destructive et érotique ayant pour objet la profanation de cadavres humains," *La lancette française: Gazette des hôpitaux civils et militaires*, 3rd series, vol. 1, no. 82 (July 14, 1849): 327 and an anonymous *"fait divers"* in *Le courrier français*, March 23, 1849.

3. Anonymous article under the rubric "Interieur" in *Le constitutionnel*, March 19, 1849 and Factum of the Bibliothèque Nationale Française, 8 Fm 3159. See also Dr. S . . . ., "Hôpital militaire du Val-de-Grâce. Service de M. Baudens. Coup de feu compliqué chez un sous-officier du 74e de ligne, soupçonné d'être l'auteur de la profanation commise au cimetière Mont-Parnasse," *La lancette française: Gazette des hôpitaux civils et militaires*, 3rd series, vol. 1, no. 36 (March 27, 1849): 144: "For several months, the Parisian newspapers had alerted the public to an unprecedented desecration committed in the Montparnasse cemetery. The public opinion attributed this desecration to a vampire, so difficult was it to believe that human intelligence could be perverted to such an extreme degree"; and Bénédicte-Auguste Morel, *Traité des maladies mentales* (Paris: Victor Masson, 1860), 413: "Bertrand belonged to a type of melancholics that is fortunately very rare today and that the history of mental illness in antiquity and the middle ages has identified under the names of *lyncanthrope, vampires*, etc."

4. "Considérations médico-légales sur un imbécile érotique convaincu de profanation de cadavres, par le docteur Morel, médecin en chef de l'asile de Saint-Yon. A M. le docteur Bédor, médecin de l'hospice civil à Troyes, Membre correspondant de l'Académie impériale de médecine, médecin du dépôt provisoire d'aliénés de l'Hôtel-Dieu de Troyes, etc. Deuxième lettre," *Gazette hébdomadaire de médecine et de chirurgie: Bulletin de l'enseignement médical* 4, no. 11 (March 13, 1857): 187. See also ibid., 184: "this final depravation, the most unprecedented of all"; and Morel, *Traité*, 413: "Although it was at first believed that Sergeant Bertrand, for such was the name of this wretched madman, was driven only by the delirium-induced and pathological need to desecrate graves, his own testimony soon demonstrated that his horrible inclination was complicated by the most dreadful deviation one can imagine." In a similar vein, the doctor Claude-François Michéa wrote that "*the attraction to human corpses* is the rarest

and most extreme deviation of the venereal appetite. . . . But of all these cases, the most monstrous and disgusting is Bertrand's" ("Des déviations maladives de l'appétit vénérien," *L'union médicale* 3, no. 85 [July 17, 1849], 339c).

5. Tardieu, *Attentats*, 114.

6. Castelnau, 327.

7. Charles-Jacob Marchal de Calvi, quoted in Ludger Lunier, "Examen médico-légal d'un cas de monomanie instinctif. Affaire du sergent Bertrand" in *Annales médico-psychologiques* (1849), 1:362.

8. Ibid., 354.

9. Ibid., 355.

10. Marchal stated: "I believe that Bertrand was under the sway of an imperious power . . . that forced him against his will to commit acts unprecedented in the annals of medicine" (Lunier, 363).

11. See Bertrand's own description from transcripts of the trial: "In checking the weapon's position, I noticed that it was aimed directly at the chest, and I had escaped these two shots as if by a miracle. Because the trip wire was loose, it allowed me to get in front of the weapon before it fired" (Castelnau, 328); and "I could not prevent myself from starting again, even though it might cost me my life. So I knew that there was a machine out there meant to kill me" (Lunier, 356).

12. "Intérieur" in *Le constitutionnel*, March 19, 1849. See also the issues from March 20–25 and *Le courrier français* from March 18–25 of the same year. Cf. Bertrand's own descriptions of the various occasions when he was fired on, cited by Castelnau, 327–28: "On November 6 [1848], at ten in the evening, someone fired a pistol at me, as I was climbing the cemetery wall. It didn't hit me. This incident didn't discourage me. I lay down on the damp earth and I slept for a couple of hours in the bitter cold. I went back into the cemetery, where I unearthed the body of a young woman who had drowned and I mutilated it. From that date until March 15, 1849, I returned to the cemetery only twice, once between December 15 and 20, and once at the beginning of January. During those two visits, I was fired at twice more. The first bullet, which wasn't at close range, went through the seam of my hood behind my back without hitting me. The second didn't touch me at all." For descriptions of the *"machine infernale"* and the wounds it inflicted on Bertrand, see Dr. S . . . ., 144.

13. See Lunier, 352.

14. "Faits divers" in *Le courrier français*, March 23, 1849.

15. Castelnau, 328. The paragraph continues: "Alas! Because of a fundamental legislative flaw, which we have already pointed out on frequent occasions and that we shall undoubtedly have to point out many more times before seeing it disappear from the code." Lunier wrote, in a similar vein: "Is it not obvious that in a case of this nature it would have been necessary to have the accused examined by specialized doctors, who alone are competent in such matters? The attorney general would undoubtedly have followed that course, if Bertrand had not been a soldier and had appeared before an ordinary tribunal" (379). See also Morel's

arguments on a similar subject: in his discussion of a case of necrophilia that he compared to that of Sergeant Bertrand, Morel wrote about the "incontestable service" that Pinel and his followers "had rendered for the cause of mental illness, when they convinced the courts to absolve madmen, who until then had been executed on the grounds that the almost completely intact state of their intelligence had made them seem entirely responsible for their actions" ("Considérations médico-légales . . . Troisième lettre *(deuxième partie)*," *Gazette hébdomadaire de médecine* 4, no. 8 (February 20, 1857): 233; and an editor's note to Morel's "Considérations médico-légales . . . Première lettre," *Gazette hébdomadaire de médecine* 4, no. 8 (February 20, 1857): 123n. About the sergeant himself, Morel wrote: "Bertrand was also considered by his doctors to be a true *erotic monomaniac*, and nonetheless he was declared guilty and condemned to a year in prison" ("Considérations médico-légales . . . Deuxième lettre," 185).

16. Lunier, 362.

17. Ibid.

18. "In the current state of science, Sergeant Bertrand's case seems to be unique, as our honorable colleague, Mr. Marchal (de Calvi) has, moreover, already stated" (Castelnau, 328).

19. "Des déviations maladives," 339. See also: "But there is more: he feels venereal passion at the sight of women's corpses, he seeks erotic pleasure in putrefaction" (ibid., 338).

20. There is excellent scholarship on the rise of doctors as a social class. On conditions just before and during the Revolution, see Jean-Charles Sournia, *La médecine révolutionnaire 1789–1799* (Paris: Payot, 1989), 11–49. On the rise of scientists in general during the late eighteenth and early nineteenth centuries, see Nicole and Jean Dhombres, *Naissance d'un nouveau pouvoir: sciences et savants en France (1793–1824)* (Paris: Payot, 1989), 171–200, 691–772. For doctors during the period 1814 to 1870, see Jacques Léonard, *La médecine entre les savoirs et les pouvoirs: Histoire intellectuelle et politique de la médecine française au XIXe siècle* (Paris: Aubier Montaigne, 1981), 201–34. On the creation of a medical elite in the nineteenth century, see George Weisz, *The Medical Mandarins: The French Academy of Medicine in the Nineteenth and Early Twentieth Centuries* (Oxford: Oxford University Press, 1995).

21. Dhombres and Dhombres, 172.

22. Ibid., 184–85.

23. Sournia, 9. The picture should be nuanced somewhat, however, since Jacques Léonard and his coauthors have demonstrated that as a whole, doctors still occupied only a modest social rank around 1810. See Jacques Léonard, Roger Darquenne, and Louis Bergeron, "Médecins et notables sous le Consulat et l'Empire," *Annales économies sociétés civilisations* 32, no. 5 (September/October 1977): 887–907.

24. Sournia, 49.

25. See Pierre Guillaume, *Médecins, église et foi depuis deux siècles* (Paris: Aubier, 1990), 75: "Doctors were able to transform their social status through the new

dignity of medical science, which was officially recognized by the jubilees or national funerals of men like Claude Bernard, Louis Pasteur, and Théodore Roussel, as well as by the opening of the new Académie de Médecine in 1902. Local studies based on an analysis of inheritances show that they began to enter the middle class, which, despite some exceptions, had previously been closed to them. In 1900, a doctor even became mayor of Bordeaux, which was at the time a bastion of the traditional elite. But above all, as Jacques Léonard has shown, they filled the republican assemblies, entered the ministries, and gave the impetus to some of the great liberal laws on divorce, education, and public assistance. And in the person of Emile Combes, they reached the level of Prime Minister."

26. Weisz, *Mandarins*, 273–74.

27. Pierre-Jean-Georges Cabanis, *Du degré de certitude de la médecine*, ed. Jean-Marc Drouin (1798; repr., Paris: Champion-Slatkine, 1989), 144.

28. Ibid., 74–92.

29. Ibid., 75.

30. Ibid., 75–76.

31. See William F. Bynum, *Science and the Practice of Medicine in the Nineteenth Century* (Cambridge: Cambridge University Press, 1994), 30, 41, 45.

32. On Broussais, see Bynum, *Science*, 45; on Bernard, see Philippe Huneman, *Bichat, la vie et la mort* (Paris: Presses Universitaires de France, 1998), 102.

33. The concept of *monomania* played a similar role in the rise of psychiatry at the same time. See "Madness between Medicine, the Law, and the Church," in chapter 2. On Bernard's *"milieu intérieur,"* see Huneman, 97–102.

34. For general descriptions of the status and structures of medical teaching prior to the Revolution, see Pierre Huard, "L'enseignement médico-chirurgical," in René Taton, ed., *Enseignement et diffusion des sciences en France au XVIIIe siècle* (Paris: Hermann, 1964), 169–236; Yves Laissus, "Le jardin du roi," in ibid., 287–341; and Bynum, *Science*, 1–24. On the state of the medical profession under the Revolution, see Sournia; and Mathew Ramsey, "Le médecin, le peuple, l'état: la question du monopole professionnel," in Vincent Barras and Micheline Louis-Courvoisier, eds., *La médecine des lumières: Tout autour de Tissot* (Geneva: Georg, 2001), esp. 33–38. On the aftermath of the Revolution and its effects on the medical profession, see William F. Bynum, "Médecine et société," in Mirko D. Grmek, ed., *Du romantisme à la science moderne*, vol. 3 of *Histoire de la pensée médicale en occident* (Paris: Seuil, 1999), 295–318. Russel C. Maulitz, *Morbid Appearances: The Anatomy of Pathology in the Early Nineteenth Century* (Cambridge: Cambridge University Press, 1987), 43–47, discusses the conflicting demands made on the Paris school of medicine between 1797 and 1801: on the one hand to certify expertise by accrediting doctors and on the other to conduct original research. Weisz, in *Mandarins*, describes the creation, structure, and importance of the French Academy of Medicine; see esp. 1–33 for a useful overview of the state of teaching in Paris during the first part of the nineteenth century. Weisz's *Divide and Conquer: A Comparative History of Medical Specialization* (Oxford:

Oxford University Press, 2006) offers a history of specialization within the medical profession during the early nineteenth century. Whereas much of what follows in my own arguments concerns tensions between doctors and other disciplines, such as the law, Weisz concentrates on the divisions *inside* the medical profession and in particular on struggles for power and dominance. Nicole and Jean Dhombres observed that at the end of the eighteenth century and the beginning of the nineteenth, medical training moved largely to the hospitals, where it was increasingly practical rather than theoretical (197).

35. Jan Goldstein, *Console and Classify: The French Psychiatric Profession in the Nineteenth Century* (Cambridge: Cambridge University Press, 1987), 15–16.

36. Sournia, 14.

37. Huard, 172.

38. Ibid.

39. Dhombres and Dhombres, 195–96. Mathew Ramsey has pointed out, however, that the enthusiasm for this deregulation was not universal and that Condorcet, in particular, made an exception for medicine when recommending that professions be liberalized. See "Le médecin, le peuple, l'état," 31.

40. Dhombres and Dhombres, 195.

41. Ibid., 196.

42. Bynum, "Médecine et société," 298.

43. Dhombres and Dhombres, 197.

44. Ibid.

45. See Weisz, *Mandarins*, 3.

46. On the professionalization of medicine, see Mathew Ramsey, "The Popularization of Medicine in France, 1650–1900," in Roy Porter, ed., *The Popularization of Medicine 1650–1850* (London: Routledge, 1992), 122, which describes a historical movement "visible in the Enlightenment and then emerging with increasing force after the Revolution [that] sharply challenged the idea of popularizing anything more than hygiene, preventive medicine, and first aid, even for educated readers. Thanks especially to the rapid growth of the periodical press, innovations in medical science were more widely reported than ever before, but the reader was meant to admire rather than emulate." Elsewhere, Ramsey describes generally unsuccessful attempts from the same period to control "secret remedies" and submit these popular panaceas to the oversight of government agencies and then, in 1813, of the Paris Faculty of Medicine. See Ramsey, "Property Rights and the Right to Health: The Regulation of Secret Remedies in France, 1789–1815," in W. F. Bynum and Roy Porter, eds., *Medical Fringe & Medical Orthodoxy 1750–1850* (London: Croom Helm, 1987), 79–105.

47. Vernon A. Rosario, *The Erotic Imagination: French Histories of Perversity* (Oxford: Oxford University Press, 1997), 60.

48. On the *Code pénal*, see André Laingui and Jean Illes, "La responsabilité du médecin dans l'ancien droit," in Didier Truchet, ed., *Etudes de droit et d'économie de la santé* (Paris: Economica, 1982), 11. See Didier Martin and Sylviane Martin, "Parcours sanitaire du code civil," in the same volume: "Health is not a major

theme of civil legislation. At least, that is the partial diagnosis an attentive examination of the 2483 articles of the current Civil Code allows us to make" (17); "Illness is literally unmentioned in the Civil Code" (19). For an overview of the relations between medicine and the legal system under the ancien régime, see André Laingui and Jean Illes; and Jean Verdier, *La jurisprudence de la médecine en France*, 2 vols. (Paris: Malassis le jeune, 1762). For the nineteenth century, see Robert Gervais, "Le microbe et la responsabilité médicale," in Claire Salomon-Bayet, ed., *Pasteur et la révolution pastorienne* (Paris: Payot, 1986), 217–75; and Paul Brouardel, *La responsabilité médicale: secret médical, déclarations de naissance, inhumations, expertises médico-légales* (Paris: J.-B. Baillière et Fils, 1898). Ruth Harris, *Murders and Madness: Medicine, Law, and Society in the* Fin de Siècle (Oxford: Clarendon Press, 1989) picks up the history at the end of the nineteenth century and contains useful sections on "Medicine, Law, and Criminology" in Italy and France (80–97) and on "The Medico-legal Debate: The Salpêtrière *v.* Nancy" (171–84).

49. Paolo Zacchia, *Quaestiones medico-legales* (Venice: M. D. Horstius, 1637).

50. Félix Vicq-d'Azyr and Jacques-Louis Moreau (de la Sarthe), *Médecine*, 13 vols. (Paris: Panckoucke, 1787–1830).

51. Brouardel, 21.

52. Quoted in and translated by Goldstein, 175.

53. The use of expert medical testimony already enjoyed a long history. In 1762, for instance, the lawyer and doctor Jean Verdier observed that "judges and jurisconsults so often need to avail themselves of the knowledge and aid of medicine, that the ministry of those who are the depositories of this art is very common among the bar. Since time immemorial, the principal tribunals of Paris have been in the habit of retaining private doctors and surgeons to perform these functions. They are the ones that Milæus terms *annuis stipendiis autorati*. The law has confirmed this custom and has even extended it to the provinces through the establishment of royal doctors and surgeons" (Verdier, 165–66). I will examine the debates about medical testimony in my discussion of madness in the next chapter.

54. Verdier, 721–22.

55. See Laingui and Illes: "Furthermore, we have noticed that [under the ancien régime] doctors escaped almost all [legal] responsibility, both for juridical reasons concerning the difficulty of proof and for social reasons, namely the highly honorable nature of their profession" (14); and Gervais, 224.

56. Laingui and Illes, 11.

57. See Gervais, 224–25. Article 1382 stated that "any act by which a person causes injury to another obliges the one whose fault it is to make reparations for it," while the article 1383 held that "each person is responsible for the damage he has caused, not only by his actions, but also by his negligence or imprudence" (quoted in Brouardel, 20–21).

58. Charles Dalboussière, "De la responsabilité médicale. Affaire Thouret-Noroy," *Annales d'hygiène publique et de médecine légale* 12, no. 2 (octobre 1834): 406, 435–36.

59. Gervais, 224n29.

60. Quoted in Brouardel, 22.

61. Quoted in ibid., 23.

62. Quoted in ibid.

63. Dalboussière, 436.

64. See Laingui and Illes, 14; Didier Truchet, "L'autorité juridique des principes d'exercice de la médecine," in Didier Truchet, ed., *Etudes de droit et d'économie de la santé* (Paris: Economica, 1982), 44; and Gervais, 224–25 and 255–56.

65. Quoted in Gervais, 244.

66. Truchet, 43.

67. Brouardel, 61.

68. Ibid., 44. See also Jacques Léonard, *Médecine*, 213–16.

69. Michel Dansel, *Le cas du sergent Bertrand: Un nécrophile conséquent* (Paris: Bibliothèque de l'homme, 1999), 114.

70. The model for this privilege can be found in the confessional and its fullest contemporary development is probably the psychiatric session. See Michel Foucault, *The History of Sexuality: Volume I: An Introduction*, trans. Robert Hurley (1978; New York: Random House, 1990), 57–70.

71. On the notion that one cures not the individual but society as a whole, see Alexis Epaulard, *Vampirisme, nécrosadisme, nécrophagie* (Lyon: A. Storck, 1901), published three years after Brouardel's *Responsabilité médicale*: "One must undertake a social prophylaxis against all of the causes that weaken our psychic state. Yes, the task of society as a whole is to take up arms against the causes of decay, against the causes of excitation such as alcohol and the convulsifying [*convulsivantes*] spirits that lead to all the crimes and perversions, for, as the aphorism of the Ecole d'anthropologie criminelle de Lyon puts it: *societies have only the criminels they deserve*" (98).

72. Conversely, for the same reasons, doctors could be mandated by law to reveal certain information about their patients, especially in the case of communicable diseases (see Gervais, 234–35, 283).

73. *Jean Santeuil*, ed. Pierre Clarac and Yves Sandre (Paris: Gallimard [Pléiade], 1971), 649.

74. For a general account of relations between scientists and the Church from 1793 to 1824, see Dhombres and Dhombres, 245–47, 256–69, 313–34. For an account of relations between the Church and medicine during the nineteenth century, see Guillaume, esp. 18–19, 42–46, 58–63. Goldstein, 197–239, describes relations between the Church and doctors in respect to mental illness, which we will discuss in more detail in the following chapter.

75. Pierre-Jean-Corneille Debreyne, *La théologie morale et les sciences médicales*, ed. A. Ferrand (Paris: Poussielgue Frères, 1884; reprint of *Essai sur la théologie morale, considérée dans ses rapports avec la physiologie et la médecine, ouvrage spécialement destiné au clergé*, 1842), ix. For Pinel and Legrand du Saulle's comments, see the first sections of the following chapter.

76. See Huard, 173.

77. Laingui and Illes, 12.

78. Sournia, 20.

79. Ibid.

80. See ibid.

81. Dhombres and Dhombres, 330.

82. Ibid., 313–34.

83. Ibid., 318–26 and Guillaume, 28–34.

84. Augustin-Louis Cauchy, *Considérations sur les ordres religieux adressées aux amis des sciences* (Paris: Poussièlgue-Rusand, 1844), 8 (quoted in Dhombres and Dhombres, 322).

85. Dhombres and Dhombres cite a particularly telling example of this reconciliation. The lessons on sciences and religion that Frayssinous gave at Saint Sulpice church in the early years of the nineteenth century attracted important figures from the medical community: "Portalis, minister of Religion, felt himself obliged to draw the Emperor's attention to the remarkable presence of polytechnicians and medical and law students, who were often accompanied by other scholars or by their professors. Among the faithful, there numbered Laennec, Régis Buisson, who was a student of Bichat, the future cardinal de Rohan, and the doctor Buté, who would soon enter the great seminary of Paris" (Dhombres and Dhombres, 322).

86. Debreyne, *Théologie*, ix.

87. Pierre Debreyne, *Etude de la mort ou Initiation du prêtre à la connaissance pratique des maladies graves et mortelles et de tout ce qui, sous ce rapport, peut se rattacher à l'exercice difficile du saint ministère* (1845; Paris: M. V. Poussielgue-Rusand, 1864), 2–3.

88. See Guillaume, 80–81.

89. See ibid., 26. See also Marie-Claude Dinet-Lecomte, *Les sœurs hospitalières en France aux XVIIe et XVIIIe siècles: La charité en action* (Paris: Honoré Champion, 2005); and Jacques Léonard, "Femmes, religion et médecine: les religieuses qui soignent," *Annales économies, sociétés civilisations* 32, no. 5 (September/October 1977): 887–907.

90. Goldstein, 21–22.

91. Guillaume, 82.

92. For example, see Jules Tillie, *Manuel de médecine à l'usage du clergé paroissial, suivi des soins à donner dans les cas urgents* (Saint-Omer: H. d'Homont, 1891); Angelo Antonio Scotti, *Le médecin chrétien, ou médecine et religion*, trans. Bernardin Gassiat (Paris: V. Palmé, 1881); and for Surbled, see Guillaume, 79, which provided the source for these references.

93. See Guillaume, 26.

94. Edouard Carrière, "De l'autorité en médecine," *L'union médicale. Journal des intérêts scientifiques et pratiques, moraux et professionnels du corps médical* 3, no. 97 (August 14, 1849): 386. I am thankful to Rosario, 63, for bringing my attention to this debate.

95. "Under the influence of the old order of things, private instruction was only a supplement, a succedaneum for the training provided by the State. Today,

however, public education has sunk to the same level as open instruction [*enseignement libre*] and can therefore no longer judge and oversee it. For the same reasons and to the same extent as all other teaching, it must therefore be supervised by a separate, independent, and impartial entity, an entity, in a word, that weighs the respective merits of all types of instruction and gives the preference only to the most useful or the best. Freedom of instruction [*enseignement libre*] thus leads to the separation of the instructional corps from the corps of students, and this is an essential point" (Amadée Latour, "Note du rédacteur en chef," *L'union médicale* 3, no. 97 [August 14, 1849]: 387).

96. Carrière, "De l'autorité en médecine," 386.

97. Ibid.

98. See Latour, "De l'autorité en médecine," *L'union médicale* 3, no. 98 (August 16 and 18, 1849): 389–90, and *L'union médicale* 3, no. 111 (September 18, 1849): 444–46.

99. Rosario, 63n.

100. On the situation between the Church and the sciences in the aftermath of Chateaubriand's *Génie*, see Dhombres and Dhombres, 265–9. On the evolution of their relations in the second half of the nineteenth century, see Guillaume, 45–101.

101. See Guillaume, 75.

102. On Pasteur, see "Rotting Waste," in chapter 4. On arguments against the possibility of progress, see Dhombres and Dhombres, 245 and 313.

103. Guillaume, 75.

104. See ibid., 81.

105. On the notion of separate truths, see Dhombres and Dhombres, 317–23, esp. 318.

106. In what follows, I will discuss the application of medical theories to a broad range of social problems, which, according to proponents of this approach, otherwise could not be adequately understood and addressed. Anne C. Vila has detailed what she terms the "medicalization of enlightenment" in *Enlightenment and Pathology: Sensibility in the Literature and Medicine of Eighteenth-Century France* (Baltimore: Johns Hopkins University Press, 1998), 80–107, where she concentrates on the figures of Antoine Le Camus and Tissot to argue that according to contemporary perceptions "the enlightenment truly *was* a medical matter" (80). Especially in *Les français et leur médecine au XIXe siècle* (Paris: Belin, 1993), Olivier Faure has described the "medicalization" of French society in the nineteenth century, contending that this revolution was as much the result of popular desires as an imposition from an educated elite who saw in it an instrument of control. Faure offers an excellent bibliography on the subject.

107. François-Emmanuel Fodéré, *Les lois éclairées par les sciences physiques, ou traité de médecine légale et d'hygiène publique*, vol. 1 (Paris: Croullebois, 1799), 1 (quoted in Léonard, *Médecine*, 54).

108. *Quelques réflexions sur la médecine légale et son état actuel en France*, (Paris: Villier, 1801), 10 (quoted in Léonard, *Médecine*, 54).

109. Cabanis, *Du degré*, 9.

110. Ibid., 10.

111. Dhombres and Dhombres, 404–6.

112. Ibid., 404–10.

113. Ibid., 406.

114. Ibid., 409–14.

115. Carrière, "De l'autorité en médecine," 385.

116. Ibid., 386.

117. Latour, "De l'autorité en médecine," 389.

118. Latour, "Note du rédacteur en chef," 387.

119. Quoted in Michel Winnock, *La France et les juifs de 1789 à nos jours* (Paris: Seuil, 2004), 111.

120. Proust, 649.

2. THE MEDICAL USES OF NONSENSE

1. Philippe Pinel, "Résultats d'observations pour servir de base aux rapports juridiques dans les cas d'aliénation mentale," *Mémoires de la Société médicale d'émulation de Paris*, vol. 8 (1817), 682. Quoted in and translated by Goldstein, 167.

2. Obliquely, Huneman makes a similar point about the relation between madness and death: "on several occasions, we have shown a communality between Pinel and Bichat, whose goal was to unearth [*mettre au jour*] figures of the negative in and through the attempt to create a natural history of man, a project that was widespread throughout French culture in the latter half of the 18th century" (124). Pinel and Bichat: madness and death. What Huneman simply calls "negativity," however, I cast in terms of nonsense, which is a specific kind of negativity with important relations to meaning and knowledge. This chapter examines some of those relations in the context of nineteenth-century medical authority.

3. Robert Castel, *The Regulation of Madness: The Origins of Incarceration in France*, trans. W. D. Halls (Berkeley: University of California Press, 1988). For Castel, the discipline and mode of thinking that are modern medicine resulted not so much from scientific imperatives as from the social forces—such as concerns about status, influence, and agency—that weighed on its practitioners. On relations between the medical profession and the courts in respect to madness during the nineteenth century, see ibid., 191–218. Ruth Harris includes useful sections on the situation in France (80–97, 125–54, 171–84) but concentrates on the period from 1880 to 1910.

4. Goldstein, 41. Michel Foucault writes: "In the classical period, it is futile to try to distinguish physical therapeutics from psychological medications, for the simple reason that psychology did not exist" (*Madness and Civilization*, 197). The mad were progressively isolated in separate institutions, but even in the 1780s, "the juridical conditions of incarceration had not changed; and although they were specifically intended for the mad, the new hospitals provided hardly any more space for medicine" (*Histoire de la folie à l'âge classique* [Paris: Gallimard,

1972], 406). Nevertheless, this separation of the mad from the general carceral population allowed, according to Foucault, for their condition to be differentiated from the more general notion of "déraison" (408) and to develop into a clinical category: "Everything is in place, from one century to the next: first, incarceration, out of which the first insane asylums will arise, and these produce the curiosity, then pity—followed by humanitarianism and social solicitude—which will lead to Pinel and Tuke. Who will, in turn, set the great reform movement in motion, with studies by commissioners and the establishment of great hospitals, which will finally usher in the age of Esquirol and a successful medical science of madness" (415).

5. For studies of hospitals before the French Revolution, see Muriel Jeorger, "La structure hospitalière en France sous l'Ancien Régime," *Annales économies sociétés civilisations* 32, no. 5 (September/October 1977): 1025–51; Colin Jones, *The Charitable Imperative: Hospitals and Nursing in Ancien Régime and Revolutionary France* (New York: Routledge, 1989); Dora B. Weiner, *The Citizen-Patient in Revolutionary and Imperial Paris* (Baltimore: Johns Hopkins University Press, 1993), 45–76; and Sournia, 51–94, 164–181. On the state of nursing in the hospital during this period, see Dinet-Lecomte, especially 309–358. For the hospitals under the Revolution, see Sournia, 51–94. For the late-eighteenth and early-nineteenth centuries, see Dora B. Weiner, *Comprendre et soigner: Philippe Pinel (1745–1826) la médecine de l'esprit* (Paris: Fayard, 1999), 191–216, which discusses conditions at the Salpêtrière; Jean Delamare and Thérèse Delamare-Riche, *Le grand renfermement: Histoire de l'hospice de Bicêtre 1657–1974* (Paris: Maloine, 1990), 95–112, 113–135; Erwin H. Ackerknecht, *Medicine at the Paris Hospital, 1794–1848* (Baltimore: Johns Hopkins Press, 1967); Olivier Faure, *Genèse de l'hôpital moderne: Les hospices civils de Lyon de 1802 à 1845* (Lyon: Presses Universitaires de Lyon, [1981]); S. Borsa and C.-R. Michel, *La vie quotidienne des hôpitaux en France au XIXe siècle* (Paris: Hachette, 1985); and "Medicine in the Hospital," in Bynum, *Science*, 25–54.

6. See Goldstein, 41–42.

7. Michel Foucault describes this transformation of the hospital as the basis for the renewal of medical thought in the late eighteenth and nineteenth centuries. See *Birth of the Clinic*, 64–87.

8. Castel, 21 (trans. modified).

9. Quoted in ibid., 158 (trans. modified); quotation cited by Castel from Ministère de l'Intérieur et des Cultes, *Législation concernant les aliénés et les enfants assistés*, vol. 1 (Paris: Berger-Lerault, 1880), 5.

10. Castel, 165–66.

11. Ibid., 165 (trans. modified).

12. "Rapport fait à la Chambre par M. le marquis de Barthélemy, au nom d'une commission spéciale chargée de l'examen du projet de loi sur les aliénés" in Ministère de l'intérieur et des Cultes, *Législation concernant les aliénés et les enfants assistés*, vol. 2 (Paris: Librairie Administrative de Berger-Levrault et Cie, 1881), 315–16. See also Castel, 168.

13. Jean-Léon Bonfils, *Essai sur la jurisprudence médicale relative aux aliénés* [*Thèse présentée et soutenue à la Faculté de Médecine de Paris, le 17 août 1826, pour obtenir le grade de Docteur en médecine*] (Paris: Didot le jeune, 1826), 8.

14. Ibid., 95.

15. Ibid., 97.

16. See, for example, Cabanis, *Du degré*, 75; Eugène Bouchut, *Traité des signes de la mort et des moyens de prévenir les enterrements prématurés* (Paris: J.-B. Baillière, 1849), 195; and Debreyne, *Mort*, 6.

17. See, for example, the entry on "*séméiotique*" in the *Encyclopédie*: "There is no part of the human body that cannot provide the enlightened observer with a sign; every action, every movement of that marvelous machine is, to his eyes, like so many mirrors in which he sees reflected depictions of the internal state, whether natural or not" (Denis Diderot, ed., *Encyclopédie ou dictionnaire raisonné des sciences et des métiers*, vol. 14 [Neufchastel: Samuel Faulche & Co., 1765], 937).

18. Debreyne, *Mort*, 8. See also Georges Canguilhem, *Ecrits sur la médecine* (Paris: Seuil, 2002): "The force that drove the idea of a medicating nature to take refuge in popular literature arose out of a conjunction of events: on the one hand, the rise of anatomo-pathology and the invention of new techniques for clinical exploration (percussion, auscultation) and, on the other, the discovery, by early 19th-century Austrian and French doctors, of the phenomena of nature's spontaneous silence. The moment that medical practitioners based their diagnoses not on the observation of spontaneous symptoms, but on an examination of the signs they were able to induce, the relations between doctors and nature abruptly separated from those between patients and nature. Because he cannot himself distinguish between signs and symptoms, the patient believes that any behavior is natural so long as it is simply guided by symptoms. But the doctor now knows that unless he uses his art to compel nature to speak, he cannot accept everything it says or the way it says it, and so he is lead to mistrust nature not only in what it says but also in what it does" (28–29). In *Birth of the Clinic*, Michel Foucault describes the difference between sign and symptom as the basis for a new relation between language and truth (95–105).

19. See Cabanis, *Du degré*: "Semiotics, or the art of recognizing the different states of the animal economy by the signs that characterize them, is undoubtedly the most difficult, but also the most important part of medicine. . . . In fact, it is by identifying, so to speak, with the patient, by taking part in his pains and by the quick action of a sensitive imagination, that he perceives the illness in a single glance [*coup-d'œil*] and grasps all of its features at once" (75–76).

20. Cabanis, *Du degré*, 145n1.

21. Bonfils, 100.

22. See Goldstein, 152–96. Marina Van Zuylen, *Monomania: The Flight from Everyday Life in Literature and Art* (Ithaca, N.Y.: Cornell University Press, 2005), revisits the monomania diagnosis, seeing it as a crucial term in a broader notion of modern life.

23. Elias Regnault, *Du degré de compétence des médecins dans les questions judici-aires relatives aux aliénations mentales, et des théories physiologiques sur la monomanie* (Paris: R.Warée fils ainé, 1828), vii.

24. Urbain Coste, "La monomanie," in *Journal universel des sciences médicales*, vol. 43 (July 1826), 53.

25. Castel, 14 (trans. modified).

26. Ibid., 180.

27. Brierre de Boismont, "Bénédicte-Auguste Morel *Etudes cliniques*" in *Annales médico-psychologiques*, 2d series, 4 (1852), 621. Quoted in and translated by Goldstein, 193.

28. *Théologie morale*, 144.

29. Ibid., 145 (emphasis added).

30. Castel, 85–88. Castel's arguments on this score are highly nuanced. Most importantly, he writes that psychiatry achieved its success as a medical specialization through a paradoxical rejection of medical science: "Paradox: in proportion to the meteoric rise of this first medical specialization [i.e. psychiatry], an increasing distance separated it from the concomitant development of medicine in general, which should have served as its foundation. . . . It was only through a very unusual model of medicine—which, unfortunately for 'science,' was already outmoded—that psychiatry could accomplish its goals, because these goals were not essentially medical. The 'choice' of this theoretical corpus seems to have been motivated less by its status as medical 'science' than by its usefulness for encoding social concerns" (87–88, trans. modified). According to Castel, the success of psychiatry in this period can be attributed, at least in part, to the fact that it facilitated "the partial rescue of the totalitarian institution [and thereby] contributed to a strategy for controlling deviant behaviors" (88, trans. modified). As I have already shown in reference to Amédée Latour's 1849 articles from the *Union médicale*, however, medicine itself did not derive its legitimacy in any straightforward way from scientific theory, and the arguments for or against it (by Brierre de Boisement, for instance, or Debreyne) are often based on utility rather than truth-value, scientific or otherwise. What Castel says about psychiatry can, in somewhat modified form, be said of medicine in general during this period.

31. Henri Legrand du Saulle, *La folie devant les tribunaux* (Paris: F. Savy, 1864), 39.

32. Ibid.

33. On Diderot, see chapter 3. In his *Du contrat social* [On the Social Contract], Rousseau wrote that life outside of the civil state was irrational and amoral: "By replacing instinct with justice in his behavior and by giving to his actions the morality that they had previously lacked, this passage from the state of nature to the civil state produces in man a very remarkable change. It is only now, when physical drives yield to the voice of duty and appetite to law, that man, who until this point had considered only himself, finds himself obliged to act on other principles and to consult his reason before heeding his penchants" (in *Social Contract, Discourse on the Virtue Most Necessary for a Hero, Political Fragments, and*

Geneva Manuscript, in *The Collected Writings of Rousseau*, vol. 4, ed. Roger D. Masters and Christopher Kelly, trans. Judith R. Bush, et al. [Hanover, New Hampshire: University Press of New England, 1994], 141, trans. modified). Before entering the state, a human being is still only an animal and not yet a man, for Rousseau describes the integration of the individual into the social contract as "the happy moment that tore him away from [his previous life] forever, and that changed him from a stupid, limited animal into an intelligent being and a man" (141).

34. Bonfils, 9. In his analysis of the law of June 30, 1838, Robert Castel wrote: "In a society founded upon contract, the insane person is the one who escapes from any type of contractual relationship. But at the same time he ceases to offend against it, since *this absence of rights constitutes his status*" (Castel, 188, emphasis added).

35. Regnault, 4.

36. Legrand du Saulle, 39. For Charcot, see Canguilhem, *Ecrits*, 28–29.

37. On the "medicalization" of death in nineteenth-century France, see the excellent historical study by Anne Carol, *Les médecins et la mort XIXe–XXe siècle* (Paris, Aubier, 2004). Carol is particularly astute in her observations about anxieties over premature burial and the relations between doctors and the Church.

38. Louis-Sébastien Mercier, *Tableau de Paris*, vol. 1 (Amsterdam [i.e. in France]: n.p., 1783–88), 76.

39. Ibid., 76–77.

40. Antoine-Alexis Cadet-De-Vaux, *Mémoire sur le méphitisme des puits, par M. Cadet de Vaux, &c. &c. lu à l'Académie royale des sciences, le 25 janvier 1783. Extrait du Journal de physique mars 1783* (n.p.: n.p., n.d.), 7. See also Robert Favre, *La mort dans la littérature et la pensée françaises au siècle des lumières* (Lyon: Presses Universitaires de Lyon, [1978]), 213: "The men of the Enlightenment offered the art of dying pleasantly and they went so far as to promise a gentle and natural death. To put the old terrors finally to rest in a world beset by quite real dangers, the principal task was clear: the best consolation against death was the struggle to fight it off." For Favre, the attempt to understand death, to confront it, and to force it back through medicine and hygiene reflects a will to dominate mortality that manifests itself through Enlightenment practice. As he remarks on Voltaire: "Death and its threats drive him into action. Promoting innoculation, praising peace to Frederick the Great, sowing, planting, draining marshlands, building, moving the cemetery away from Ferney, protecting the young parishioners in Moëns from the whims of their priest, throwing himself into great disputes in order to save Admirial Byng or to defend Calas, it's all one and the same thing to him" (394). Still, as Favre points out, "it still remains very easy to die in the 18th century" (59), and although the *philosophes* had wanted to cure human beings of their *factice*, or artificial fear of death, they became increasingly troubled by the possibility that such fear was perhaps innate and natural (see 363–411). The scope of the project and the extraordinary optimism it produced can be glimpsed in the sheer idea that modern science's real and stunning gains over mortality could be

considered a failure. For a statistical analysis of the triumph over death in the eighteenth and nineteenth centuries, see Vovelle, 367–72.

41. André Pichot has argued, however, that Bichat's physiological theories about death relied on certain principles of contemporary chemistry, even if he never explicitly referred to or fully grasped them: "Life is thus defined by its opposition to the forces of death; it is indeed a form of vitalism. The forces of death are of two kinds. The first are the various external agents that constantly attack the living being. The second are the physical forces that work on the living being's matter from within and tend to decompose it. The latter are less explicitly discussed by Bichat, but they are implicit in much of his physiology. The chemistry by which Stahl explained the corruptibility of bodies had just been discredited by Lavoisier. Since Bichat was not a chemist, he could not pass judgment on the chemical notion of corruptibility that replaced it, even though his conception of life required it" ("Présentation" in Xavier Bichat, *Recherches physiologiques sur la vie et la mort (première partie) et autres textes*, ed. André Pichot [Paris: GF-Flammarion, 1994], 28).

42. For the importance of Paris in the history of modern medicine and the iconic role of Bichat in that history, see Ackerknecht, *Hospital*, xi. On Bichat himself and his influence, see the slim but very useful volume by Philippe Huneman. Maulitz, 9–105, details the influence of Bichat on the Paris school. Omar Keel, "L'essor de l'anatomie pathologique et de la clinique en Europe de 1750 à 1800: Nouveau bilan," in Vincent Barras and Micheline Louis-Courvoisier, 69–92, describes the conditions surrounding the rise of pathology up until the death of Bichat. William Coleman, *Biology in the Nineteenth Century: Problems of Form, Function, and Transformation* (Cambridge: Cambridge University Press, 1971) retraces the role of Bichat and physiology in relation to the debates about biology in the nineteenth century and argues that the most interesting definitions of life came from the physiologists. Interesting responses to Bichat from the early nineteenth century can be found in F.-R. Buisson, "Additions aux recherches sur la vie et la mort. De la division la plus naturelle des phénomènes physiques," in Alibert, et al. eds., *Encyclopédie des sciences médicales*, Division 1, vol. 4 (1802; Paris: Bureau de l'Encyclopédie, 1835), 121–214; and César-Julien-Jean Legallois, "Expériences sur le principe de la vie, notamment sur celui des mouvements du cœur, et sur le siége de ce principe," in Alibert, et al., 215–327. I will return to Bichat's notions of life when I discuss theoretical relations between materiality, sentience, and death in chapter 3.

43. Xavier Bichat, *Physiological Researches on Life and Death* in *Significant Contributions to the History of Psychology 1750–1920*, vol. 2, ed. Daniel N. Robinson, trans. F. Gold (Washington, D.C.: University Publications of America, 1978), 10–11 (trans. modified).

44. Ibid., 10 (trans. modified).

45. Or as Claude Bernard would put it: "life is the whole of *vital* properties which resist the *physical* properties" (quoted in and translated by George Mora, "Cabanis, Neurology and Psychiatry" in Pierre-Jean-George Cabanis, *On the*

Relations Between the Physical and Moral Aspects of Man, vol. 1, ed. George Mora, intros. Sergio Moravia and George Mora, trans. Margaret Duggan Saidi (Baltimore: Johns Hopkins University Press, 1981), lxx.

46. See Huneman, 91–121.

47. See Sigmund Freud's *Beyond the Pleasure Principle*, in *The Standard Edition of the Complete Psychological Works of Sigmund Freud*, vol. 18, ed. and trans. James Strachey (London: Hogarth Press, 1955), 34–43. Freud writes: "These germ-cells, therefore, work against the death of the living substance and succeed in winning for it what we can only regard as a potential immortality, though that may mean no more than a lengthening of the road to death" (40). Freud distinguished between two drives, one toward life and the other toward death, but unlike Bichat, who understood the animate and the inanimate to be separated by their mutual antagonism, Freud located both drives—*eros* and *thanatos*—in the living organism itself. Rather than death against life, Freud understood *thanatos* to be life against itself. Drives, as Freud understood them, are conservative by nature, always tending to reestablish a preexisting condition, and therefore "the elementary living entity would from its very beginning have had no wish to change" (38). But the condition of life itself is not primordial. Inorganic matter precedes the organic, and the impulse to return to an inanimate state is therefore "the first instinct" (38). That inorganic aspect thus remains as a residue in the organic, orienting its most fundamental inclination as a paradoxical memory of unconsciousness (although Freud does not use the word *memory*). There is, in short, some sort of awareness of a primordial unawareness on the part of the living organism and this paradoxical memory is what propels the death drive. In this sense, it is the will of the inorganic, as expressed by the organic, that motivates *thanatos*, and this comes close to reconciling Freud's scenario with Bichat's. For somewhat similar observations, cf. Huneman, 125.

48. Auguste Comte, *Système de politique positive ou traité de sociologie instituant la religion de l'humanité*, vol. 1 (1851; Paris: G. Crès, 1912 [4th ed.]), 440.

49. Bichat himself had emphasized the variability in organic matter, although he was a little more circumspect about it than his follower Comte. "A double movement also occurs in organic life," he wrote. "One tendency constantly composes while the other decomposes the animal. As the ancients and several of their modern followers have observed, the animal's manner of being is such that at any given moment it ceases to be what it had been before. Its organization always remains the same, but its elements constantly change. The nutritive molecules, in turn absorbed and expelled, pass from the animal to the plant, from the latter to elementary matter, return to the animal, and are then expelled. Organic life is adapted to this circulation" (*Recherches*, 62–63). Although he argues that organic life is shaped by its nutritive relation to the inorganic, he does not go so far as to pronounce explicitly on the question of whether the organization of living bodies derives from the stability of their lifeless surroundings, as Comte contended.

50. Comte, 1:615 and 4:439.

51. Félix Gannal, *Moyens de distinguer la mort réelle de la mort apparente* (Paris: Jules-Juteau et Fils, 1868), 4. See also: "Death is the end of life. These few

words should suffice at least to indicate what life is, if the authors could agree" (ibid., 3).

52. Bouchut, iv.

53. See D. A. Miller, *The Novel and the Police* (Berkeley: University of California Press, 1988).

54. As Tardieu wrote in a review of Bouchut's *Traité des signes de la mort*, the issue had become popularized: "The very subject of his book counts among those that will always command the public's interest. Everything that touches on the mystery of death piques the scholar's curiosity for the same reasons that it does the layman's. And although ample allowance must be made for credulousness, there is also room for the doubts, or at least the controversies of science. The fear of being buried alive will not be banished from the popular imagination until the signs of death are established with absolute certainty and the verification of these signs is guaranteed everywhere and for all" (*"Traité des signes de la mort* d'Eugène Bouchut," in *Annales d'hygiène publique et de médecine légale*, vol. 41 [January 1849], 474). For a slightly earlier treatise on the same subject, see Léonce Lenormand, *Des inhumations précipités* (Mâcon: D. Ceville, 1843).

55. Robert Vovelle argues that a pervasive fear of premature burial began around 1760 (see Vovelle, 455). Claudio Milanesi, *Mort apparente, mort imparfaite: Médecine et mentalités au XVIIIe siècle* (Paris: Payot, 1991) argues that such anxieties were not particularly characteristic of the mid-eighteenth to mid-nineteenth centuries, but were, instead, "a sort of constant in our culture" since Democritus (11). On the other hand, Huneman (64–66), citing Philippe Ariès, corroborates my general impression that there was an increased anxiety about premature burial in the period following 1740. For examples of the literature on the subject from the eighteenth century, see Antoine Louis, *Lettres sur la certitude des signes de la mort, où l'on rassure les citoyens de la crainte d'être enterrés vivans avec des observations et des expériences sur les noyés* (Paris: M. Lambert, 1752); and Jacob Benignus Winslow, *Dissertation sur l'incertitude des signes de la mort et l'abus des enterremens et embaumemens précipités*, trans. Jacques-Jean Bruhier (Paris: C.-F. Simon, fils, 1742).

56. See Edgar Allan Poe, "The Premature Burial" in *Poetry and Tales*, ed. Patrick F. Quinn (New York: Library of America, 1984), 666–679. Poe also wrote what is considered to be the first example of the detective genre in a story whose title—"The Murders on the Rue Morgue"—referred to a then novel institution embodying the cooperation of medicine and law (397–431).

57. See Brouardel, 226–27.

58. Caroline Hannaway and Owen Hannaway, "La fermeture du cimetière des Innocents" in *XVIIIe siècle* (1977), 189.

59. Brouardel, 226–27.

60. Favre, 358. On this point, see in general 335–62.

61. Quoted in Daniel Arasse, *The Guillotine and the Terror*, trans. Christopher Miller (London: Allen Lane, 1989), 11.

62. Pierre-Jean-George Cabanis, *Note sur le supplice de la guillotine* (Périgueux: Fanlac, 2002; repr. of "Note sur l'opinion de MM. Œlsner et Sœmmering, et du

citoyen Sue, touchant le Supplice de la Guillotine," 1795), 26. On the importance of the guillotine as an emblem of the Revolution, or at least of the Terror, see Jules Michelet, *Histoire de la révolution*, vol. 2, ed. Gérard Walter (Paris: Gallimard [Pléiade], 1952), 922: "The guillotine rolled along, eating its fill. The meat for this butchery came in by the cartloads, the tumbrils always returning full. It was a sort of routine, a mechanism set up in advance. Everyone seemed to have grown accustomed to the spectacle. Was it from surfeit or from shock? What is certain is that the man who turned the wheel, Fouquier-Tinville, started to get stunned. It is said that he considered setting the guillotine up at the tribunal itself. The Committees asked him if he had gone mad."

63. *Guillotine*, 24.

64. See Jonathan Strauss, *Subjects of Terror: Nerval, Hegel, and the Modern Self* (Stanford, Calif.: Stanford University Press, 1998), 26–37.

65. *Guillotine*, 14n, 19.

66. On the importance of "death-based subjectivity" during this period, see Strauss, *Subjects*, 23–73.

67. The importance of death in the relations between medical practitioners and the law was so central and persistent that even as late as 1962, the doctor Christiane Vitani could look back on the history of forensic medicine and affirm that "although in its current state the medico-legal discipline extends to multiple services within the city, from justice to deontology, from the social safety-net to criminology, so that thanatological problems now occupy only a small part of its ministry, the encounter with death nonetheless remains its primary vocation" (*Législation de la mort: Travail de l'association lyonnaise de médecine légale* [Paris: Masson & Cie, 1962], vii).

68. *Guillotine*, 24.

69. Robert Favre documents these attempts at freeing humanity from the "artificial" fear of of death. See esp. 184–213.

70. Favre, 362, 337. Auguste Comte, as we have seen, held a similar attitude about the legislative force of death and the need for all living things to fight against it. For an argument against the proposition that death is an ahistorical absolute, see Jonathan Strauss, "After Death" in *Diacritics* 30, no. 3 [Fall 2000]): 90–104.

71. Carrière, 442.

72. On Bertrand's sentence, see Lunier, 365 and Dansel, 140–46.

73. Lunier, 362. Similarly, in England, it had proven difficult to prosecute body snatchers or "ressurrectionists." Since corpses were not considered property, they could not be stolen, and grave robbers were therefore brought to trial on incidental grounds, such as stealing the clothes that the deceased was wearing. See Ruth Richardson, *Death, Dissection and the Destitute* (Chicago: University of Chicago Press, 2000), 58–59.

74. On the *idéologues*, and especially their relation to medicine, see Sophie Audidière et al., eds., *Matérialistes français du XVIIIe siècle: La Mettrie, Helvétius, d'Holbach* (Paris: Presses Universitaires de France, 2006).

75. Antoine-Louis-Claude Destutt de Tracy, *Eléments d'idéologie*, vol. 3 (Brussels: n.p., 1826), 751, quoted in Sergio Moravia, "Cabanis and His Contemporaries" trans. George Mora, in Cabanis, *On the Relations Between the Physical and Moral Aspects of Man*, vol. 1, ed. George Mora, intros. Sergio Moravia and George Mora, trans. Margaret Duggan Saidi (Baltimore: Johns Hopkins University Press, 1981), xxxvi (trans. modified).

76. According to George Mora, these included Lamarck, J. S. Mill, Darwin, Spencer, Taine, Saint Simon, Claude Bernard, Ribot, Schopenhauer, Sainte-Beuve, De Vigny, Stendhal, and Flaubert (see lxxiv–v). Thomas Kselman traces nineteenth-century opposition to belief in God and the soul back to La Mettrie, Holback, Diderot, and Condorcet (132–33). For a general description of atheist and antitheist currents in nineteenth-century France, see Kselman, 125–62.

77. Debreyne, *Mort*, 2.

78. "Mémoire des curés de Paris à l'occasion des arrêts du 12 mars 1763, 21 mai, 23 septembre 1765 sur le déplacement des cimetières" (Bibliothèque Nationale, Fonds Joly de Fleury, 1207, fol. 18). The same volume (Joly de Fleury, 1207) contains numerous other documents from the same period concerning the exclusion of sepulchers from the city.

79. "Mémoire des curés de Paris," fol. 19.

80. See Kselman, 222–90.

81. Quoted. in ibid., 271.

82. Quoted. in ibid., 277.

83. Quoted. in ibid., 280.

84. Pierre Desrosières, "A propos d'un cas de nécrophilie: Place du corps mort dans les perversions: Nécrophilie, nécrosadisme et vampirisme," (doctoral thesis in medicine, Université de Paris, Val de Marne, Faculté de Médecine de Créteil, 1974, no. 37), 67–68.

85. Desrosières, however, conflates two very different registers when he assimilates a denial of death to the denial of sexual difference, for the first concerns ontological and the latter ethical issues. For a discussion of some of the problems and perversities involved in such conflations, see preface to Strauss, ed. *Diacritics* 30, 8–9.

86. Lunier, 353–54.

87. It is difficult, at moments, to determine what were really Bertrand's own words and what, for one reason or another, was attributed to him by others. A letter by the sergeant detailing his activities seems indisputably his since it was read in his presence at the trail and copied into the official transcript of the proceedings. What I am referring to now, in the body of my text, is another, lengthier document, also supposedly by Bertrand, which was included in Ambroise Tardieu's 1878 *Etude-médico légale sur les attentats aux mœurs*. Its provenance, however, is unclear and its authenticity uncertain: the events described correspond more or less to those recorded in the trial, and the tone is familiar, but there are some discrepancies in the dates. Still, in his account of the court-martial, Lunier had referred to a "piece written by the accused himself" that

contained all of the principal information laid out in the evidence brought against him, and it does seem likely that this document is the one included in Tardieu's volume (see Lunier, 352).

88. Tardieu, *Attentats*, 122–23. Expert opinions were divided about the fundamental orientation of Bertrand's pathology. Marchal, Castelnau, Lunier, and Morel believed it to be a "destructive monomania complicated by erotic monomania," as Lunier put it (367), whereas others, such as Cl.-F. Michéa, argued, again in Lunier's words, that "erotic monomania was the basis for that monstrous insanity" (368.). See also Morel, "Considérations médico-légales . . . Deuxième lettre," 185, and Michéa, 338a–339c.

89. On Nerval's *Aurélia*, see Strauss, *Subjects of Terror*, 209–10.

90. Tardieu, *Attentats*, 123.

91. Emmanuel Levinas based his notion of subjectivity on the absolute difference that joins human beings in an ethical relationship. Only this relationship, for him, was truly free and only from it, therefore, could genuine acts of goodness result. "The absolutely foreign [*étranger*] alone can instruct us," he wrote. "And it is only man who could be absolutely foreign to me—refractory to every typology, to every genus, to every characterology, to every classification—and consequently the term of a 'knowledge' finally penetrating beyond the object. The strangeness of the Other, his very freedom! Free beings alone can be strangers to one another. Their freedom which is 'common' to them is precisely what separates them. As a 'pure knowledge' language consists in the relationship with a being that in a certain sense is not by relation to me, or, if one likes, that is in a relationship with me only inasmuch as he is wholly by relation to himself, *kath'autó*, a being that stands beyond every attribute, which would precisely have as its effect to qualify him, that is, to reduce him to what is common to him and other beings—a being, consequently, completely naked" (*Totality and Infinity: An Essay on Exteriority*, trans. Alphonso Lingis [Pittsburgh: Duquesne University Press, 1969], 73–74).

92. A contemporary report described the scenes left behind by Bertrand in the following terms: "We are now able to complete the monstrous details [of the crimes] that were repeatedly perpetrated inside the Mont-Parnasse cemetery. We recall that on several occasions the cemetery guards had advised the authorities that tombs had been desecrated during the night under circumstances that belonged more to novels than to reality. Twice the unearthed corpses were found lying on the ground and horribly mutilated. The diabolical genius that committed these monstrosities had thrust his hands into the body of these corpses and had scattered about bits of flesh that could be seen on the ground and hanging from the funerary trees of the adjacent tombs. The vigilance of the guards and the enormous dogs who patrol the cemetery at night had been unable to discover the perpetrator of these odious desecrations" (Factum of the Bibliothèque Nationale de France, 8 Fm 3159, 1).

93. Jacques Derrida described death as a gift, the "*mysterium tremendum*" that terrifies and subjectifies an individual in the act of sacrifice (*The Gift of Death:*

Second Edition & Literature in Secret, trans. David Wills [Chicago: University of Chicago Press, 2008], 8). But Derrida was writing about *death*, the terrifying abstraction at the base of history and subjectivity in the Christian West, while Bertrand's gift was his relation to the *dead* as an aesthetic and emotional category.

94. Foucault, *Birth of the Clinic*, 145 (trans. modified).

95. "Avant-propos," in *Anatomie générale*, vol. 1 (Paris: Brosson, Gabon, et Cie. 1801), xcix.

96. In 1861, Jean-Antoine Villemin compared the "era when the anatomical sciences were in their infancy" to the practices of his own period. He summarized the revolution in clinical pathology that divided those two epochs in terms that echo Bichat's: "A disease was formed by grouping together a certain number of symptoms, out of which a body or individuality was abstracted. All of medical science consisted in thus establishing morbid species and in applying to each of them a specific, empirical remedy. Medicine was an art and a profession, but not a science. Later, illnesses were characterized by an anatomical lesion. The principal goal of medicine was to succeed in identifying that lesion. Palpation, percussion, ausculation, etc. were born. Corpses were opened, their organs examined, and pathological anatomy was created. By connecting organic alterations with the symptoms observed during the patient's life, it was possible to establish a diagnosis" (*Du tubercule au point de vue de son siége, de son évolution et de sa nature* [Paris: J.B. Baillière et fils, 1861], 3). Two elements, therefore, to the revolution: the identification of an underlying pathological disorder or lesion that organized the various symptoms into a coherent system and the use of cadavers to translate those symptoms into expressions, or signs, of that lesion. See also Villemin's thesis for the *agrégation*: *Du rôle de la lésion organique dans les maladies* (Strasbourg: Vve Berger-Levrault, 1862).

97. *Birth of the Clinic*, 145, 141 (trans. modified).

98. Ibid., 144.

99. Buisson, 137. Also quoted in Foucault, *Birth of the Clinic*, 145.

100. See G. W. F. Hegel, *Phenomenology of Spirit*, trans. A. V. Miller (Oxford: Oxford University Press, 1981), 19. It is, however, somewhat unclear why Hegel should call that force of negativity death, since it supposes a continuing subjectivity. He seems, moreover, to incorporate a conflicting conception of death into his master/slave dialectic (114–15). In the latter passage, death has no progressive force and seems to correspond more closely to biological notions of the end of life. For an analysis of these passages, see Strauss, "After Death," 91–92.

3. A HOSTILE ENVIRONMENT

1. One of the articles on death in the *Encyclopédie* includes the startlingly optimistic promise: "We dare affirm, however, based on a knowledge of the structure and properties of the human body and on a large number of observations, that it is possible to *cure death*" (Diderot, *Encyclopédie*, 10:726).

2. Ibid., 716. Michel Foucault noted that for Xavier Bichat and the physiologists, there was a similar "permeability of life by death" and that "death is therefore multiple, and dispersed in time: it is not that absolute and privileged point

at which time stops and moves back; like disease itself, it has a teeming presence that analysis may divide into time and space" (*Birth of the Clinic*, 142).

3. Rodenbach wrote of "mute analogies! The reciprocal penetration of the spirit and physical things! We enter into them, while they penetrate into us" (*Bruges-la-morte*, trans. Philip Mosley [Scranton, Penn.: University of Scranton Press, 2007], 73, trans. modified). Death took on a tangible quality in the symbolic urban universe of the Belgian city: "It could truly be said that there one walked in death" (76). Indeed, the rhetorical trope (analogy or symbol) seems to have functioned for Rodenbach as an allegory for the relation between the conceptual nonbeing of death and the physical presence of things. Death could be "present" in certain places much the same way that abstract meanings could be figured in language or images. Cf. the discussion of *ptomaines* in J.-K. Huysmans, *Becalmed*, trans. Terry Hale (London: Atlas, 1992), 122–25.

4. Octave Mirbeau, *Torture Garden*, trans. Michael Richardson (Sawtry: Dedalus, 1995), 189.

5. See, for example, Jacques-Hippolyte Ronesse, *Vues sur la propreté de Paris* (n.p.: n.p., 1782): "This truth has no need of proof. It has been acknowledged in all periods. Consider how Francis I expressed it in his edict of the month of November, 1529. 'The city of Paris is so foul and full of muds, dung, rubble and other rubbish, that each has left and placed commonly before his door, against reason and against ordinances, that it is a great horror and a most great displeasure to all persons of good and honor: and so are things . . . to the harm and prejudice of the human creatures residing in and frequenting our said city and suburbs, which, by the infection and infestation of the said muds, dung, and other rubbish, have suffered in past times from grievous maladies, mortalities and infirmities of the body, to our great displeasure and not without cause'" (13n).

6. Ibid., 12. Ronesse cites, as an example of this newly increased involvement, the sections of the "Ordonnance de Police" of November 8, 1778 concerning street sweeping.

7. Mercier, 1:73–79.

8. Ibid., 77.

9. Ibid.

10. Lachaise, 14.

11. Ibid.

12. On the rise of public hygiene in France, see Bernard P. Lécuyer, "L'hygiène en France avant Pasteur 1750–1850," in Salomon-Bayet, 65–142 and Erwin H. Ackerknecht, "Hygiene in France, 1815–1848," *Bulletin of the History of Medicine* 22 (March/April 1948): 117–55. Sournia includes a very useful section on public hygiene during and just after the Revolution (192–200). Gérard Jorland's *Une société à soigner: Hygiène et salubrité publiques en France au XIXe siècle* (Paris: Gallimard, 2010), describes the evolution of hygiene as a public policy in nineteenth-century France. William Coleman's *Death is a Social Disease: Public Health and Political Economy in Early Industrial France* (Madison: University of Wisconsin Press, 1982) focuses on the career of Louis-René Villermé and his seminal work

on the relations between illness and social conditions. Robert Carvais's "La maladie, la loi, et les mœurs," in Salmon Bayet, 279–330 describes legal aspects of public health and the movement to create an international hygienic policy in the second half of the nineteenth century. Georges Vigarello, *Concepts of Cleanliness: Changing Attitudes in France since the Middle Ages*, trans. Jean Birrell (Cambridge: Cambridge University Press, 1988), discusses how water acquired a central role in early nineteenth-century discussions of public hygiene and, in a Bachelardian vein, examines some of the imaginary structures involved in that development (165–225).

13. See Sournia, 195–99.

14. See Lécuyer, "Hygiène," 67.

15. See ibid., 69–71 and Sournia, 163, 194–95.

16. See Sournia, 196.

17. Ibid., 197.

18. Ibid.

19. Lécuyer, "Hygiène," 73–74.

20. On Villermé, see Coleman, *Death* and Bynum, "Médecine et société," 308. On statistical methods in hygiene during this period, see Lécuyer, "Hygiène," 80–92 and Sournia, 193.

21. Lécuyer, "Hygiène," 83–92.

22. Quoted in ibid., 100.

23. Royer-Collard, *Cours d'hygiène professé à la Faculté de médecine* (Paris: Lacrampe, 1846), 2.

24. Ibid., 4.

25. Ibid., 5.

26. Ibid., 9–10.

27. Ibid., 10.

28. Ibid., 12–13.

29. Bruno Latour has described the pre-Pasteurian approach to hygiene as a "combat tous azimuts" or a battle on all fronts (*The Pasteurization of France*, trans. Alan Sheridan and John Law [Cambridge, Mass.: Harvard University Press, 1988], 19–22). He attributes this anxious and granular vigilance to the fact that hygienists lacked a central argument to organize their field (20).

30. Royer-Collard, 12.

31. On the idea of a "tame death," see Philippe Ariès, *The Hour of Our Death*, trans. Helen Weaver (New York: Knopf, 1981), 3–28.

32. "Medical Observations Concerning the History and Cure of Acute Diseases" in *The Works of Thomas Sydenham, M.D.*, vol. 1, trans. R. G. Latham (London: Sydenham Society, 1848), 31. Such *"skiey influences"* were, according to Sydenham, the cause of epidemic diseases (32).

33. See Stephen Hales, "Experiments, Whereby to Prove, That a Considerable Quantity of Air Is Inspired by Plants" in *Vegetable Staticks: or, an Account of Some Statical Experiments on the Sap in Vegetables: Being an Essay Towards a Natural History of Vegetation* (London: W. & J. Innys, 1727), 177–84, and Stephen Hales,

A Treatise on Ventilators: Wherein an Account Is Given of the Happy Effects of the Several Trials That Have Been Made of Them (London: Richard Manby, 1758). For more general accounts of these developments in gas theory, see David L. Swift, "Priestley and Lavoisier: Oxygen and Carbon Dioxide" in Donald F. Proctor, ed., *A History of Breathing Physiology* (New York: M. Dekker, 1995), 223–38; Hannaway and Hannaway; Alain Corbin, *The Foul and the Fragrant: Odor and the French Social Imagination*, trans. Miriam L. Kochan, Roy Porter, and Christopher Prendergast (Cambridge, Mass.: Harvard University Press, 1986), 29–30; and Vigarello, 144–45, 147–48.

34. Concerning cemeteries and latrines, Michel du Tennetar condemned "their infected vapors, dangerous at all times and in all places" (Michel du Tennetar, *Mémoire sur l'état de l'atmosphère à Metz et ses effets sur les habitans de cette ville, ou réflexions sur les dangers d'une atmosphère habituellement froide et humide, et les moyens de les prévenir* [Nancy: C.-S. Lamort, 1778], 23). Some three years before the French Revolution, Mathieu Géraud writes: "The vapor from privies corrupts every kind of meat, and . . . this corruption occurs when the putrid exhalations of the latrine absorb the constituant air of the meat" (*Essai sur la suppression des fosses d'aisances et de toute espèce de voirie, sur la manière de convertir en combustibles les substances qu'on y renferme* (Amsterdam: n.p., 1786), 55. See also Mercier, 11:55.

35. Mercier, 1:78.

36. Vicq d'Azyr, "Discours préliminaire," cxxxi.

37. See Jacques de Horne, *Mémoire sur quelques objets qui intéressent plus particulièrement la salubrité de la ville de Paris* (Paris: J.-C. Dessaint, 1788), 4.

38. Hannaway and Hannaway, 183–84.

39. P. Charles Gabriel Porée, *Lettres sur la sépulture dans les églises. A Monsieur de C. . . .* (Caen: Jean-Claude Pyron, 1745), 23. For similar arguments, see also H. Haguenot, *Mémoires sur les dangers des inhumations* (n.p.: n.p., 1744); Jean-Philibert Maret, *Mémoire sur l'usage où l'on est d'enterrer les morts dans les églises et dans l'enceinte des villes* (Dijon: Cause, 1773).

40. Maret, 22–23.

41. Ibid., 23.

42. In the last thirty years, this literature has been rediscovered and commented on by historians such as Arlette Farge (for example, "Signe de vie, risque de mort. Essai sur le sang et la ville au XVIIIe siècle," *Urbi*, no. 2 [December 1979]: xviii) and Richard Etlin (31).

43. Piattoli, 13–14.

44. Jean-Baptiste Banau and François Turben, *Mémoire sur les épidémies du Languedoc, adressé aux états de cette province* (Paris: Banau, 1786), 12–13.

45. On the mechanical properties of air, see Piattoli, 113.

46. "Discours préliminaire," cxxix.

47. Ibid., cxxxixn.

48. Cadet-De-Vaux, *Innocents*, 5.

49. Ibid.

50. Ibid., 5–6.
51. Ibid., 7.
52. Ibid., 7–8.
53. Bernardin de Saint-Pierre proposed that the dead be interred in wooded cemeteries outside the city. "First of all, I would want no citizen to be buried inside a church," he wrote and then argued that natural settings "inspire a deep and gentle melancholy, not only by the natural effect of their decoration, but by the moral sentiment that tombs inspire in us" (Henri Bernardin de Saint-Pierre, *Etudes de la nature* [Paris: Deterville, 1804], 378–79). He also wrote that priests would be only too happy to bury their parishioners in the countryside, because "as they sit in their stalls, they would not have to breathe the revolting odor of corpses throughout the year" (376–77).
54. Hippolite Cloquet, *Osphrésiologie ou traité des odeurs, du sens et des organes de l'olfaction; avec l'histoire détaillée des maladies du nez et des fosses nasales, et des opérations qui leur conviennent* (Paris: Méquignon-Marvis, 1821), 87–88.
55. Lachaise, 144.
56. Ibid., 144–45.
57. "Petition from the inhabitants of the faubourg Saint Michel to the mayor, June 25, 1832," Municiple Archives Angers, 37 M 10, quoted in and translated by Kselman, 175.
58. "Observations sur les gaz méphitiques des caveaux mortuaires des cimetières de Paris" *Annales d'hygiène publique* 41 (January, 1849): 128.
59. Ibid.
60. "Notes sur le mémoire précédent," *Annales d'hygiène publique* 41 (January, 1849): 141.
61. Eugène Belgrand, *Préfecture du département de la Seine. Direction des eaux et égouts. Rapport du directeur sur les emplacements proposés pour de nouveaux cimetières* (Paris: Imprimérie centrale des chemins de fer, A. Chaix et Co., 1876), 8.
62. de Horne, 1.
63. In 1822, Lachaise still complained about the management of human excreta in Paris, noting in particular the effects produced on the city's air by the vast reservoirs of fecal material stored in open tanks at Montfaucon, where the contents of urban latrines were dumped and held until they could be dried for use as fertilizer. "Is this the best location to store the fecal matters of such a populous city?" he asked. "When we examine the wind charts . . . we immediately see it is not" (138).
64. Belgrand, 9.
65. Ibid.
66. Kselman, 26. The cholera outbreak of 1832 in particular has received significant scholarly attention. For statistical information and a sociological approach, see Louis Chevalier's classic "Paris," in Louis Chevalier, ed., *Le choléra: La première épidémie du XIXe siècle* (La Roche-sur-Yon: Imprimerie Centrale de l'Ouest, 1958), 1–46. François Delaporte, *Disease and Civilization: The Cholera in Paris, 1832*, trans. Arthur Goldhammer (Cambridge, Mass.: MIT Press, 1986),

picks up on the social issues in Chevalier's work and concludes that "the epidemic of 1832 surely marks a historical watershed: the moment when the need to *import* into the exploited class a health apparatus forged by and for the bourgeoisie became evident" (199–200). William Coleman's chapter on "Inequality before Death: Paris" in *Death* (149–80) uses statistics, maps, and tables similar to Chevalier's to describe economic/class differences, especially in relation to cholera outbreaks in the nineteenth century. Olivier Faure's *Histoire sociale de la médecine* (Paris: Anthropos-Economica, 1994) describes how the cholera outbreak of 1832 marked a psychologically important failure of medical progress, especially in respect to campaigns for vaccination, and synthesizes some of the debate about contagion and infection (135–52). Catherine J. Kudlick's *Cholera in Post-Revolutionary Paris: A Cultural History* (Berkeley: University of California Press, 1996) explains the difference between reactions to the 1832 and 1849 cholera epidemics in Paris by arguing that in the earlier outbreak, the disease was connected to revolution and class disturbances.

67. For a concise overview of the principal scholarship on the contagionist debate (and whether it actually occurred at all), see Lécuyer, "Hygiène," 71–72, 95–96. Generally, the contagionists believed that disease spread through direct physical contact, while the infectionists (or anticontagionists as they are sometimes called) emphasized environmental and social factors. According to Lécuyer, the 1832 cholera outbreak cemented the success of the latter. The quarantines and *cordons sanitaires* set up to prevent dissemination through physical contact proved ineffective, and hygienists focused instead on living conditions. "At the end of the cholera epidemic," Lécuyer writes, "the commission met in 1834 to draw some conclusions about the epidemic in Paris. These conclusions were mixed. On the one hand, cholera was judged not to be contagious (transmissible). On the other hand, although it was generally associated with insalubrious living *conditions* (a connection that was, however, neither necessary nor general), it was equally associated with unsatisfactory living *standards*" (97).

68. Honoré de Balzac, "Ferragus: Chief of the Companions of Duty" in *History of the Thirteen*, trans. Herbert J. Hunt (New York: Penguin, 1974), 32 (trans. modified).

69. A manual published some seven years later explained the human body's need for light: "We have said that light passes through atmospheric air. Apparently, everything that has received the principle of life needs this agent to exist in a state of health and to fulfill the functions that nature has attributed to it. . . . So it is for men who take up sedentary occupations and etiolate in the narrow streets where sunlight never penetrates. Their vital functions lose their activity, their face grows sallow, their circulation slows, and the children born to these incomplete individuals bear the marks of a sickly and bastard constitution. . . . The intensification of illnesses that is often observed at night has been attributed to the absence of light. It is noteworthy that for every twenty sick people who die, at least two-thirds expire at nightfall or during the night" (M. L. N**., *L'hygiène, ou l'art de conserver la santé* [Chatillon-sur-Seine: C. Cornillac, 1840], 44–45). The author also confirmed the need for unpolluted air (33–49).

70. François-Marc Moreau, *Histoire statistique du choléra-morbus dans le quartier du faubourg Saint-Denis (5e arrondissement), pendant les mois d'avril, mai, juin, juillet, août et septembre* (Paris: Chez l'auteur, 1833), 29.

71. Ibid., 41.

72. "One can also understand why certain houses present a larger number of cholera cases and deaths, if one remembers that these houses generally . . . stand out for their dirtiness, their insalubriousness, the poor location of their site, and the indigence of their inhabitants" (ibid., 53–54.

73. Ibid., 57.

74. Lachaise, 203.

75. Ibid., 203–4.

76. "Rapport de M. Emile Trélat sur l'évacuation des vidanges par la voie publique," in Emile Trélat, A. Hudelo, and Henri Gueneau de Mussy, *De l'évacuation des vidanges dans la ville de Paris* (Paris: G. Masson, 1882), 18.

77. Antoine Alexis Cadet-De-Vaux, Laborie, and Antoine-Augustin Parmentier, *Observations sur les fosses d'aisances et moyens de prévenir les inconvéniens de leur vuidange* (Paris: P.-D. Pierres, 1778), 6.

78. Lachaise, 265.

4. DEATH COMES ALIVE

1. Mercier, 1:75.

2. Ibid.

3. Hippolyte du Roselle, *Les eaux, les égouts et les fosses d'aisances dans leurs rapports avec les épidémies* (Amiens: T. Jeunet, 1867), 18–19. In 1876, Eugène Belgrand expressed similar concerns about the effects of dead bodies on the Parisian water supply: "It seems that the authors of these projects deem the effects of cemeteries on the earth and subterranean waters to be negligible and feel that the violent opposition of the population to any new establishments is based on simple prejudice, namely, the fear, more chimerical than justified, of drinking water contaminated by human detritus. This fear is unfortunately only too legitimate" (Belgrand, 8).

4. Trélat, 19.

5. Ibid., 42.

6. Ibid.

7. Ibid., 18.

8. "Discours préliminaire," clii–cliii.

9. Cadet-De-Vaux, *Innocents*, 6.

10. Cloquet, 17. How to translate this strange piece of unexpected poetry? *Bousiers* are dung-beetles. *Necrophores*, which live in decaying animal flesh, *escarbots*—the word comes from scarab under the influence of *escargot*—*sphéridies*, which are forms of dung-beetles (*sphaeridia*), *dermestres* (or larder beetles), and *ptines* are all coleoptera, whose species include beetles, weevils, and fireflies. *Sylphes* are insects, but also, of course, mythological creatures of the air.

11. Ambroise Tardieu, *Voiries et cimetières: Thèse présentée au concours pour la chaire d'hygiène à la faculté de médecine de Paris, et soutenue le 1er mars 1852* (Paris: J.-B. Baillière, 1852), 5.

12. Félix Gannal, *Cimetières*, 155.

13. Porée, 24.

14. Pierre Bertholon, *De la salubrité de l'air des villes et en particulier des moyens de la procurer* (Montpellier: J. Martel aîné, 1786), 72.

15. Emile-Louis Bertherand, *Mémoire sur la vidange des latrines et des urinoirs publics au point de vue hygiénique, agricole et commercial* (Lille: Lefebvre-Ducrocq, 1858), 4.

16. Quoted in du Roselle, 15.

17. Ibid., 15–16.

18. In *Pasteur sans la légende* (Paris: Géraldine Billon, 1994), François Dagognet has argued that Pasteur's interest in amylic alcohol has long been misunderstood. According to Dagognet, Pasteur's work on fermentation did not result from happenstance—the needs of a certain brewer, named Bigo, in Lille—but rather from the internal theoretical needs of a scientific project (see esp. 150–51). On Pasteur's work in general and its significance, see also Dagognet's earlier *Méthodes et doctrine dans l'œuvre de Pasteur* (Paris: Presses Universitaires de France, 1967) and Salomon-Bayet.

19. Quoted in Trélat, 38.

20. Quoted in ibid., 39.

21. Dagognet, *Légende*, 150–51.

22. Quoted in ibid., 156.

23. See ibid., 189.

24. Louis-Auguste Cadet, *Hygiène, exhumation, crémation ou incinération des corps* (Paris: Baillière, 1877), 11 (quoted in Carol, 236).

25. See Claude Bernard, *Leçons sur les phénomènes de la vie communs aux animaux et aux végétaux*, preface by Georges Canguilhem (1878; Paris: J. Vrin, 1966), 176. Fermentation as a whole remained similarly obscure: "Chemists and physiologists have never agreed, and still do not agree, on what is be understood by the term 'fermentation'" (158).

26. "It has always been known that after death the materials constituting animal bodies begin to alter, to be transformed and to decompose into various principles, among which are substances with a strong and putrid odor. From this comes the term 'putrefaction'" (Bernard, 173). See also 157 and 178 on the relations between fermentation and putrefaction and the latter's effects on organic matter. As a measure of how these concepts had penetrated into government discussions of hygiene, cf. an 1877 report to the Conseil d'hygiène du Nord: "it is unwise to linger near cesspools [*fosses*] when then they are in a state of putrid fermentation or to spend time in the close proximity of a cemetery, for fear of potentially serious accidents" (in Du Mesnil, *Rapport de la commission d'assainissement des cimetières*, December 24, 1880, VII/27, Archives de Paris [quoted in Carol, 251–52]).

27. Bernard, 176. See also 177.

28. Ibid., 178.

29. As Georges Canguilhem has put it: "According to Claude Bernard, . . . the functioning of an organ is a physico-chemical phenomenon, it is death. We can grasp and characterize these phenomena, and it is this death that we mistakenly call life [*c'est cette mort que nous sommes portés illusoirement à appeler la vie*]" (preface in Bernard, 1).

30. Foucault, *Birth of the Clinic*, 140 (trans. modified).

31. On the rise and significance of pathology, see Keel, 69–92; Maulitz, 60–82; Foucault's *Birth of the Clinic*, esp. 124–48, which discuss the importance of pathological anatomy in relation to physiology; and Ackerknecht, *Hospital*. Coleman, *Biology* discusses the rise of biology, but his descriptions show that the most interesting definitions of life came from the physiologists.

32. Ackerknecht, *Hospital*, xiii.

33. Ibid., xi.

34. Historians seem to enjoy using physical aspects of Bichat's death and commemoration to make larger points about the history of medicine. Maulitz discusses the handling of his corpse (1–5) as emblematic of contemporary theoretical questions. For the centrality of Bichat's role and his influence on later physiologists, see Huneman and, again, Foucault's *Birth of the Clinic*, esp. 124–48. Nicolas Dobo and André Role, *Bichat: La vie fulgurante d'un génie* (Paris: Perrin, 1989) contains a helpful biography. L. S. Jacyna, "Romantic Thought and the Origins of Cell Theory," in Andrew Cunningham and Nicholas Jardine, eds., *Romanticism and the Sciences* (Cambridge: Cambridge University Press, 1990), 161–68, describes some of the important elements missing from Bichat's methods and theories and how those lacunae were subsequently addressed.

35. Huneman makes a similar observation about Bichat's instrumentalization of poisons and the role of death in isolating vital functions for both Bichat and Claude Bernard (109–11).

36. Bichat, *Physiological Researches*, 59–65.

37. Ibid., 10–11.

38. Ibid., 10 (trans. modified).

39. Buisson, 137. Foucault has commented on this passage, in *Birth of the Clinic*, 145. A similar objection, in almost the same terms as Buisson's, was raised by André Pichot, who edited a recent edition of Bichat's book: "So there really is a vicious circle in this definition" (Bichat, *Recherches*, 57n).

40. Bichat, *Physiological Researches*, 10–11, 14–16.

41. Ibid., 163 (trans. modified).

42. Buisson, 126–27.

43. Ibid., 129.

44. Ibid., 129.

45. Legallois, 215–327.

46. Ibid., 217–18, 221.

47. François Broussais, *De l'irritation et de la folie* (1839; Fayard, 1986). On Broussais's influence on medical materialism and Auguste Comte, see Jean-François Braunstein, *Broussais et le matérialisme: Médecine et philosophie au XIXe siècle* (Paris: Klincksieck, 1986). See also Ackerknecht, *Hospital*, 61–82.

48. Francisque Bouillier, *Du principe vital et de l'âme pensante ou examen des diverses doctrines médicales et psychologiques sur les rapports de l'âme et de la vie* (Paris: Baillière et fils, 1862), 42–43, 378.

49. Ibid., 396–98.

50. On Claude Bernard as a continuator of Bichat's physiology, see Huneman, 96–121.

51. Bernard, 343, 125, 127, 128, 157, 347–49.

52. Ibid., 125: "We have shown two aspects that characterize the existence of living beings: *life*, or organic creation, and *death*, or organic destruction. It is now necessary to prove this division and to show that it is the basis for general physiology."

53. Ibid., 136–42.

54. Ibid., 142–43.

55. Ibid., 143–44.

56. Ibid., 132.

57. Ibid., 144. Cf. 292 on irritability and sensitivity.

58. Ibid., 292–93.

59. Ibid., 350.

60. Ibid., 300–18, 344–45.

61. Ibid., 345. A little later, Bernard rephrased this idea in somewhat different terms: "Life is, for us, the result of a conflict between the organism and the outside world" (346). Here, he conceives of life not as the conflict itself but rather its result.

62. Ibid., 347. Georges Canguilhem has remarked on the surprising nature of life in Bernard's theories: "The functioning of an organ was a physicochemical phenomenon, that is, death. We can grasp such phenomena, we can understand and characterize them, and so we are inclined, misleadingly, to apply the name 'life' to what is in fact a form of death" (*A Vital Rationalist: Selected Writings from Georges Canguilhem*, ed. François Delaporte, trans. Arthur Goldhammer, intro. Paul Rabinow [New York: Zone, 1994], 313).

63. George J. Romanes, *Animal Intelligence* (London: Kegan Paul, Trench, & Co., 1882), 25.

64. Ibid., 25.

65. Ibid., 25n.

66. Ibid., 28: "I incline to Mr. Darwin's opinion that the facts can only be explained by supposing them due to intelligence on the part of the snails. Thus considered, these facts are no doubt very remarkable; for they would appear to indicate not merely accurate memory of direction and locality for twenty-four hours, but also no small degree of something akin to 'permanent attachment,' and sympathetic desire that another should share in the good things which one has found."

67. Latour, "De l'autorité en médecine," in *L'union médicale. Journal des inté-rêts scientifiques et pratiques, moraux et professionnels du corps médical* 3, no. 112 (September 20, 1849): 446. The oyster did have an iconographic role in the Christian tradition, but it was very different from the use Latour makes of it here. According to medieval Catholic writers, pearls were created by dew falling into the oyster and symbolized the immaculate conception of Jesus. See Stephen Manning, "I Sing of a Myden" in *PMLA* 75 (1960): 8–12; Costantino Vona, "La *Margarita Pretiosa* nella interpretazione di alcuni scrittori ecclesiastici" in *Divinitas* 1 (1957): 118–60; Albert the Great, *Man and the Beasts: de Animalibus (Books 22–26)*, trans. James J. Scanlan (Binghamton: MRTS, 1987), 361 (this text also contains a wonderful section on the conception of pearls and a description of oysters emerging in droves from the water to receive dew); and Thomas Usk, *The Testament of Love*, ed. R. Allen Shoaf (Kalamazoo, Michigan: Medieval Institute Publications, 1998), appendix I. Closer to Latour's conception of mollusk consciousness is a passage from Plato's *Timaeus*, which describes the various orders of animals, the lowest of which was populated by the oyster: "The fourth class were the inhabitants of the water; these were made out of the most entirely senseless and ignorant of all. . . . And hence arose the race of fishes and oysters [*ostreon*], and other aquatic animals, which have received the most remote habitations as a punishment of their outlandish ignorance" (91d–92c, trans. Benjamin Jowett, in Plato, *Collected Dialogues*, 1210–11).

68. M. L. N**., *L'hygiène*, 81.

69. Ibid., 81.

70. See Carol, 143–61, 199–205, 211–31.

71. Gannal, *Moyens de distinguer*, 11.

72. Cloquet, 9.

73. Ibid., 13, 15–16.

74. Ibid., 34.

75. Bouchut, 196 and Gannal, *Moyens de distinguer*, 17. Similarly, in the *Encyclopédie*, putrefaction is taken as the sole sign of irreversible death: "[W]e dare affirm, however, based on a knowledge of the structure and properties of the human body and on a large number of observations, that it is possible to *cure death*, which is to say, bring back the interrupted movement of the blood and vessels, until putrefaction shows us that *death is absolute*" (10:726). Cf. 720, where the author describes the dangers of interring bodies "without, above all, waiting until the appearance of putrefaction has determined their *death* to be irrevocable."

76. Bouchut, 176–77.

77. Cloquet, 25, 28–29, 37.

78. Ibid., 25.

79. Ibid., 24–25, 61.

80. Ibid., 8.

81. Etienne de Condillac, *Condillac's Treatise on the Sensations*, trans. Geraldine Carr (Los Angeles: University of Southern California, School of Philosophy, 1930), 3 (trans. modified).

82. Ibid., 6 and 30 (trans. modified).
83. Ibid., 6 (trans. modified).
84. Ibid., 43 (trans. modified).
85. Ibid. (trans. modified).
86. Ibid., 44n (trans. modified).
87. Cloquet, 24.
88. Ibid., 20.
89. Ibid., 25.
90. Condillac, 36 (trans. modified).
91. Koch published his findings in 1876 as *Die Aetiologie der Milzbrandkrankheit, begrundet auf die Entwicklungsgeschichte des Bacillus Anthracis* in Ferdinand Cohn, ed., *Beiträge zur Biologie der Pflanzen*, vol. 2, no. 2 (Breslau: J. U. Kerns, 1876), 277–310.
92. Quoted in Walter Benjamin, "On Some Motifs in Baudelaire" in *Illuminations*, trans. Harry Zohn, ed. Hannah Arendt (New York: Schocken, 1969), 158.
93. Ibid., 159.
94. Ibid., 184.
95. Ibid.
96. Ibid., 158.
97. Ibid., 184
98. Ibid., 184, 159.
99. Ibid., 184.
100. Ibid., 184–85.
101. Ibid., 185.
102. Ibid.
103. Ibid.
104. Rousseau, *Discourse on the Origins of Inequality* in *Discourse on the Origins of Inequality (Second Discourse), Polemics, and Political Economy* in *The Collected Writings of Rousseau*, vol. 3, ed. Roger D. Masters and Christopher Kelly, trans. Judith R. Bush et al. (Hanover, New Hampshire: University Press of New England, 1992), 43 (trans. modified).
105. See Strauss, *Subjects of Terror*, 23–73 and "After Death."
106. *Social Contract*, 139n (trans. modified).

5. PLEASURE IN REVOLT

1. Peter Stallybrass and Allon White, *The Politics and Poetics of Transgression* (Ithaca, N.Y.: Cornell University Press, 1986), 191.
2. Royer-Collard, 7.
3. Ibid., 8.
4. Ibid.
5. Ibid.
6. On Zacchia and Garmann, see Ariès, 353–61.
7. Ibid., 358 (trans. modified).
8. See Favre, 339–40.

9. This idea that life depends on death persists into Claude Bernard's last writings, where they form the core of his approach to biology. "There is no life without death," he writes. "There is no death without life" (128). He then adds, "nature engenders life only through death, creation only through destruction" (147). Cf. 127, 148, 157.

10. Etienne-Louis Boullée, "Architecture: Essai sur l'art" in Etienne-Louis Boullée, *L'architecte visionnaire et néoclassique*, ed. J.-M. Pérouse de Montclos (Paris: Hermann, 1993), 162. The most useful recent study on Boullée's funerary architecture can be found in Etlin, 108–44, to which I am deeply indebted for my own reading of the architect. Jean-Marie Pérouse de Montclos, *Etienne-Louis Boullée* (Paris: Flammarion, 1994), also contains a chapter on funerary projects, in which the author traces the origins of Boullée's ideas and contests his claims of originality. Surprisingly, despite the central position that Boullée himself attributed to the architecture of death, critics and historians have given little attention to its peculiar role in his aesthetics. The classic study by Emil Kaufmann, *Three Revolutionary Architects, Boullée, Ledoux, and Lequeu* in *Transactions of the American Philosophical Society*, new series, vol. 42 (1952), 429–564, makes no mention of the question, and with the exception of Etlin more recent works seem to have added little to an understanding of this aspect of Boullée's theories.

11. Boullée, 162.

12. Ibid., 140–41. Christophe Henry, "'De la fumée surgit la lumière.' Sources théoriques et fonctions poétiques du clair-obscur boulléen" in *Claude Nicolas Ledoux et le livre d'architecture en français. Etienne Louis Boullée l'utopie et la poésie de l'art*, ed. Daniel Rabreau and Dominique Massounie, (Paris: Editions du patrimoine, 2006), 278–99, traces the origins of Boullée's *chiaroscuro* to traditions in painting. It is worth remarking that neither his article nor the volume that contains it gives much attention to the role of death in the work of either Ledoux or Boullée.

13. Boullée, 144, 162.

14. Ibid., 137.

15. Ibid.

16. Ibid.

17. Ibid., 138.

18. Cf. Kant's description of the pyramids in the "Mathematically Sublime" section of the *Critique of Judgement*, trans. James Creed Meredith (Oxford: Oxford University Press, 1952): "In order to get the full emotional effect of the size of the Pyramids we must avoid coming too near just as much as remaining too far away. For in the latter case the representation of the apprehended parts (the tiers of stones) is but obscure, and produces no effect upon the aesthetic judgement of the subject. In the former, however, it takes the eye some time to complete the apprehension from the base to the summit; but in this interval the first tiers always in part disappear before the imagination has taken in the last, and so the comprehension is never complete" (99–100). By thus standing in just the right place, the viewer experiences a feeling of the sublime: "For here a feeling comes home to him of the inadequacy of his imagination for presenting the

idea of a whole within which that imagination attains its maximum, and, in its fruitless efforts to extend this limit, recoils upon itself, but in so doing succumbs to an emotional delight" (100). This delight comes, according to Kant, from the imagination's "want of finality for our judgement in the estimation of magnitude" (100). Kant's assertion that the delight of such sublime moments comes in the imagination's recognizing a higher, mathematical kind of thinking beyond its own powers is very different from the notion of the sublime that Boullée describes in his buried pyramids. The power of Kant's model is so great, however, that it is difficult to appreciate that the sunkenness of Boullée's structures is not merely a technique to create a sublime viewpoint through physical means and to intimate the infinite through them but instead derives from the idiosyncratic notions of natural and material embeddedness that Boullée adumbrates throughout his essay.

19. Boullée, 139.

20. Claude-Nicolas Ledoux, *L'architecture considéré sous le rapport de l'art, des moeurs et de la léglislation,* vol. 1 (Paris: chez l'auteur, 1804), 8 (quoted in and translated by Etlin, 146). One should note that Ledoux is actually talking about clouds in this passage, but that he is doing so in the context of tombs—and as a metaphor for them—in a way that plays off other passages in the same volume. The "chaotic" nature of clouds, for example, relates them to Ledoux's description of his "Elévation du cimetière de la ville de Chaux" (Ledoux, vol. 1, plate 100), in which the "chaos" of the tomb replicates the original chaos of the universe (195); the echos between these two passages are further reinforced by the way that the author imagines tombs as stains on the "globe's mass" (8), an image that supposes the sort of view from outer space that he depicts only, but quite strikingly, in the "Elévation du cimetière de Chaux [Elevation of the Chaux Cemetery]." The principal contemporary work on Ledoux is Anthony Vidler's *Claude-Nicolas Ledoux: Architectural Reform at the End of the Ancien Régime* (Cambridge, Mass.: MIT University Press, 1990), but Vidler's discussion of cemeteries and funerary architecture by Ledoux concentrates mostly on hygienic questions, such as the prevention of miasmas (272–74). Daniel Rabreau's more recent *Claude-Nicolas Ledoux (1736–1806). L'architecture et les fastes du temps* (Paris: Centre Ledoux, Unviersité de Paris-I Pathéon-Sorbonne, 2000) contains intriguing sections on Ledoux's metaphysical and mystical tendencies but virtually nothing on his attitudes about the dead. Again, it is to Etlin's *Architecture of Death*—and especially to a highly suggestive quotation (146, cited above)—that I am indebted for my own interest in Ledoux.

21. See Etlin, 229–301.

22. Légouvé, "La sépulture" in *Gazette nationale ou le moniteur universel*, no. 42 (November 2, 1796), 166. I am indebted to Etlin (254) for this quotation, which Etlin, curiously, attributes to A. Jourdan, who did, however, write an article on inhumations for the July 6, 1796, issue of the *Moniteur.*

23. Andrieux, "Fable. Les passagers et le pilote," *Gazette nationale ou le moniteur universel*, no. 134 (February 3, 1796): 533.

24. Le citoyen Piis, "La pâque naturelle: Hymne à l'usage des philosophes" in *Gazette nationale ou le moniteur universel*, no.190 (March 30, 1796): 757–58.

25. A. Jourdan, "Mélanges," *Gazette mationale ou le moniteur universel*, no. 288 (July 6, 1796): 1130.

26. See Etlin, 294.

27. Jacques Fernand, *Les cimetières. Supprimer la fosse commune et les fosses temporaires. Pétition adressée à l'assemblée nationale au conseil de Paris et aux autres conseils municipaux pour supprimer les fosses temporaires et la fosse commune, et donner gratis aux pauvres le repos et le terrain à perpétuité, les riches paieront plus chers* (Paris: C. Vanier, 1874), 14.

28. Dissimulated in Fernand's metaphorics of food and corpse is probably the idea of funerary anthropophagy, an archaic practice that Jacques Derrida still sees at work in Hegel's readings of Sophocles's *Antigone*. The unconscious desire to eat the dead would, according to Derrida, motivate the heroine's actions, since they are part of a process of introjection and mourning. A similar fantasmatic desire can be imagined for Fernand. See Derrida, *Glas*, trans. John P. Leavey, Jr. and Richard Rand (Lincoln, Nebraska: University of Nebraska Press, 1986), 144–45. Suggestive as it is, however, Derrida's reading does minimize the action of what Hegel calls an "abstract essence" at work in decomposition, replacing it with psychological processes. But to minimize that action, Derrida must dismiss Hegel's explicit interpretation of Antigone's behavior—he understands it to express a concern about the return of the organic to the inorganic—as "banal" (164) and explain it as the displacement of a deeper, but unavowable concern (unavowable by Hegel, as well as by Sophocles and Antigone) about introjection. The stakes are higher than they seem, however, since Hegel's reading of *Antigone* works through concerns about the relation between the living and the dead that structure his dialectical project as a whole and that parallel contemporary scientific anxieties. To read Hegel's analysis of *Antigone* as Derrida does, one would have to see the whole relation between phenomena and spirit in Hegel's work, and indeed contemporaries' anxieties about the limits between the organic and the inorganic, as expressions of a psychological process of mourning. This is a seductive idea, since it redefines ostensibly biological and ontological questions as questions about interpersonal relations, and thereby recasts them as ethical issues. On the relation between corpses and the state in Sophocles's *Antigone*, see Jonathan Strauss, "Antigone et l'état cadavérique," in *La hontologie*, ed. Bruno Chaouat (Lyon: Presses Universitaires de Lyon, 2007), 185–206.

29. Thomas Robert Malthus, *An Essay on the Principle of Population, as it Affects the Future Improvement of Society with Remarks on the Speculations of Mr. Godwin, M. Condorcet, and Other Writers* (London: J. Johnson, 1798), 1–2. For a recent study of the ethical aspects of Malthus's theories, see Albino Barrera, *God and the Evil of Scarcity: Moral Foundations of Economic Agency* (Notre Dame, Ind.: University of Notre Dame Press, 2005). For the nineteenth-century reception of Malthus's writings, see Andrew Pyle, ed., *Population: Contemporary Responses to Thomas Malthus* (Bristol: Thoemmes Press, 1994), which reprints reviews of the *Essay on*

Population in journals form 1798 to 1827. Catherine Gallagher's *The Body Economic: Life, Death, and Sensation in Political Economy and the Victorian Novel* (Princeton: Princeton University Press, 2006) devotes significant sections to Malthus, but within the context of the Victorian novel. It should be noted that Pierre Leroux has not been treated as an indispensable reference by scholars of Malthus. The classic study, James Bonar's *Malthus and His Work* (1885; Frank Cass, 1966) makes no mention of Leroux. Geoffrey Gilbert's *Malthus: Critical Responses*, 4 vols. (New York: Routledge, 1998), contains some sixty-six reactions to Malthus, including five from France, but nothing by Leroux. Antoinette Fauve-Chamoux, ed., *Malthus hier et aujourd'hui: Congrès international de démographie historique CNRS, mai 1980* (Paris: CNRS, 1984) tends more toward citations of Keynes, Ricardo, Spengler, and Darwin, but does include a solitary article on Leroux: Bernard Pierre Lécuyer's "Pierre Leroux pourfendeur de Malthus inspirateur de Lacordaire dans *Malthus et les économistes, ou y aura-t-il toujours des pauvres?*" (349–55). Useful as it is for an appreciation of Leroux's relation to Malthus, Lécuyer's approach concentrates on the more classically mathematical and ethical aspects of Leroux's response and omits any mention of the fertilizers and feces we will be discussing below.

30. Malthus, 11.

31. Ibid., 14.

32. Ibid., 16.

33. See part 2 of Immanuel Kant, *The Conflict of the Faculties: Der Streit der Fakultäten*, trans. Mary J. Gregor (New York: Abaris Books, 1979), 140–71.

34. Pierre-Henri Leroux, *Malthus et les économistes, ou y aura-t-il toujours des pauvres*, vol. 1 (Paris: Librairie de la Bibliothèque nationale, 1897), 171. For a general study of Leroux's thought, see Paul Bénichou, *Le temps des prophètes* (Paris: Gallimard, 1977), 330–58. More recent monographs include Miguel Abensour, *Le procès des maîtres rêveurs; suivi de Pierre Leroux et l'utopie* (Arles: Sulliver, 2000); Georges Navet, *Pierre Leroux, politique, socialisme et philosophie* (Paris: Publications de la Société P.-J. Proudhon, 1994); and Vincent Peillon, *Pierre Leroux et le socialisme républicain* (Latresne: Le Bord de l'eau, 2003). For an analysis of Leroux's *Malthus et les économistes*, see Bernard Lécuyer's "Pierre Leroux." Donald Reid's *Paris Sewers and Sewermen: Realities and Representations* (Cambridge, Mass.: Harvard University Press, 1991) discusses Leroux's notion of circulus, describing its historical antecedents and repercussions, including the filtration systems that were established in the late nineteenth century to purify the waste waters of Paris (see 54–59).

35. Jules Leroux, "Préface" in Pierre-Henri Leroux, *Malthus*, 1:6–7.

36. *Malthus*, 1:156.

37. Ibid., 2:43, 51.

38. Ibid., 51–3.

39. Bertherand, 13. Cf. also 13–14.

40. du Roselle, 24.

41. *Aux états de Jersey, sur un moyen de quintupler, pour ne pas dire plus, la production agricole du pays, par Pierre Leroux* (London: Universal Library, 1853), 51. Cf.

39n.: "[Justus von] Liebig's followers have gone so far as to claim that human manure is *ten to twelve times more useful for the production of grains than the manure from herbivores.*" Cf. also 53–54: "ask these scholars, and they will tell you that human manure is the most fertilizing of all and that the quantity of this manure produced by human beings would be sufficient to fertilize all the lands necessary to feed the entire human species with grain, since each man provides enough of it to generate the amount of wheat needed for his own nourishment."

42. Bertherand, 14.

43. du Roselle, 23, 25. For an example of a more humble application of the principle of circulus, see Jean-Pierre-Joseph d'Arcet, *Latrines modèles, construites sous un colombier, ventilées au moyen de la chaleur des pigeons, et servant à la préparation de l'engrais* (Paris: L. Mathias, 1843). In d'Arcet's plan, the warmth generated by the doves would create a current of air to draw off the unpleasant smells created by the excrements deposited in the latrine below. Those excrements would be allowed to accumulate and, once dried, could be used as "an excellent fertilizer at a nominal price" (12). Not only does the author imagine recycling human waste, but he takes the principle even further by attempting to capture a profit from animal heat loss. His project represents, in this way, a tendency toward recuperating not merely feces and urine, but all that is fleeting in the animal body, indeed, toward recapturing life itself.

44. Leroux, *Jersey*, 44.

45. Ibid., 63.

46. Ibid., 44–45.

47. Ibid., 45.

48. Ibid., 71.

49. Victor Hugo, *Les Misérables*, trans. Charles E. Wilbour (New York: Modern Library, n.d.), 1054 (trans. modified).

50. Ibid. (trans. modified).

51. Ibid., 1055 (trans. modified).

52. Ibid., 1054 (trans. modified).

53. Ibid., 1054–55 (trans. modified).

54. Hugo writes that this is no metaphor. In "Medical Mapping: the Thames, the Body and Our Mutual Friend" (in William A. Cohen and Ryan Johnson, eds. *Filth: Dirt, Disgust, and Modern Life* [Minneapolis: University or Minnesota Press, 2005]), David L. Pike understands Hugo to mean that "the sewers did in fact contain grains, herbs and cattle, the 'warm blood' and the life of the French countryside within their tunnels, transmuted into waste through the excretory systems of the city's inhabitants. It required not an alchemical process but a simple change in perspective for the filth described in the first half of this passage to transmute into the pastoral vision purportedly its opposite" (60). The nonmetaphorical transmutation Pike describes, however, moves in a direction opposite from that described by Hugo (i.e. Pike speaks of the transmutation of the pastoral scene into feces, while Hugo speaks of the transmutation of human wastes into meadows) and Pike's "simple change of perspective" would seem to be a shift, in

fact, from the literal to the metaphorical. I propose reading "no metaphor" to mean that what Hugo describes is happening in the text: it is not about what is meant or described by the words but what is occurring on the page itself, literally, linguistically, in front of the reader.

55. Quoted in Trélat, 52.

56. Geoffrey Bennington is a notable exception to this refusal. Commenting on a passage in which Terry Eagleton describes Hegel's method as "eternally replete but constantly absorptive, like a grazing cow," Bennington writes: "What such a description leaves out (and in leaving it out it is doubtless true to the discourse it describes) is any notion that a body not only absorbs but also excretes: add that function, and the characterisation will do as a description of the 'body' of 'Marxism,' which both secures and compromises its unity and integrity as a body by ingesting and expelling or excreting, leaving behind it a trail of what it was in the form of the waste-product, the *déchet*, the dropping. The history of what Marxism itself expels as its own 'deviations' (due to the absorption of foreign bodies) or its own 'vulgar' version (generated by internal or intestinal malfunctions) could persuasively be read, in eminently materialist terms, as a history of digestion and eventually of shit" ("Demanding History" in *Post-structuralism and the Question of History*, ed. Derek Attridge, Geoffrey Bennington, and Robert Young [Cambridge: Cambridge University Press, 1987]). Despite his willingness to use excretion as a conceptual paradigm for understanding materialist history, Bennington has not yet, to my knowledge, taken this proposal any further. In his analysis of eating as a metaphor and organizing principle in Hegel's philosophy, Werner Hamacher, does, on the other hand, address the issue of indigestible remainders as part of an excursus on the philosophical value of nausea: "It is the very law of the dialectic that the circular reappropriation of the selfsame, for which the totality of the organism and the totality of the system is designed, remains unaccomplished. To suckle at its own breast, to eat its own cadaver, to consume itself as its own result, this represents at once the telos of the dialectical operations of the corporeal system and the unsurpassable limit of that system. . . . Like the organism, time too must accomplish what it cannot accomplish: to digest once again what has already been digested, in order to have digested itself utterly and to have enlivened everything other, everything dead and done with, into utter presence" (*Pleroma: Reading in Hegel*, trans. Nicholas Walker and Simon Jarvis [Stanford, Calif.: Stanford University Press, 1998], 268–69).

57. *Jersey*, 32.

58. On the importance of emblems and the symbolic for Leroux, see Bénichou, 339–40.

59. Leroux imagined the distribution of fertilizer to operate like that of gas: "You can arrange things so that all of your farmers have nitrogen-rich [human] manure, which is the best of all fertilizers, *in their home, in the same way that all of your shopkeepers have gas*" (*Jersey*, 51).

60. On homes as imaginary spaces that fantasmatically express the material world's organization, see Gaston Bachelard, "La maison natale et la maison oniri-que" in *La terre et les rêveries du repos: Essai sur les images de l'intimité* (Paris: José

Corti, 1948), 95–128. J.-K. Huysmans imagined a similar inversion of the human digestive tract in his novel *A rebours* (Against Nature), in which a stomach ailment forces the principal character, des Esseintes, to sustain himself through a "nourishing enema": "the operation was a success, and des Esseintes could not resist congratulating himself on this event which, in a certain sense, represented the crowning glory of the existence he had created for himself. Almost by accident, his penchant for the artificial had now reached its culmination. He could take it no further. Absorbing food in this way was, without a doubt, the ultimate deviation that one could commit" (*Against Nature* [*A rebours*], trans. Robert Baldick [New York: Penguin, 2003], 193). This enema represents the *summum* of the aesthetic program outlined in the novel, such that the very notion of art presented in it can best be understood as an inversion of the digestive tract. The artist eats with his anus, thereby freeing himself from the constraints imposed by nature and asserting his creative liberty. While des Esseintes's enema is a refusal of nature, Leroux's fantasies of transformed houses and human bodies represent, on the other hand, an attempt to better understand the plasticity created by the laws of nature themselves. In both cases, however, the inversion of the digestive tract constitutes a crucial liberatory act.

61. Leroux, *Malthus*, 2:44. See also the following passage: "The economists delight in observing that 'Nature's fertility is such that if the seeds she produces did not almost all abort, and if the vast majority of beings did not die from malnutrition almost immediately after being born, in no time at all a single species of plant would suffice to cover the entire earth and a single species of animal to populate it.' They make a great show of science and facts, always with the intention of proving that because Nature, 'which is solely concerned with species, and not with individuals, has sown the seeds of living beings with such prodigious generosity, it is unwise to attempt to multiply the individuals of the human race and better to recognize that our species is subject to the same law as all others, which calls for the destruction of seeds and individuals.' From these arguments, some, like Malthus, deduce the necessity for celibacy and artificial checks, while others conclude in favor of a *laissez faire* attitude" (43–44).

62. Ibid., 46–47.

63. Ibid., 46.

64. Ibid., 55 (original emphasis).

65. Ibid.

66. Leroux, *Jersey*, 11n.

67. For Leroux, "these secretions are actually, from Nature's point of view, the price of the individual's nourishment, since they are intended for others in the same way that the secretions of other beings are intended for the individual" (*Jersey*, 10–11).

68. Ibid., 11n.

69. Ibid., 12.

70. Leroux, *Malthus*, 2:58.

71. See, for instance, Eugène Sue's *Les Mystères de Paris*, ed. Francis Lacassin (Paris: Robert Laffont [Bouquins], 1989), and the discussion of the novel in the section "The Reign of Terror against the Anarchy of Horror" in chapter 7.

72. Leroux, *Jersey*, 10.

73. See Favre: "It falls upon the philosopher to *explain* the necessity of death. Since the quantity of matter in the 'universal storehouse' is thought to be invariable, life is made up of its circulation, or 'vicissitudes,' as Holbach and Diderot, inspired by *Telliamed*, put it. This is the principle underlying all the analyses that justify death on the basis of its necessary function" (339). And: "the doctrine of necessity is replaced by a certain providentialism of sacralized nature. The blunt assertion that 'some must die so that others can be born' yields to a formulation that emphasizes the finalism implicit in those words. And one can always sense the underlying notion that there is a fixed and finite quantity of alimentary substances, of material available for life. The world, in other words, is stable and closed" (340).

74. Leroux, *Jersey*, 23.

75. Ibid., 10.

76. Bichat, *Physiological Researches*, 10 (trans. modified).

77. On the relation between sewers and prostitution in the work of Parent-Duchâtelet, see Charles Bernheimer, *Figures of Ill Repute: Representing Prostitution in Nineteenth-Century France* (Cambridge, Mass.: Harvard University Press, 1989), 8–33. For another, landmark study on the subject of prostitution in nineteenth-century Paris, see Alain Corbin, *Women for Hire: Prostitution and Sexuality in France after 1850*, trans. Alan Sheridan (Cambridge, Mass.: Harvard University Press, 1990). Also very useful is Jill Harsin's *Policing Prostitution in Nineteenth-Century Paris* (Princeton: Princeton University Press, 1985), which describes the life of prostitutes along with the theories and mechanisms devised for their control and repression.

78. See, for example, Hollis Clayson, *Painted Love: Prostitution in French Art of the Impressionist Era* (New Haven: Yale University Press, 1991). In *Scenes of Seduction: Prostitution, Hysteria, and Reading Difference in Nineteenth-Century France* (New York: Columbia University Press, 1994), Jann Matlock attempts to demonstrate and demystify the male fantasms of seduction that she argues were overlaid onto prostitutes.

79. Yves Guyot, *La prostitution* (Paris: G. Charpentier, 1882), 215.

80. According to Alain Corbin, Parent-Duchâtelet treated prostitution as an "indispensable excremental phenomenon" (*Women for Hire*, 4). In *Les vierges folles* (Paris: Auguste Le Galloir, 1840), Alphonse Esquiros wrote that "prostitution has always been a necessary evil" (6).

81. *La femme, le mariage et le divorce: Etude de physiologie et de sociologie* (Paris: Germer Baillière et Cie, 1880), 112.

82. "The double curtains veiling the windows indicate, by their mystery, that these are houses of shame where nameless things occur" (Esquiros, 19–20).

83. See Corbin, *Women for Hire*, 10. Charles Bernheimer describes efforts to "render the prostitute invisible through the precise regulation of her availability" (17–20).

84. See Corbin, *Women for Hire*, 234.

85. Jill Harsin addresses this question in her first chapter, "Bringing Order into Disorder" (3–55), from the perspective of the authoritarian system established to police prostitutes' behavior. What I am focusing on is, however, the disorder of the prostitute's *being* and the abjection that such a subjectivity represented for contemporary hygienists.

86. Alexandre-Jean-Baptiste Parent-Duchâtelet, *De la prostitution dans la ville de Paris considérée sous le rapport de l'hygiène publique, de la morale et de l'administration*, vol. 1 (1836; Paris: J.-B. Baillière, 1837), 26–27, 90. Of the *pierreuses*, or the lowest order of prostitutes, he wrote: "to prevent disorder, the government must constantly pursue them" (189).

87. Ibid., 115, 117. Parent-Duchâtelet held that a predisposition to *débauche*, or debauchery, was the consequence of early family conditions, which included a "lowly origin" and subjection, as a child, to "disorder at home" (94–95). Similarly, Alphonse Esquiros argued that the prostitute's behavior often resulted from hereditary predispositions: "In short, one must recognize a sad and wretched truth, which is that many of these girls have inherited from their parents a taste for riffraff, libertinage, drunkenness, and debauchery that makes society shun them. Conceived in the midst of an orgy, most of them have prostitution in their blood. . . . There is a terrible law, written somewhere in the Bible and confirmed by experience, that at birth, children will carry in their organs the marks of their parents' vice" (39).

88. Ibid., 76. See also 55–56: "This need for love, which bestial, brutal, and disordered lust could not satisfy, leaves the *fille* vague and aimless."

89. Cited from various contemporary journalistic reactions to Manet's painting in T. J. Clark, *The Painting of Modern Life: Paris in the Art of Manet and His Followers* (New York: Alfred A. Knopf, 1985), 92n48.

90. Corbin, *Women for Hire*, 221.

91. Ibid., 222.

92. Ibid., 223.

93. See Guyot, 245–59.

94. "Semaines littéraires" in *La gazette de France*, 11 June 1865. At the other end of the social scale, the *filles à soldats* exhibited a similar resemblance to other, acceptable, members of society: "Since they do not troll for customers, nothing distinguishes them from other workers, and since many of them still hold jobs, how is one to recognize and arrest them?" (Parent-Duchâtelet, 1:187).

95. Mireur, *Syphilis*, 279. Quoted in Guyot, 223.

96. Esquiros, 229–30.

97. Ibid., 100.

98. Parent-Duchâtelet, 1:116. Cf. Balzac, *Splendors and Miseries of Courtesans*, vol. 1 (London: Caxton, 1895): "Prostitutes are fundamentally mobile beings,

who pass for no reason from the most stubborn defiance to an absolute trust. They are, in this respect, beneath animals" (47, trans. modified).

99. Esquiros, 89. Cf. Hippolyte Mireur on the recording of prostitutes in the police registers and their possible subsequent removal from those lists in *La syphilis et la prostitution dans leurs rapports avec l'hygiène, la morale et la loi* (Paris: Masson, 1888), 284: "A wide range of circumstances can, at certain times, lead to their removal [from the lists] and permit a woman, who is today marked with infamy, to regain tomorrow all the rights belonging to members of society." Like Esquiros, but in somewhat more measured terms, Mireur thus recognized that the prostitute lost her rights as a member of society. Parent-Duchâtelet himself was explicit: "Public debauchery feeds public prostitution. It is the transition from an honest life to the abject state of a class entirely separated from society along with the renunciation of that society. By its scandalous habits, which it flaunts constantly and shamelessly in public, this class abjures society and the communal laws that govern it" (1:26–27).

100. Esquiros, 82–83.

101. On Saint-Just, Robespierre, and Diderot, see chapter 7.

102. Parent-Duchâtelet, 1:27.

103. Guyot, 236. The quotation from Hippolyte Mireur is found in *La prostitution à Marseille: Histoire, administration et police, hygiène* (Paris: E. Dentu, 1882), 130.

104. F.-F.-A. Béraud, *Les filles publiques de Paris et la police qui les régit*, vol. 1 (Paris & Leipzig: Desforges et Cie., 1839), 41–42.

105. Guyot, 236, 223.

106. Mireur, *Syphilis*, 280.

107. Esquiros, 47, 124. Esquiros saw a homology between sewer workers and prostitutes: "The laborers to whom these women attach themselves are, for the most part, cesspool cleaners, street sweepers, and sewermen: one kind of filth [*fange*] purifies the other" (70). For a discussion of the assimilation of prostitutes to sewers in Parent-Duchâtelet's writings, see Bernheimer, 15–17. More generally for the functioning of houses of prostitution as *égouts séminaux*, or seminal sewers, see Corbin, *Women for Hire*, 53–84.

108. Guyot, 207.

109. Esquiros, 5, 74.

110. Ibid., 80.

111. Ibid., 126. Other passages establish similar analogies between prostitutes and the dead: "[T]hey sign a cross on the registers where the police inscribe their surname. And, in fact, it is a fitting sign to mark the name of these wretches, for they are henceforth dead to honor, to love, and society: one places a cross on the tomb of the deceased" (37); and "after having shared her bed for so long with all the world, she feels at last the need to have a bed for her alone, cold, solitary, and chaste, where she might rest. This bed is the girl's coffin." (73). As the coffin was the true bed of the prostitute, so did the common grave represent, according to Esquiros, her true society: "only the cemetery, more fair in this than the city,

takes her to its breast like any other and confuses her with the poor of the common grave" (75). Even on a physical level, the prostitute functioned analogously to a corpse. Like the vapors of the dead that Cadet-De-Vaux studied in the houses adjoining the Saints-Innocents cemetery, prostitutes "decomposed" the health of those who came into contact with them: "The prostitute grows old before her age. After a few months, the brightest eyes grow dull and watery. The shapeliest features decompose. The atmosphere characteristic of brothels darkly lines and tarnishes the freshest complexions" (49).

112. See Alain Corbin, "Présentation" in Alexandre Parent-Duchâtelet, *La prostitution à Paris au XIXe siècle*, ed. Alain Corbin (Paris: Seuil, 1981), 21–23.

113. Guyot, 7.

114. Mireur, *Syphilis*, 279. On the childlike quality of the prostitute's impersonality, see Esquiros: "The practice of vice makes some of them fall imperceptibly into a sort of infancy, which is undoubtedly the origin of the nickname, 'foolish girls,' that was given them in the middle ages. Theirs are the weakest and the happiest of minds. They are less aware than others of the horrors attaching to their condition" (69) and Corbin, *Women for Hire*, 7n35. Esquiros cited the inherent goodness of the prostitute's character, which Parent-Duchâtelet had already remarked on, and noted that when that goodness failed, the prostitute generally fell back, once again, into a state of childishness: "Mr. Parent Duchâtelet observes, moreover, that prostitutes are usually of a good, distinguished, and powerful nature. It is true that they need an uncommon force of character to endure the sufferings and humiliations that they must swallow. This is, however, uncommon" (69). Generally speaking, insofar as the prostitute had a self, it was good, to the extent that she lacked one, she was innocent.

115. Esquiros, 121.

116. See Jacques Lacan, *On Feminine Sexuality: The Limits of Love and Knowledge: Book XX: Encore 1972–1973*, trans. Bruce Fink (New York: W. W. Norton, 1998), 1–13, 62–63, and 71–89; "Radiophonie" in *Scilicet*, vol. 2/3 (Paris: Seuil, 1970), 65; and "Pour une logique du fantasme" in *Scilicet*, vol. 2/3, 247–255. On the connection between *jouissance* and subjectivity in the relation between the sexes, and particularly during the sexual act, see especially *Scilicet*, vol. 2/3, 264–26. "There can be no sexual act," Lacan writes, "unless it is in the signifying reference that can alone constitute it as an act. Now, far from involving the two natural entities—the male and the female—this signifying reference, by the sheer fact of its dominance, introduces these beings as a function of the subject. But the effect of that subject is precisely the disjunction of the body and *jouissance*, and the signifying intervention is there only to attempt to resolve the aporia that this disjunction produces. It succeeds in this only by making of the other's body the metaphor for my own *jouissance*. But there is no overlap [*entrecroisement*]: this chiasmus that would make of each body the metaphor for the *jouissance* of the other remains in suspense, so that we can only observe the movement that makes one *jouissance* depend on the body of the other while the *jouissance* of the other consequently remains adrift" (265–66).

117. Matlock, *Scenes*, 7–8.

118. According to Lacan, "the most anodyne fantasm has the characteristic of being more unavowable than anything at all" (*Scilicet*, vol. 2/3, 271–72). For an idiosyncratic and very illuminating discussion of Lacan's notion of the fantasm, see J.-D. Nasio, *Le fantasme: Le plaisir de lire Lacan* (Paris: Payot, 1992). Nasio describes the fantasm as an "invisible scene" that "repeats itself . . . without ever being clearly [*nettement*] and consciously perceived" (14). The qualification *"nettement"* is important, since the fantasmatic scene, according to Nasio, can be glimpsed, although only imperfectly, by the subject. Its significance, however, escapes and exceeds the subject: it is "the event of an utterance made by the patient *without his knowing* what he has said" (29). Hygienists and reformers were able to formulate an image that equated prostitutes with sewers, but that image was never sufficiently clear as to become entirely conscious, and what remained most hidden, I would argue, was its significance as an expression of desire. On the relations between conscious and unconscious fantasms, both topologically in the structures of the psyche and historically in the development of Freud's theories, see Jean Laplanche and J.-B. Pontalis, *Fantasme originaire fantasme des origines origines du fantasme* (1964; Paris: Hachette, 1985). For a fuller discussion of fantasms in relation to abjection, see chapter 7.

6. MONSTERS AND ARTISTS

1. Preface to *Cromwell*, in *Théâtre complet*, ed. J.-J. Thierry and Josette Mélèze (Paris: Gallimard [Pléiade], 1963), 414. For an overview of necrophilic culture in the early nineteenth century, see Vovelle, 574–604.

2. On the issue of death in Chateaubriand's *Mémoires d'outre-tombe* see Marie-Hélène Huet, "Chateaubriand and the Politics of (Im)mortality" in *Post-Mortem*, 28–39, and Bruno Chaouat, *"Je meurs par morceaux": Chateaubriand* (Villeneuve-d'Ascq: Presses Universitaires du Septentrion, 1999).

3. See Jann Matlock, "Ghostly Politics" in *Diacritics* 30, 53–71, and Jean de Mutigny, *Victor Hugo et le spiritisme* (Paris: Fernand Nathan, 1981).

4. On Jean Valjean's simulated burial, see Hugo, *Les Misérables*, 459–76.

5. See Enid Starkie, *Petrus Borel the Lycanthrope: His Life and Times* (London: Faber and Faber, 1954), 89–90. See also a description of this same group, sometimes called the Jeunes-France, in a contemporary newspaper: "The *Jeune-France* is gay, but with a putrid gaity. During the day, he has visited the Catacombs, Père Lachaise cemetery, and the Chamber of Peers in the Senate. He holds forth on Montfaucon and the anatomist's office. He shows a bone to the young ladies and tells them: 'You've got the same thing under your gauzes and veils. You're always walking with a skeleton, you have death under your skirt. Let's see that death" ("Les Jeunes France," in *Le Figaro*, August 30, 1831).

6. See Philothée O'Neddy (pseudonym for Théophile Dondey), "Succube" in *Feu et flamme*, ed. Marcel Hervier (1833; repr., Paris: Editions des Presses Françaises, 1926), 31–33.

7. On Baudelaire's necrophilia, see Lisa Downing, *Desiring the Dead: Necrophilia and Nineteenth-Century French Literature* (Oxford: Legenda, 2003), 67–91.

8. *Les derniers des Beaumanoirs, ou la tour d'Helvin*, 4 vols. (Paris: Bossange frères, 1825), cited by Lunier (378) and Morel ("Considérations médico-légales . . . Deuxième lettre," 186).

9. The French school of Spiritism took shape largely as a rejection of theories that had been propounded by Mesmer's disciples. The latter had seen in somnambulistic trances and the apparent miracles that accompanied them the expression of physical laws hitherto undisclosed. The visible, material world was shot through, according to their beliefs, by a subtle electrical fluid that, when played upon, could transfer thought and will across seemingly empty space. This fluid carried in it a powerful vital force that could be communicated to animate and inanimate objects—to people, trees, and iron rods, for instance. In human beings, this force was capable of inducing convulsions, curing diseases, or revealing the thoughts of others. The Mesmerists explained the phenomena of their séances through recourse to a model of life principles that closely resembled those being worked out by contemporary physiologists like Condillac, Bichat, and Cabanis. Life was a physical property that spread itself subtly but materially, and it was this vital force which Mesmerism sought to harness. In 1857, however, Hippolyte Rivail, under the pseudonym of Allan Kardec, published the first and most important volume on what came to be known as Spiritism, *Le livre des esprits* (The Book of Spirits) (1857; repr., Paris: Didier et Cie, 1867), which he claimed had been dictated to him by voices of the deceased. On the basis of this volume, and several that followed, Kardec quickly became the leading force in French Spiritism. In *Le livre des esprits* he broke firmly with the materialist tradition that had previously dominated explanations of psychic phenomena. The occurrences that marked somnambulistic trances, he argued, could not be explained by physical causes, but rather through the intervention of spirit forces, namely the souls of the dead. In this sense Spiritism was, according to him, a science of the transcendental, of the infinite (see *Le livre des esprits*, xxxi), the sublime (xxxvi), and the abstract (2). For a concise history and useful bibliography of French Spiritism, see Matlock, "Ghostly Politics."

10. See Alphonse Devergie, *Notions générales sur la morgue de Paris: Sa description, son système hygiénique; de l'autopsie judiciaire comparée à l'autopsie pathologique* (Paris: F. Malteste, 1877), 11. On the popularity of the morgue, see also Vanessa R. Schwartz, *Spectacular Realities: Early Mass Culture in Fin-de-Siècle Paris* (Berkeley: University of California Press, 1998), 45–88.

11. See Devergie, 10. Because she wants to avoid such scrutiny, a character in one of Balzac's novels travels far downstream before throwing herself in the river, past the nets that the popular imagination believed to stretch across the Seine at Neuilly in order to catch the bodies of the drowned. See Balzac, *Ferragus*, 126.

12. See the description of Camille's corpse in Emile Zola, *Thérèse Raquin* (London: William Heinemann, 1955), 75. Cf. descriptions of the passage du Pont-Neuf (1), of the boutique (3), of Thérèse (4), and Camille (28–9, 32, 66).

13. Ibid., 18–19 (trans. modified).

14. Ibid., 72 (trans. modified).

15. Ibid., 19 (trans. modified).

16. Ibid., 72–73 (trans. modified). A symmetrical version of this scene can be found in a description of Thérèse just before the crime: "Her lover gazed on her, half frightened to see her so motionless and mute beneath his caresses. That dead, white face, drowned among the folds of her skirts, inspired in him a sort of dread, filled with burning desire" (56, trans. modified). Again, desire blends with fear as Laurent feels himself sexually excited by what seems to be the corpse of his lover. The reciprocity between these two descriptions—one of a living woman who appears to be dead, the other of a corpse that seems to live—indicates a continuity between the worlds of the animate and the inanimate and the inherent sexual attractiveness of the dead *as* dead.

17. Ibid., 74 (trans. modified).

18. "In all respects, I intend to fall back on the authority of Claude Bernard. Most often, I will need only replace the word 'doctor' with the word 'novelist' to convey my thoughts clearly and to bring to them the rigor of scientific truth" (Emile Zola, *Le roman expérimental*, in *Œuvres complètes*, 10:1175).

19. Théophile Gautier, *Romans, contes et nouvelles*, vol. 1, ed. Pierre Laubriet *et al.* (Paris: Gallimard [Pléiade], 2002), 7.

20. Ibid., 527. For an example of the similarities between scientific and literary discourses during this period, one can compare the final graveyard scene from Gautier's "La morte amoureuse [*The Dead Woman in Love*]" (ibid., 550–52) to an anecdote recounted by Bouchut, 323–24. In both cases a man opens the tomb of his supposedly deceased lover and is amazed to find that she is untouched by any signs of decomposition. This similarity attests to the pervasive and interdisciplinary quality of certain fantasies about the dead.

21. Gautier, 1:529.

22. Tardieu, *Attentats*, 117.

23. Gautier, 2:310.

24. Ibid., 292. On Gautier's life-long horror of decomposition, see Pierre Laubriet's note to this passage in ibid., 1301–2.

25. J.-K. Huysmans, *L'Art moderne* in *Œuvres complètes françaises*, vol. 6 (Paris: G. Crès, 1929), 300.

26. On social issues and folkloric material in Redon's work, see Stephen, F. Eisenman, *The Temptation of Saint Redon: Biography, Ideology, and Style in the* Noirs *of Odilon Redon* (Chicago: University of Chicago Press, 1992). Redon's contemporaries Huysmans, Emile Hennequin, and André Mellerio all discussed the importance of recent science in the artist's work, a theme subsequently developed at greater length in Sven Sandström's *Le monde imaginaire d'Odilon Redon: Etude iconologique* (Lund: n.p., 1955) and in Douglas W. Druick and Peter Kort Zegers, "In the Public Eye," in *Odilon Redon: Prince of Dreams, 1840–1916*, ed. Douglas W. Druick (Chicago: The Art Institute of Chicago in association with Harry N. Abrams, 1994), 137–45. The scientific sources of Redon's imaginary have

attracted particular attention recently, with several significant publications exploring the significance of those relations. See Martha Lucy, "The Evolutionary Body" (PhD diss. New York University, 2004); Barbara Larson, *The Dark Side of Nature: Science, Society, and the Fantastic in the Work of Odilon Redon* (University Park, Penn.: Pennsylvania State University Press, 2005); and Marina Van Zuylen, "The Secret Life of Monsters" in Jodi Hauptman, *Beyond the Visible: The Art of Odilon Redon* (New York: Museum of Modern Art, New York, 2005), 57–73. Jerome Viola disputed the influence of science in general, and evolutionism in particular, on Redon's work in his "Redon, Darwin and the Ascent of Man," *Marsyas* 11 (1962–64): 42–57. In what follows, I have been particularly indebted to the work of two individuals. It was a characteristically brilliant and idiosyncratic talk by Marina Van Zuylen that first brought my attention to Redon's artworks. Barbara Larson's *The Dark Side of Nature* not only confirmed my intuitions but also showed the extent to which the artist was aware of contemporary scientific debates. Larson's volume masterfully works the difficult zone between the history of science and artistic analysis and has offered invaluable material for my own study. Many of the quotations in what follows, especially from Mellerio, derive from her own research.

27. Odilon Redon, *A soi-même: journal 1867–1915: Notes sur la vie, l'air et les artistes* (Paris: José Corti, 1961), 100. See also: "As far as I am concerned, I believe I have created an expressive, suggestive, and indeterminate art. Suggestive art is the irradiation of divine, plastic elements that have been brought together and combined in order to provoke reveries that it illuminates and exalts while stimulating the thought processes" (ibid., 116).

28. "A thought cannot become a work of art, except in literature. Art borrows nothing from philosophy either" (ibid., 93). "I am not speaking to metaphysical minds here, nor to pedagogues, because they have not gazed constantly enough on the beauties of nature. The habits of their thinking keep them too far removed from the intermediary ideas that bind sensations to thoughts: their mind is too occupied by abstractions for them to fully share and taste the pleasures of art, which always demand a relation between the soul and real, external objects. I speak to those who yield docilely, and without the aid of sterile explanations, to the secret and mysterious laws of feelings and the heart" (ibid., 115).

29. On Clavaud, see H. D. Schotsman, "Clavaud, sa vie, son œuvre" in *Bulletin du Centre de Recherches Scientifiques de Biarritz* 8, no. 4 (May 2, 1881): 335–36 and Larson, 5–13.

30. Redon, *A soi-même*, 18.

31. "I believe that I have followed the guidance of instinct in creating certain monsters. They do not derive, as Huysmans has insinuated, from the findings of the microscope, when it is focused on the frightening world of the infinitely small. No. In making them, I was concerned with the more important issue of organizing their structures" (ibid., 28).

32. See André Mellerio, *Odilon Redon* (1913; repr. New York: Da Capo Press, 1968), 29. For a detailed analysis of Redon's relation to medicine and the sciences, see Larson, esp. 49–106.

33. See, for instance, the interview between Redon and his biographer André Mellerio from November 30, 1891 (Mellerio General Research Notes in the André Mellerio Archive, Art Institute of Chicago).

34. André Mellerio, *Odilon Redon, peintre, dessinateur et graveur* (Paris: H. Floury, 1923), 155n3. See also Mellerio, *Odilon Redon*, 16. It should be noted that no letter to Redon figures in Pasteur's collected correspondance (see *Correspondance de Pasteur 1840–1895*, ed. Pasteur Vallery-Radot, 4 vols. [Paris: Flammarion, 1951]).

35. See Charles E. Hoffhaus, "A Homogeneous Theory of the Origin of Vertebrates" in *Journal of Paleontology* 37, no. 2 (March, 1963): 465. There was, however, debate on this idea, even among the figures who influenced Redon. Georges Cuvier, Saint-Hilaire's contemporary and colleague, rejected the notion of transitional species, believing instead that the fossil record attested to a series of deluges followed by new animal forms.

36. Redon, *A soi-même*, 18. Redon was probably also familiar with the teaching of Paul Gervais, a professor of comparative anatomy, since the latter gave public lectures in the amphitheater of the Muséum d'Histoire Naturelle and was involved in curating its osteology collection at the same time that Redon was frequenting its galleries. Gervais spoke, according to Barbara Larson, on "the similarity between plant and animal forms at lower levels" (see Larson, 55).

37. Huysmans, *L'art moderne*, 299.

38. See Redon, *A soi-même*, 28. For images of vibrio-type creatures see "Then there appears a singular being, having the head of a man on the body of a fish (Oannes)" (plate 5 from *The Temptation of Saint Anthony*, 1888, lithograph, Elizabeth Hamond Stickney Collection, The Art Institute of Chicago, in Larson, 57), "That eyes without heads were floating like mollusks" (plate 13 from *The Temptation of Saint Anthony*, 1896, lithograph, Elizabeth Hammond Stickney Collection, The Art Institute of Chicago, in Larson, 59), "Phantom" (1885, charcoal, Kunsthandel Wolfgang Werner, KG Bremin/Berlin, in Larson, 89), and "And all manner of frightful creatures arise" (plate 8 from *The Temptation of Saint Anthony*, 1888, lithograph, Charles Stickney Colletion, The Art Institute of Chicago, in Larson, 102). Since all of these images date from *after* Huysmans's 1882 review, it would seem less that the critic was describing forms that he actually saw than situating Redon's imagery within what he understood to be its iconographic context. It is possible that it was Huysmans's review, in fact, that inspired Redon to introduce comma-shaped bacillus forms in his later works, especially the Saint Anthony series. For a partial reconstruction of the 1882 *Gaulois* show, see Druick and Zegers, 134–35.

39. Lorrain described them as "nightmares crawling with vibrios and volvoxes, all of these animalcules that are revealed by the microscope" in "Un étrange jongleur" in *L'écho de Paris*, April 10, 1894, n.p. (quoted in and translated by Larson, 89). Larson quotes other reactions to the show that use a similar vocabulary, including the essay by André Mellerio, who wrote that the world represented in Redon's art "was from Darwinian epochs. . . . In the protoplasm of

strange spurting bacilli, of unknown cells coming into being" ("Odilon Redon," preface to *Exposition Odilon Redon*, exhibition catalogue, Galeries Durand-Ruel, Paris, 1894, 6, quoted in and translated by Larson, 89); the review by Gérard Beauregard, who wrote that "[i]t is alright to exhibit again the fantastic and terrible . . . but why these microbes [. . .] these 'vibrios'?" ("Notes d'art: Exposition de M. Odilon Redon" in *La patrie*, April 2, 1894, n.p., quoted in and translated by Larson, 89); and the reaction of Auguste Barbey: "In the obscure depths of marshes illuminated suddenly by a phosphorescent glow, vibrios and germs, bacilli and infusoria, big with human faces, sad or inexpressive, produce a dreadful effect" ("Odilon Redon" in *Mémorial artistique*, April 7, 1894, n.p., quoted in and translated by Larson, 89).

40. See Larson, 89.

41. Emile Hennequin, "Beaux-arts: Odilon Redon," *Revue littéraire et artistique* 5 (March 4, 1882): 136–38. Quoted and translated in Henri Dorra, ed. *Symbolist Art Theories: A Critical Anthology* (Berkeley: University of California Press, 1994), 50.

42. "The Marshflower" in plate 1 was published as part of the series *Origins* in 1883. Redon produced an almost identical charcoal sketch under the same title in 1882 (Collection State Museum Kröller-Müller, Otterlo, the Netherlands, in Larson, 65). A similar charcoal entitled "The Marshflower" appeared around 1880, two years before the show at the *Gaulois* reviewed by Hennequin (see Eisenman, 110; and Jacques Chaban-Delmas, ed. *Odilon Redon: 1840–1916* [Bordeaux: Galérie des Beaux-Arts exhibition catalogue, 1985], 112).

43. For the "Spirit of the Forest," also called "The Skeleton Man," (c. 1880 or 1886, charcoal and black and white chalk on wove paper, Ian Woodner Family Collection, New York), see Van Zuylen, 63; for "Cactus Man" (c. 1880, Charcoal, Ian Woodner Family Collection), see Eisenman, 195; for "A Flower with a Child's Face" (c. 1885, charcoal, The Art Institute of Chicago), see Eisenman, 111.

44. Jean-Paul Sartre, *Being and Nothingness: An Essay on Phenomenological Ontology*, trans. Hazel E. Barnes (New York: Philosophical Library, 1956), 607 (trans. modified).

45. "Premier frontispiece pour Fables et contes de Thierry-Faletans," 1868, Lithograph, in Hippolyte de Thierry de Faletans, *Fables et contes: essais* (Paris: Lemercier et Cie, 1871) in Eisenman, 59.

46. Redon, *A Soi-même*, 128.

47. On Redon's lithographic techniques, see Starr Figura, "Redon and the Lithographed Portfolio" in Hauptman, *Beyond the Visible*, 76–95, esp. 89. In a similar vein, Redon wrote that his lithographs emerged out of their materials themselves: "All of my plates, from the first to the last, have been nothing but the fruit of a curious, attentive, anxious, and passionate analysis of the power of expression contained in the lithographer's grease pencil, as it is aided by paper and stone. I am astonished that artists have not gone farther with this supple and rich art, which obeys the subtlest impulses of the sensibilities" (Redon, *A Soi-même*, 129).

48. Redon, *A soi-même*, 21, 111.

49. Ibid., 127.

50. "When the painter draws from his dreams, do not forget the action of those secret lineaments that bind and hold him to the earth with a lucid and wakeful mind" (ibid., 129). "In the course of daily life, the artist is the receptacle of ambiant things. From outside himself, he receives sensations that he transforms along a necessary, inexorable, and tenacious path, which is his alone. One never really produces without having something to say, without the need to expand. I will go so far as to say that the seasons act on him. They activate and dull his sap [*sève*]. Anything that he tries to achieve outside of these influences, which his gropings and experiences reveal to him, will be fruitless for him, if he neglects them" (ibid., 23).

51. Plate 1 from *To Edgar Poe*, 1882, lithograph (Paris: G. Fischbacher, 1882), in Hauptman, *Beyond the Visible*, 119.

52. *A soi-même*, 131.

53. Lithograph on chine appliqué, 1896, in Gustave Flaubert, *La tentation de Saint Antoine* (The Temptation of Saint Anthony) (Paris: Ambroise Vollard, 1938), facing 136. In Hauptman, *Beyond the Visible*, 176.

54. ". . . And Eyes without Heads Were Floating Like Mollusks" (Plate 13 from *Temptation of Saint Anthony*, 1896, lithography, Elisabeth Hamond Stickney Collection, the Art Institute of Chicago, in Larson, 82).

55. On the oyster and other mollusks, see "Living Death" in chapter 4.

56. In a letter to Haeckel from December 27, 1871, Darwin wrote "I shall continue to work as long as I can, but when I stop there are so many good men fully capable of carrying on our work and of these you rank as the first."

57. Ernst Haeckel, *Generelle Morphologie der Organismen: allgemeine Grundzüge der organischen Formen-Wissenschaft: mechanisch begründet durch die von Charles Darwin reformirte Descendenz-Theorie*, vol. 1 (Berlin: G. Reimer, 1866), pl. 1.

58. Ernst Haeckel, *The Wonders of Life: A Popular Study of Biological Philosophy*, trans. Joseph McCabe (New York: Harper & Row, 1904), 27–28. Perhaps as important, for the study of Odilon Redon, is the fact that Haeckel was also a successful artist, whose drawings of plants and animals were intended to demonstrate the beauty and plastic intelligibility of the living world. He tried to make the case for the aesthetic significance of living beings and for an inherent relation between them and artistic production in his lavishly illustrated volume, *Kunstformen der Natur (Art Forms of Nature)*, 2 vols. (Leipzig and Vienna, 1899–1904).

59. *The Power of Movement in Plants*, vol. 27 of *The Works of Charles Darwin*, ed. Paul H. Barrett & R. B. Freeman (London: William Pickering, 1989), 418.

60. Ibid., 419.

61. Ibid.

62. Plate 6 from *Rêves*, 1891, Lithograph on chine appliqué, in Hauptman, *Beyond the Visible*, 152.

63. *A soi-même*, 64, 77.

64. Ibid., 184.

65. Ibid., 28–29.

66. Interview between Redon and his biographer André Mellerio from November 30, 1891 (Mellerio General Research Notes in the André Mellerio Archive, Art Institute of Chicago; quoted in Druick and Zegers, 138n49).

67. André Mellerio, "Les artistes à l'atelier: Odilon Redon" in *L'art dans les deux mondes*, July 4, 1891, and notes for *Odilon Redon*, André Mellerio Archive, Art Institute of Chicago (quoted in Larson, 88n). Cf. Mellerio's description of *In the Primeval Mud*, from when it was reexhibited in Redon's 1894 retrospective: what the painting depicted "was from Darwinian epochs. . . . In the protoplasm of strange spurting bacilli, of unknown cells coming into being. It is the terrible in the infinitely small. Then silhouettes begin vaguely to form, in a painful unconscious effort of matter in the direction of organized being" (André Mellerio, "Odilon Redon" in *Exposition Odilon Redon*, 6, quoted in and translated by Larson, 88).

68. Hennequin, 137, quoted in and translated by Larson, 89.

69. *A soi-même*, 28–29. On fermentation, see "Rotting Waste," in chapter 4.

70. *A soi-même*, 137–38.

71. Ibid., 81.

72. Cf. also another description: "A landscape of antique gold, a solemn peacefulness, leaves thick underfoot . . . O melancholy odor of the dead leaves that evoke in autumnal gardens the memories of vanished life . . . that sad and funereal charm, in which death would seem sweet, blended in this way with everything that goes away and bids us farewell . . ." (*ibid.*, 105). The apostrophe is addressed here not to death itself but to the dead leaves, which combine the notions of the vegetal and the dead.

73. Plate 3 of *To Gustave Flaubert*, 1889, Lithograph, Art Institute of Chicago, in Eisenman, 214.

74. *A soi-même*, 89.

75. Ibid., 115, 184.

76. Ibid., 25.

77. Ibid., 81.

78. It is from this perspective that Jann Matlock reads *La cousine Bette* in *Scenes of Seduction*. The relation between aesthetics and class structures in the novel has been discussed, most notably by Fredric R. Jameson in "*La cousine Bette* and Allegorical Realism," *PMLA* 86 (1971): 241–54. In *The Myth of the French Bourgeoisie: An Essay on the Social Imaginary 1750–1850* (Cambridge, Mass.: Harvard University Press, 2003), Sarah C. Maza responds to Marxist readers of Balzac, such as Jameson and Lukács (see *Studies in European Realism: A Sociological Survey of the Writings of Balzac, Stendhal, Zola, Tolstoy, Gorki, and Others*, trans. Edith Bone [1950; repr., London: Merlin Press, 1978]), to argue that "[f]ar from an eccentric right-wing point of view, Balzac's disgust with the bourgeois as embodied by Crevel [in *La cousine Bette*] was a standard attitude in a culture which glorified universalism and transcendence" (190). The relation between materialism and disgust, which Maza describes, is worth noting, since it seems to take its

most acute and exposed form in the novel's descriptions of putrefaction, thereby tying social issues into questions of death. Issues of sexuality in *La cousine Bette*—especially insofar as they concern heteronormativity and the fluidity of gender—have received significant attention in recent years, particularly in Dorothy Kelly, *Fictional Genders: Role & Representation in Nineteenth-Century French Narrative* (Lincoln: University of Nebraska Press, 1989), 44–57; Diana Knight, "Reading as an Old Maid: *La cousine Bette* and Compulsory Heterosexuality," in *Quinquereme* 12, no. 1 (1989): 67–79; and Michael Lucey, *The Misfit of the Family: Balzac and the Social Forms of Sexuality* (Durham: Duke University Press, 2003), 154–71. The medical aspects of Balzac's novels have been discussed by Patrice Boussel in his untitled introduction to *Balzac et la médecine de son temps*, exhibition catalogue (Paris: Ville de Paris, Maison de Balzac, 1976) and by Pierre Laubriet, *L'intelligence de l'art chez Balzac* (1961; repr., Paris: Slatkine Reprints, 1980), 274–86. Useful, if somewhat dated bibliographies on the subject can be found in René Cruchet, *La médecine dans la littérature française* (Baton Rouge, La.: n.p. 1939), 234–36, and Moïse Le Yaouanc, *Nosographie de l'humanité balzacienne* (Paris: Librairie Maloine, 1959), 31–39. Studies on Balzac's theories of artistic creation in *Bette* tend to be more descriptive than analytical and to have fallen, as a genre, from favor, but the following are still useful: Marc Eigeldinger, *La philosophie de l'art chez Balzac* (1957; repr., Geneva: Slatkine Reprints, 1998), 48–52, and Laubriet, 152–74, 503–13. All this is to say that, to my knowledge, the current analysis of *Bette* is substantially different from all of the studies that have so far been devoted to it. The closest point of approach is undoubtedly to be found in discussions of sexuality and gender, but, as in my discussion of prostitution, sexuality in my own reading is taken as a displacement of other concerns.

79. Honoré de Balzac, *Cousin Bette: Part One of Poor Relations*, trans. Marion Ayton Crawford (New York: Penguin Books, 1965), 33. In his introduction to the novel, André Lorant remarks on the importance of mud for its narrative structure (Honoré de Balzac, *La cousine Bette*, ed. André Lorant [Paris: GF Flammarion, 1977], 20).

80. Balzac, *Cousin Bette*, 289 (trans. modified), 64.

81. Ibid., 431, (trans. modified).

82. Hippolyte Taine, *Essais de critique et d'histoire* (Paris: Hachette, 1858) (quoted by André Lorant in Balzac, *La cousine Bette*, 496).

83. Balzac, *Cousin Bette*, 223 (trans. modified).

84. Ibid., 423 (trans. modified).

85. Ibid., 422 (trans. modified).

86. Ibid., 421. Cf. also: "—'Oh!' said Bianchon, 'the cause is a rapid transformation of the blood, which is decomposing at a frightening speed. I'm hoping to attack the disease in the blood. I am on my way home to pick up the result of a blood analysis made by my friend Professor Duval, the famous chemist, before attempting one of those desparate gambles that we sometimes try against death'" (ibid., 420; trans. modified).

87. Ibid., 423 (trans. modified). One finds another example of a living corpse at the end of the novel, when Balzac describes Adeline Hulot's death: "And, a

phenomenon that must be rare, tears were seen to fall from a dead woman's eyes" (ibid., 443).

88. When Madame de Merteuil is disfigured by smallpox in Pierre Choderlos de Laclos's *Les liaisons dangereuses*, trans. Douglas Parmée (Oxford: Oxford University Press, 1995), another character moralizes on the disease: "I was surely correct when I said that it would be a blessing for her to die of smallpox. It is true that she has recovered but she is terribly disfigured. . . . The Marquis de----, who never misses a chance to say something unkind, when talking of her yesterday said that her illness had turned her inside out and that now her soul was showing on her face. Unfortunately everyone thought that the remark was apt" (370). Similarly, Zola draws a moral from his character Nana's death by smallpox: "And around this grotesque and horrible mask of death, the hair, the beautiful hair, still blazed like sunlight and flowed in a stream of gold. Venus was decomposing. It was as if the poison that she had picked up in the gutters, from the carcasses left there by the roadside, that ferment with which she had poisoned a whole people, had now risen to her face and rotted it" (*Nana*, trans. George Holden, [New York: Penguin, 1972], 470).

89. "'A true doctor,' Bianchon replied, 'takes a passionate interest in science. He sustains himself by this feeling and by the certainty of his usefulness to society. For example, at this very moment, you find me in a sort of scientific ecstasy. . . . Tomorrow, I am going to announce a discovery to the Académie de Médecine. I am currently observing a long-lost disease" (*Cousin Bette*, 419). The illness in question is the one that is ravaging Valérie Marneffe and her new husband, Augustin Crevel.

90. Ibid., 9 (trans. modified), 10. In *Le roman expérimental*, Zola cites *La cousine Bette* as an example of how medical principles can usefully be applied to the construction of novels: "Here, it is almost always an experiment 'to see,' as Claude Bernard calls it. I shall take as an example the figure of Baron Hulot, in Balzac's *La cousine Bette*" (1178). Balzac compared himself to Buffon, Zola to Bernard. Zola contentrated on the pathology of Baron Hulot, while I have been focusing on Valérie Marneffe. The underlying principle is, however, the same in all cases: *La cousine Bette* is a medical document.

91. Balzac, *Cousin Bette*, 224, 431 (trans. modified).

92. Ibid., 214.

93. Ibid., 215 (trans. modified).

94. In his "Lettres satiriques et critiques," the critic Hippolyte Babon summarized this "Rabelaisian" perception of Balzac, addressing the novelist with the following words: "Whether you agree or not, you have, moreover, philosophical principles that do not fit well with the cult of abstraction. I recognize in you a cleric from Tours, a monk from the abbey of Thélème, governed by the Reverend Father Alcofribas Nasier" (*La revue nouvelle*, February 1, 1847).

95. "Whenever Wenceslas was about to head off to the studio at Gros-Caillou to work the clay [*glaise*] and finish the model, either the Prince's clock would demand his presence at the studio of Florent and de Chanor, where its figures

were being carved, or . . ." (Balzac, *Cousin Bette*, 217 [trans. modified]). A few pages later, the sculptor's wife will use the same term, *glaise*, to designate the laborious aspect of artistic creation: "To tell you the truth, if Wenceslas doesn't get to work," she says, "I don't know what's going to become of us. Oh! If I could only learn to make statues, how I would get the clay [*glaise*] moving!" (Balzac, *Cousin Bette*, 221 [trans. modified]).

96. See ibid., 215: "But to produce! To give birth! To raise a child by the sweat of your brow, putting him to bed every evening gorged with milk, kissing him every morning with the unfailing heart of a mother, licking him clean when he's dirty, dressing him a hundred times in the prettiest smocks just so he can tear them to shreds; not to flinch at the upheavals of this mad existence and make of it the living masterpiece that speaks to every beholder's eye in sculpture, to every intelligence in literature, to every memory in painting, to every heart in music—this is Execution and its labors" (trans. modified).

97. On the significance of such "illuminations," see Simone Delattre, *Les douze heures noires: La nuit à Paris au XIXe siècle* (Paris: Albin Michel, 2003), 155–57.

98. Philippe Vigier, *La vie quotidienne en province et à Paris pendant les journées de 1848: 1847–1851* (Paris: Hachette, 1982), 67.

99. The final death toll would rise to 52. See Albert Crémieux, *La révolution de février: Etude critique sur les journées des 21, 22, 23 et 24 février 1848* (Paris: Edouard Cornély, 1912), 194–95.

100. Although the most distinguished of the contemporary commentators on the events, Karl Marx and Alexis de Tocqueville, make no mention of the procession of cadavers, most other accounts of February 1848 identify it as the precipitating cause for the downfall of the monarchy and the installation of the Republic. Among contemporary accounts see Alphonse de Lamartine, *Histoire de la révolution de 1848*, vol. 1 (Paris: Perrotin, 1849), 99–100; and Louis-Antoine Garnier-Pagès, *Histoire de la révolution de 1848*, vol. 1 (Paris: Degorce-Cadot, 1868), 150–51. For important subsequent analyses, see Crémieux and Vigier as well as Charles Seignobos, *Histoire de la France contemporaine depuis la révolution jusqu'à la paix de 1919*, vol. 6, ed. Ernest Lavisse (Paris: Hachette, 1921); G.A.S. Grenville, *Europe Reshaped: 1848–1878* (Oxford: Blackwell, 2000); Maurice Agulhon, *The Republican Experiment, 1848–1852*, trans. Janet Lloyd (Cambridge: Cambridge University Press, 1983); Peter N. Stearns, *1848: The Revolutionary Tide in Europe* (New York: W.W. Norton, 1974); Jean Sigmann, *1848: The Romantic and Democratic Revolutions in Europe*, trans. Lovette F. Edwards (New York: Harper & Row, 1973); William L. Langer, *Political and Social Upheaval: 1832–1852* (New York: Harper & Row, 1969); and Georges Duveau, *1848: The Making of a Revolution*, trans. Anne Carter (New York: Random House, 1967). Marx's commentary on the events is contained principally in "The Eighteenth Brumaire of Louis Bonaparte" in Karl Marx and Frederick Engels, *Collected Works*, vol. 11, ed. James S. Allen et al. (New York: International Publishers, 1979), 99–197. For de Tocqueville, see *Souvenirs* in *Œuvres*, vol. 3, ed. François Furet and Françoise Mélonio (Paris: Gallimard [Pléiade], 2004), 739–823.

101. See *Le National*, February 24, 1848 (quoted in Crémieux, 200–1).

102. Marx, 300.

103. Tocqueville, vol. 3, 768–69.

104. Maxime Du Camp, *Souvenirs de l'année 1848: La révolution de février, le 15 mai, l'insurrection de juin* (Paris: Hachette, 1876), 74.

105. Marx, 300, 302.

106. Gustave Flaubert, *Correspondance*, vol. 1, ed. Jean Bruneau (Paris: Gallimard [Pléiade], 1973), 491.

107. For a reading of the relations between history and fiction in *L'éducation sentimentale*, see notably Jay Bernstein, *The Philosophy of the Novel: Lukács, Marxism and the Dialectics of Form* (Brighton: The Harvester Press, 1984), 109–46 and Pierre Bourdieu, *The Rules of Art: Genesis and Structure of the Literary Field*, trans. Susan Emanuel (Stanford: Stanford University Press, 1995), 1–43.

108. Gustave Flaubert, *Sentimental Eduction*, trans. Robert Baldick (New York: Penguin, 2004), 306.

109. Ibid., 311.

110. Ibid., 306.

111. Ibid., 302.

112. Ibid., 303 (trans. modified).

113. Letter of November 7, 1847 in *Correspondance*, 1:482.

114. *Correspondance*, 1:476.

115. Ibid., 479. In his correspondence with Colet, Flaubert regularly referred to Cousin as "the philosopher" (e.g. ibid., 487).

116. Ibid., 470.

117. *Le salon de 1847 précédé d'une lettre à Firmin Barrion* (Paris: Alliance des Arts, 1847), 66. Quoted in the editor's notes to Flaubert, *Correspondance*, 1:1036.

118. Flaubert, *Correspondance*, 1:470.

119. Ibid., 471. Flaubert's elipsis.

120. Ibid., 826. Letter of February 21, 1847. For a brilliant reading of Flaubert's plastic use of time, see Elissa Marder, *Dead Time: Temporal Disorders in the Wake of Modernity (Baudelaire and Flaubert)* (Stanford, Calif.: Stanford University Press, 2001).

121. Flaubert, *Correspondance*, 1:482. Letter of November 7, 1847.

122. Flaubert, *Sentimental Education*, 303–4 (trans. modified).

123. Whether or not the connection between *Colot* and *Colet* was intentional, it was undoubtedly significant for Flaubert, who was extremely careful in choosing names for his characters. Before finally going ahead with *Moreau*, for example, he had one of his relatives make sure that no Moreaus lived in Nogent-sur-Seine, the town that his protagonist inhabited. He was informed that there were none, but much later his relative wrote back asking him to change the character's name since there were in fact Moreaus in the town. Flaubert refused, explaining that "the time has passed for me to change it. A proper noun is a very important thing in a novel, a *capital* thing. You can't change a character's name any more than you can change his skin. . . . Too bad for the Moreaus who live in Nogent"

(*Correspondance*, 1:1033). The letter indicates that Flaubert was extremely careful about the connections between the names of his fictional creations and other identifiable people. It seems that one as obvious as Colet/Colot could not have escaped him and would have become a "capital" element in his character's identity.

124. Ibid., 493.

125. Ibid., 474.

126. Ibid., 491.

127. See, for example, ibid., 465–46, 471, 493–95.

128. Ibid., 493.

129. Ibid., 494.

130. Maxime Du Camp, *Souvenirs littéraires, Tome I: 1822–1850* (Paris: L'Harmattan, 1993), 272. The punctuation and many words are altered in Du Camp's version of the letter. The word *horriblement*, for instance, is replaced by *affreusement*.

131. *Correspondance*, 1:449.

132. Ibid., 494.

133. Du Camp, *Souvenirs littéraires*, 273. See also 274, where Du Camp develops the reasons for this conviction at greater length.

134. Robiano de Borsbeek, 41.

135. "The sign is some immediate intuition, representing a totally different import from what naturally belongs to it; it is a pyramid into which a foreign soul has been conveyed, and where it is conserved" (G. W. F. Hegel, *Hegel's Philosophy of Mind: Part Three of the Encyclopaedia of the Philosophical Sciences*, trans. William Wallace [Oxford: Clarendon Press, 1971], para 458, 213). For a reading of this figure, see Jacques Derrida, "The Pit and the Pyramid: Introduction to Hegel's Semiology" in *Margins of Philosophy*, trans. Alan Bass (Chicago: University of Chicago Press, 1982), 81–87. What is unsettling in Hegel's description is that it complicates a long-standing tradition that sees the relation between sign and meaning as that between body and soul. For while the pyramid seems to replace the body, it historically contained a preserved corpse rather than a pure soul—in fact, pyramids are remarkable for the attention given in them to preserving the physical remains of the deceased. In this sense, Hegel's figure puts the corpse in the place of the soul and makes of meaning a dead body rather than a living spirit. This substitution of a preserved or mummified corpse for a soul reappears in Paul de Man's reference to this passage, when he uses it to interpret Baudelaire's "Spleen": "Baudelaire . . . uses 'pyramid,' which connotes, of course, Egypt, monument and crypt, but which also connects, to a reader of Hegel, the emblem of the sign as opposed to the symbol. . . . Baudelaire, who in all likelihood never heard of Hegel, happens to hit on the same emblematic sequence to say something very similar. The decapitated painter lies, as a corpse, in the crypt of recollection" ("Reading History" in *The Resistance to Theory* [Minneapolis: University of Minnesota Press, 1986], 69–70). By replacing the term *soul* with *corpse*, De Man's misreading (or miscollection) of Hegel's text makes explicit what is only implicit in the original.

136. Auguste-Hilarion Kératry, *De l'âme humaine et de la vie future* (*Extrait de la Revue contemporaine, liv. du 15 décembre*) (Paris: La Revue contemporaine, 1852), 16.

137. Ibid., 17.

138. Auguste-Hilarion Kératry, *Examen philosophique des considérations sur le sentiment du sublime et du beau, dans le rapport des caractères, des tempéraments, des sexes, des climats, et des religions, d'Emmanuel Kant* (Paris: Bossange frères, 1823). Kératry was also the author of a work on ontology entitled *Inductions morales et physiologiques* (Paris: C. Gosselin, 1841).

139. For example, *Les derniers des Beaumanoirs* is cited by Morel in "Considérations médico-légales . . . Deuxième lettre," 186; and by Lunier, 352. The novel was based on a supposedly real incident that is recounted in another article on Bertrand, by Dr. Alexandre Jacques François Brierre de Boismont: "Remarques médico-légales sur la perversion de l'instinct génésique," *Gazette médicale de Paris*, no. 29 (July 21, 1849): 555–64.

140. Fernand, 13.

141. On the relation between death and historiography, see Michel de Certeau, *The Writing of History*, trans. Tom Conley (New York: Columbia University Press, 1988). De Certeau summarizes the situation: "Discourse about the past has the status of being the discourse of the dead" (46), and his point of departure is Michelet's unpublished draft of a preface for the *Histoire de France* (ibid., 1).

142. Jules Michelet, *Œuvres complètes*, vol. 4, ed. Paul Viallaneix (Paris: Flammarion, 1974), 34.

143. Ibid., 727. The persistence of Michelet's necrophilic historiographical imagination can be seen in the fact that the scholars who recently reissued an obscure eighteenth-century medical volume used this passage as an epigraph to their preface (Rodolphe Trouilleux and Jean-Michel Roy, "Préface" in Robert Ducreux, *Le médecin radoteur ou les pots pourris et autres textes*, ed. Rodolphe Trouilleux et Jean-Michel Roy [Paris: Honoré Champion, 1999], 13). On the other hand, some of the violence and strangeness of Michelet's metaphorics can be judged by comparing his descriptions to those of Ducreux's editors: "The discovery of forgotten texts is always a moving and exceptional event," they write. "When, furthermore, these writings, mishandled by earlier generations, also reappear in the form of an illegible puzzle, the experience is very exciting. The historian then becomes a little more of a detective than he usually is" (20). Michelet's necrophilia is replaced by the affective neutrality of the detective, while the ontological ravaging of time reveals itself as a "puzzle" rather than putrefaction. In *Le goût de l'archive* (Paris: Seuil, 1997), Arlette Farge emphasizes the materiality of documents and their repositories, the sensuousness already indicated in her title. "The archive is unlike texts, or printed documents, or 'accounts,' or correspondence, or newspapers, or even autobiographies," she writes. "It is difficult because of its materiality" (10). And once again, for Farge as for Michelet, the archive is remarkable for the immediacy with which its contents signify lost existences, the "naked trace of lives that never sought to tell

their tale" (12). In them, she finds a language of the inexpressible, since, by recording what was never meant to be read, "they yield something unspoken [*un non-dit*]" (13). As the language of unspeakable lives, the archives exist, according to Farge's conception, in a state that fundamentally betrays the existences they seem to represent. Their documents are signs marked by an infinite distance and so constitute another version of the mystery of the past, embodied in the very nature of words.

144. *Œuvres complètes*, 4:26. See also the formulation of his historiographical method in the 1833 version of his preface to the *Histoire de France*: "And as I breathed upon their ashes," he wrote, "I could see them rising up. They dragged from the tomb here a hand, there a head, like in Michelangelo's Last Judgment or the Dance of the Dead. They circled about me in a galvanic round, and that is what I have tried to capture in this book" (ibid., 727).

145. Bouchut described putrefaction as "the most certain of all the signs of death" (196). Similarly, Félix Gannal wrote that "only one [sign] is certain in itself, which is to say that it is sufficient to characterize death, and that is putrefaction" (*Moyens de distinguer*, 17).

146. Michelet, *Œuvres complètes*, 4:727.

147. On Blanchot's analysis of the relation between language and the corpse, see the discussion of "La Littérature et le droit à la mort" in chapter 8.

148. See Paul De Man, Allegories of Reading: Figural Language in Rousseau, Nietzsche, Rilke, and Proust (New Haven and London: Yale University Press, 1979).

7. ABSTRACTING DESIRE

1. The notion that scientific truth is shaped by nonscientific forces has gained increasing currency since the 1980s. In his study of Pasteur, for instance, Bruno Latour writes: "In fact, 'science' is never explained by itself alone. It is an ill-made entity that excludes most of the elements that give it existence. . . . The social movement in which Pasteur was situated . . . was *exclusively* responsible for the effectiveness that was attributed to his demonstrations" (34–35). Steven Shapin has recently argued: "you could say that science happens within, not outside of, historical time, that it has a deep historicity, and that whatever transcendence it possesses is itself a historical accomplishment" (*Never Pure: Historical Studies of Science as if It Was Produced by People with Bodies, Situated in Time, Space, Culture, and Society, and Struggling for Credibility and Authority* [Baltimore: Johns Hopkins University Press, 2010], 5). Similarly, François Delaporte describes the effects of "*fantasmes*" on the evolution of medical thought (*Figures de la médecine*, [Paris: Cerf, 2009]). His readings of particular cases reveal the influence of non-medical conditions and ideas on key conceptual breakthroughs, but it is not clear why he chose the term *fantasme* or what he means by it.

2. See Bruce Gordon and Peter Marshall, "Introduction: Placing the Dead in Late Medieval and Early Modern Europe" in Bruce Gordon and Peter Marshall, eds., *The Place of the Dead: Death and Remembrance in Late Medieval and Early*

Modern Europe (Cambridge: Cambridge University Press, 2000), 9. Thomas Kselman has argued that it was because of this resistance, this ongoing desire to preserve the Christian community between the living and the dead, that Paris was allowed to reincorporate its cemeteries little more than half a century after having so laboriously removed them (177–78).

3. Porée, 1–26, 38–43.

4. "But we can easily offer detailed proof that this new arrangement outrages the people, undermines the religious cult of funerals, ruins the *fabriques*, and threatens the whole city with an infection more contagious than the one the decree is intended to prevent" ("Mémoire des curés de Paris," 16 recto-verso).

5. Ibid., 16 recto.

6. Robiano de Borsbeek, 41.

7. See Hannaway and Hannaway: "Decidedly, the reasons that led to the closing of the Saints-Innocents cemetery were theoretically heterogeneous" (189), and: "The project of a vast natural history of disease, illustrated by numerical indices, like the one that Sydenham and the *Encyclopédie* had wished for and the Société Royale de Médecine had subsequently attempted, was doomed to failure in the 18th century. The period lacked a theory of probability that would have allowed it to establish significant correlations among statistical data that was gathered with more zeal than method. In the clinical field, singular cases could still be endlessly opposed to each other" (190). For exceptions to this, notably Villermé, see the section on hygiene in chapter 3.

8. Cadet-De-Vaux, *Innocents*, 1.

9. Ibid., 2 and Cadet-De-Vaux, *Méphitisme*, 4. See also his *Innocents*, 2: "I shall not enter here into the details of my experiments," and 4; and *Méphitisme*, 2: "I tried few experiments."

10. Cadet-De-Vaux, *Innocents*, 4–5. Cf. his *Méphitisme*: "My intention was to conduct some experiments. To that end, I lowered into the pit an apparatus containing several reactive agents, among them lime water and sugar of Saturn, which immediately decomposed, but I little insisted on these physical details. It is hardly possible to indulge coolly in experimentation when faced with the imperious demands of another person's danger, and when one is surrounded by asphyxiated or even dead people, as happens in these unfortunate circumstances. Moreover, when personally exposed to the dangerous effects of these vapors, one would rather fight them than seek to understand them better, for one never breathes them with impunity, and I have always been more or less acutely affected by them in such cases. Ultimately, in the present instance, I was no longer able to resist my impatience to see if the methods for which I had recently congratulated myself would be confirmed by new successes, and if I would be able to identify definitive principles concerning the demephitization of wells, as did in fact happen" (4).

11. "Des cimetières de la terreur" in *Histoire de la révolution*, vol. 2, ed. Gérard Walter (Paris: Gallimard [Pléiade], 1952), 923.

12. Ibid. See Marie-Hélène Huet's commentary on this passage in *Mourning Glory: The Will of the French Revolution* (Philadelphia: University of Pennsylvania

Press, 1997), 139. The general argument of Huet's book is powerful and characteristically brilliant. According to her, the ideology of the Revolution was based on the aesthetics of the sublime, especially as described by Kant in the *Critique of Judgement*. As Huet observes, however, the sublime is a formulation of unrepresentability, and the leaders of the Revolution were attempting to create a representational democracy (see, for example, 76). The role of her extended analysis of graveyards in this argument is a little unclear to me, but I understand her to mean that the impasse of this political aesthetics played itself out in an ideology and praxis of death. Although Huet herself does not do so, this impasse could be usefully reformulated in Hegelian terms as the aporia of immediacy between individual and universal, which would put it more directly into dialogue with certain other analyses of death in the Revolution. In a section of the *Phenomenology of Spirit* devoted to the Terror, Hegel, for instance, understood the guillotine to have functioned as an attempt to resolve this aporia by annihilating the individual as such; for him, the guillotine served as an acting out of an ideology of selflessness and death, something that Alexandre Kojève would later, and quite perversely, call a "political right to death." See G. W. F. Hegel, *Phenomenology of Spirit*, 355–63; Alexandre Kojève, *Introduction à la lecture de Hegel: Leçons sur la Phénoménologie de l'Esprit professées de 1933 à 1939 à l'Ecole des Hautes Etudes*, ed. Raymond Queneau (Paris: Gallimard, 1947), 557–58; Maurice Blanchot, "Literature and the Right to Death" in *The Work of Fire*, trans. Lydia Davis (Stanford: Stanford University Press, 1995), 300–44; and Strauss, *Subjects of Terror*, 54–63. The importance of language in terrorist sublimation is analyzed in ibid., 16–22. Similarly, in *Terror and Its Discontents: Suspect Words In Revolutionary France* (Minneapolis: University of Minnesota Press, 2003), Caroline Weber further pursues Huet's central insights into the sublimity of the revolutionary projects, emphasizing their linguistic aspects and the inherent forces in words, such as "language's polyvalent possibilities" (xvi), that resist those projects.

13. Like Michelet, a more recent author, Marcel Colin, has argued that there is an irrational component to the desire to expel the corpse from the city and has speculated on the subconscious drives that this desire translates: *"by its exile, the corpse redeems all the urbanist's remorse*. You can follow step by step the stages of rejection that carried it outside the ramparts" ("L'anthropologie et la mort" in Christiane Vitani, *Législation de la mort: Travail de l'association lyonnaise de médecine légale* [Paris: Masson & Cie, 1962], xi); and "not all of the legislation about death can be deduced from the weakly rationalist abstract principles that claim to have guided its regulations. Its roots reach down through centuries of human tradition and drink from the hidden wells of sub-conscious motivations" (xv).

14. Among the scholarship on Robertson, Max Milner's *La fantasmagorie: Essai sur l'optique fantastique* (Paris: Presses Universitaires de France, 1982), 9–23, comes closest to our own approach, with its attempt to read the fantasmagoria as a representation of irrational aspects of the psyche. Milner's discussion of Robertson is part of a historically based analysis of the relation between the use of optical devices in fantastic literature and the optical within Freud's theory of the psyche,

especially as revisited by Lacan. Milner argues for the importance of scientific models in the creative imaginary while recognizing, conversely, the role of the irrational in the development of science (see, for example, his reference to Bachelard, 5). Most significantly, he contends that the fantasmagoria represented a dreamlike imaginative state that could not otherwise be depicted and, as such, constituted a breakthrough in the perception—if not understanding—of the unconscious (see 23). Somewhat similarly, Terry Castle's *The Female Thermometer: Eighteenth-Century Culture and the Invention of the Uncanny* (Oxford: Oxford University Press, 1995) includes discussions of Robertson's fantasmagoria (see esp. 140–67), which Castle views as a step in the reconceptualization of ghosts from objective phenomena to subjective hallucinations and, subsequently, elements of the Freudian unconscious. "The rationalists did not so much negate the traditional spirit world," she writes, "as displace it into the realm of psychology" (161). From the other scholarship on Robertson, one should cite Françoise Levie's biography, *Etienne-Gaspard Robertson: La vie d'un fantasmagore* (Paris: Editions du Préambule, 1990). Maurice Samuels, *The Spectacular Past: Popular History and the Novel in Nineteenth-Century France* (Ithaca: Cornell University Press, 2004) discusses the representation of history in Robertson's shows as part of a larger argument concerning the role of the spectacular in the determination of realism as an aesthetic category. I am indebted, in particular, to his bibliography on Robertson on p. 26. Jann Matlock has worked on Robertson, but mostly in reference to another of his spectacles, the "invisible woman," for which one should see "Reading Invisibility," in Marjorie Garber, Paul B. Franklin, and Rebecca L. Walkowitz, eds., *Field Work: Sites in Literary and Cultural Studies* (New York: Routledge, 1996), 183–95. A more developed version of similar arguments can be found in "The Invisible Woman and Her Secrets Unveiled," in *Yale Journal of Criticism* 9, no. 2 (1996): 175–221. In "Voir aux limites du corps: Fantasmagories et femmes invisibles dans les spectacles de Robertson," in Ségolène Le Men et al., eds., *Lanternes magiques, tableaux transparents* (Paris: Réunion des Musées nationaux, 1995), 85–99, Matlock speaks of Robertson's spectacles as a response to the need for transgressive "fantasms," but unlike Milner or—to a lesser extent—Castle, her interest is not in the psychoanalytic significance of those fantasms but in the way they represent a longing to "believe in a reality beyond the flesh" at a time of scientific scepticism (96).

15. Etienne-Gaspard Robertson, *Mémoires récréatifs, scientifiques et anecdotiques d'un physicien-aéronaute. I. La fantasmagorie* (1831–1833; Langres: Café, Clima, 1985), 130.

16. This idea of demystification does, however, permeate all of Robertson's thinking, which suggests that he did take it in earnest. For instance, the progress from superstition to disabused rationality that the spectators were promised was in some ways a recapitulation of Robertson's own experiences. In an autobiographical sketch, he described his background in the sciences as a movement away from his previous fascination with the occult toward a more enlightened fascination with the powers of reason. "The knowledge that I derived from the

study of physics and, in particular, the phenomena of light," he wrote, "had much earlier transformed my eccentric ideas about sorcery into more rational studies on fantastic effects. I had a particular taste for experiments with the solar microscope" (ibid., 121). As Dhombres and Dhombres have observed, one of the primary values of the sciences, for contemporaries of Robertson, was to demystify superstitions (403). In this vein, an early nineteenth-century guide to Paris, F.-M. Marchant's *Le conducteur de l'étranger à Paris* (Paris: Moronval, 1811), describes a fantasmagoria run by a certain M. Le Breton as a demystification of the "tricks used by pagan sibyls and priests to gain control over the masses" (164–65). Contemporaries, moreover, used the term *fantômes*, or fantoms, to refer to the irrational beliefs that science was expected to overturn. In *Du degré de certitude de la médecine*, for instance, Cabanis wrote: "Just like all the other physical sciences and all the other arts that depend on the detailed observation of nature, [medicine] directly serves to dissipate the fantoms that fascinate and torment the imagination" (10–11).

17. Articles quoted in Robertson, 128–129.

18. Quoted in ibid., 129.

19. Ibid., 183.

20. This idea that fantasms were products of language goes back at least to Plato, as can be seen from a passage in the *Sophist*: "Stranger: And is it not inevitable that, after a long enough time, as these young hearers advance in age and, coming into closer touch with realities, are forced by experience to apprehend things clearly as they are, most of them should abandon those former beliefs [*doxas*], so that what seemed important will now appear trifling and what seemed easy, difficult, and all the illusions created in discourse [*ta en tois logois phantasmata*] will be completely overturned by the realities which encounter them in the actual conduct of life?" ("Sophist" 234d–e, trans. F. M. Cornford in *Collected Dialogues*, 977). In ancient Athenian funeral orations, Nicole Loraux observed a conflation between real and fantasmatic cities that recalls—or rather, foreshadows—the one that Robertson observed in the Paris of the year VII: "The funeral oration thus broke down the barriers separating the real from the imaginary and, by excessively trying to concentrate on Athens, which it transformed into a spectacle or mirage, it ended up moving Athens outside itself and replacing the real city with a fantom of the ideal polis, or a *utopia*. Citizens of nowhere, the dazzled Athenians were enthralled by the hallowest of all fantasms" (*The Invention of Athens: The Funeral Oration in the Classical City*, trans. Alan Sheridan [Cambridge, Mass.: Harvard University Press, 1986], 267, trans. modified). In both cases—Robertson's and the Athenians'—the dead create a privileged transitional space between the fantasmatic and something else, which Loraux calls the "real."

21. In an analysis of *Antigone* that sees the heroine's reverence for the dead as characteristically female, Hegel describes women as "the irony [in the life] of the community." This notion that concern for the dead is linked to a figural status (for irony is a trope) echoes Robertson's conflation of death and metaphor while elevating it to a social condition. See *Phenomenology of Spirit*, 288.

22. Marie Hélène Huet has argued that the post-Revolutionary period was marked by fears that those killed during the Revolution would return to exact vengeance. See *Mourning Glory*, 125–48, esp. 139–40.

23. On the powerfulness of that instrument, see Milner, 9–23.

24. "The Narcissistic Evaluation of Excretory Processes in Dreams and Neurosis" in *Selected Papers of Karl Abraham M.D.*, intro. Ernest Jones, trans. Douglas Bryan and Alix Strachey (London: Hogarth Press, 1949), 319.

25. Ibid., 321, and "Contributions to the Theory of the Anal Character" in Abraham, *Selected Papers*, 371.

26. See Abraham, "Excretory Processes" in *Selected Papers*, 319–22, and "Contributions" in ibid., 377.

27. Ernest Jones, *Papers on Psycho-analysis* (New York: William Wood & Co., 1923), 698–99. Similarly, Freud wrote of the positive and affectionate significance that feces can have in his discussion of the "Wolfman" case, but unlike Jones, he viewed that positive aspect as primary and the negative aspect as derivative: "like every other child, he was making use of the content of the intestines in one of its earliest and most primitive meanings. Faeces are the child's first *gift*, the first sacrifice on behalf of his affection, a portion of his own body which he is ready to part with, but only for the sake of some one he loves. To use faeces as an expression of defiance . . . is merely to turn this earlier 'gift' meaning into the negative" (Sigmund Freud, *From the History of an Infantile Neurosis* in *Standard Edition*, 17:81 [original emphasis]; cf. Freud, "On Transformations of Instinct as Exemplified in Anal Erotism" in *Standard Edition*, 17:130).

28. Jones, 699.

29. *Purity and Danger: An Analysis of the Concepts of Pollution and Taboo* (1966; London: Routledge, 1996), 36–37.

30. Ibid., 57.

31. Abraham, "The Narcissistic Evaluation of the Excretory Processes" in *Selected Papers*, 319.

32. Jean Laplanche and J.-B. Pontalis, 46; and Jean-Paul Valabrega, *Phantasme, mythe, corps et sens: Une théorie psychanalytique de la connaissance* (1980; Paris: Payot, 1992), 21.

33. René Kaës, "Quatre études sur la fantasmatique de la formation et le désir de former" in René Kaës, et al., *Fantasme et formation* (1979; Paris: Dunod, 2001), 2; and Lacan, "Fantasme," 272–73.

34. Lacan does, in fact, speak of neurotics in his discussions of the fantasm, but that is because he sees in them a paradigm for *all* fantasmatics and therefore as a significant access to its more general structures and meanings. On the relation between the fantasm and perversion, see, for instance, Lacan, "Fantasme," 266.

35. See Lacan, "Fantasme," 272–73. On the relation of the phallus to language and the subject in Lacan, see Strauss, *Subjects of Terror*, 259–65. In his own analysis of the fantasm, Valabrega returns to Lacan's logico-linguistic model, asserting: "Ontologically speaking, meaning *is not*" (49). In *De la horde à l'état:*

Essai de psychanalyse du lien social (Paris: Gallimard, 1983), Eugène Enriquez attempts to establish the general applicability of Freudian psychic structures from a different perspective, arguing for their foundational role in society.

36. Lacan, "Fantasme," 234–36.

37. Ibid., 270.

38. Ibid., 266.

39. See Nasio, 14–16; and Laplanche and Pontalis on the *Urphantasien*, 59–69. Since fantasms derive from the Oedipal complex, according to Lacan, they are consequently fundamentally incestuous (see "Fantasme," *passim*).

40. See Laplanche and Pontalis, 88–97.

41. Lacan, "Fantasme," 247–50.

42. Nasio, 81.

43. Ibid.

44. Ibid., 89. "Kant with Sade" in *Ecrits: The First Complete Translation in English*, trans. Bruce Fink et al. (New York: W.W. Norton, 2002), 659 and "The Subversion of the Subject and the Dialectic of Desire in the Freudian Unconscious," esp. 691.

45. Lacan, "Fantasme," 255.

46. On the importance of detumescence, see ibid., 258, 260–61, 267.

47. Ibid., 239. See also 255 and 262.

48. Nasio, 51.

49. Ibid., 90.

50. Ibid., 92.

51. See *The Seminar of Jacques Lacan Book VII: The Ethics of Psychoanalysis*, ed. Jacques-Alain Miller, trans. Dennis Porter (New York: W. W. Norton, 1992), 279–83, especially 279: "This value comes essentially from language. Outside of language, it could not even be conceived, and the being of him who had lived could not therefore be detached from everything—good and evil, destiny, consequences for others, feelings for himself—for which he had been a vessel. This purity, this separation of a being from all the characteristics of the historical drama that it has traversed, is itself the limit, the *ex nihilo*, around which Antigone holds herself. It is nothing other than the split that the very presence of language institutes in a man's life" (trans. modified).

52. See "The Language of Abjection" in chapter 8.

53. Nasio., 83. On putting-to-death in fantasmatics, see also Kaës, 25; on fantasms involving cadavers, see Kaës, 38; and on the fantasmatic need to expel death and excrements from social spaces, see Kaës, 53–54.

54. See Piera Aulagnier, *La violence de l'interprétation: Du pictogramme à l'énoncé* (Paris: Presses Universitaires de France, 1974), 226–32.

55. "Myth and origin are one and the same thing. . . . Every myth refers to an origin. Every question of origin inevitably opens onto a myth" (Valabrega, 52).

56. Lacan, "Fantasme," 272–73.

57. Valabrega, 52.

58. See ibid., 64: "For this reason, we can observe that far from belonging in the museum of past errors and horrors that we have left behind, sophisms have never produced such abundant and flourishing vegetation as in theoretical thought, in the human, social, and political sciences, in the City, and in contemporary ideology." The City, in this discussion of the originary fantasm, is taken as synonymous with theoretical thought and human science, the agencies, we have been arguing, that organize the hygienic imagination as a refusal of the abject.

59. See "Athens and Jerusalem," in *Mourning Becomes the Law: Philosophy and Representation* (Cambridge: Cambridge University Press, 1996), 15–39.

60. Plato, "The Parmenides" 130c–d, trans. F. M. Cornford, in *Collected Dialogues*, 924 (trans. modified).

61. Ibid., 130e, 924–5.

62. "Protagoras" 322b–c, trans. W. K. C. Guthrie, in *Collected Dialogues*, 319.

63. "Now Epimetheus . . . had used up all the available powers on the brute beasts [*ta aloga*]" (ibid. 321b–c, 319).

64. Ibid. 322c, 320 (trans. modified).

65. Ibid. 322d, 320.

66. On the influence of Newton on the *philosophes*, see Ernst Cassirer, *The Philosophy of the Enlightenment* (Princeton: Princeton University Press, 1951), 3–92. For an overview of the problem of applying the laws of nature to human behavior, see Lorainne Daston and Fernando Vidal, "Introduction: Doing What Comes Naturally," in Lorraine Daston and Fernando Vidal, eds., *The Moral Authority of Nature* (Chicago: University of Chicago Press, 2004), 1–20. Daston and Vidal focus on the movement from *is* to *should*: what happens in nature, in other words, *should* happen in human behavior, with the result that natural laws do not merely exist but also prescribe.

67. "Droit naturel (morale)" in *Encyclopédie*, 5:115.

68. Ibid., 116.

69. "To begin with, I observe something that seems to me to be accepted by both good and wicked men, which is that one must use reason in all things, since man is not only an animal, but an animal that reasons; that the means therefore exist by which we can discover the truth in the present inquiry; that the man who refuses to seek the truth abdicates his status as man and must be treated by the rest of his species as a wild beast; and that once the truth has been discovered, whoever refuses to conform to it is mad or morally wicked"; and "all of these consequences are obvious to whoever reasons, and whoever does not want to reason, by thus abdicating his status as man must be treated as a degenerate [*dénaturé*] being" (ibid.).

70. Ibid.

71. Ibid. "What shall we say in response to our violent reasoner, before snuffing him out [*avant que de l'étouffer*]?" (ibid.).

72. While Rousseau also based the social contract on reason, describing "the moral person of the State as a being produced by reason" (*Social Contract*, 141)

and as an expression of the "general will" (ibid., 138–39), he differed from Diderot in refusing to see natural laws as the basis for human ones: "The social order is a sacred right that serves as a basis for all the others. However this right does not come from nature; it is therefore based on conventions" (ibid., 131). Still, the laws of nature are a constant reference point in his political theories and often justify his arguments about convention, as when he observes that "under the law of reason nothing is done without a cause, any more than [is the case] under the law of nature" (ibid., 148). Like Diderot, he spoke of the need for all human beings to be integrated into the social pact and viewed it as intolerable for a single one to remain outside. He was explicit on the need to put violators to death (see ibid., 150–51). On the complexity of Rousseau's idea of nature in relation to the general will, see Jonathan Strauss, "Political Force and the Grounds of Identity From Rousseau to Flaubert" in *MLN* 117, no. 4 (September 2002), esp. 812–826.

73. In *On Jean-Jacques Rousseau Considered as One of the First Authors of the Revolution* (Stanford, Calif.: Stanford University Press, 2000), James Swenson analyzes some of the problems raised by the notion of historical derivation and, in particular, by attempts to determine Rousseau's influence on the French Revolution. Addressing the issue through the notion of authorship and literary techniques of reading, Swenson finds that Rousseau's writings were less a cause of the Revolution than a way of making them intelligible, an approach that I am happy to adopt in my own readings not only of Rousseau and the Revolution, but also of the relation between Platonic texts and Enlightenment political theories. Michael Walzer, *Régicide et révolution: Le procès de Louis XVI*, trans. J. Debouzy (Paris: Payot, 1989) reproduces the principal documents concerning the trial, including transcripts from debates (159–349). There was, however, disagreement over the historical and political significance of the King's death between Walzer and Ferenc Fehér, who is given space, at the end of the volume, to present his own case ("Justice révolutionnaire," 351–80; see also Fehér, *The Frozen Revolution: An Essay on Jacobinism* [Cambridge: Cambridge University Press, 1987], esp. 97–112). Walzer argued for, Fehér against. What is important to my own interpretation, however, is not the political efficacy of the trial and execution, which is what interests Walzer and Fehér, but rather their significance in an imaginary of social justice: the way in which the theories of judicial exclusion and inclusion that were elaborated in the debate about Louis borrowed, on the one hand, from Rousseau (and others) and subsequently reappeared, on the other, in the establishment of summary justice.

74. Louis-Antoine-Léon Saint-Just, *Discours et rapports*, ed. Albert Soboul (Paris: Editions Sociales, 1957), 68.

75. Maximilien Robespierre, *Pour le bonheur et pour la liberté: Discours*, ed. Yannick Bosc, Florence Gauthier, Sophie Wahnich (Paris: La Fabrique, 2000), 196.

76. Saint-Just, 66.

77. Ibid., 64.

78. Ibid., 67.

79. Robespierre, *Bonheur*, 195.

80. On the relation between Saint-Just's arguments and summary revolutionary justice, see Fehér, "Justice," 377. On what constituted suspicious, and therefore punishable behavior, see ibid., 375–77.

81. On the Law of Suspects, see Weber, 80–83.

82. *Social Contract*, 150–52.

83. "Droit naturel," in *Encyclopédie*, 5:115.

84. Hegel explained the peremptory judgments of the revolutionary tribunals in a different but not incompatible way by arguing that the death of any individual citizen was immaterial, since as citizen he had identified with the general will and had already, therefore, negated his own individual existence. See *Phenomenology of Spirit*, 360.

85. Robespierre, *Bonheur*, 202. I have blended Robespierre's arguments with Saint-Just's, although they differed in certain, important respects. Ferenc Fehér, for instance, notes divergences between the two legislators in relation to the applicability of natural law to justice ("Justice," 369–71), with Robespierre being more reserved on the question. These differences are not, however, significant to my own argument, and Fehér himself recognizes an eventual reconciliation between the two approaches, noting that Robespierre ultimately perceived the Revolution as a state of nature and therefore subject to its laws, as Saint-Just had argued (ibid., 371).

86. Robespierre, *Bonheur*, 203. Cf. Robespierre's speech of May 30, 1791 to the Constituent Assembly: "I want to prove two principal propositions: the first is that capital punishment is essentially unjust; the second it that it is not the most dissuasive of punishments and that it contributes more to the multiplication of crimes than to their prevention" (ibid., 208).

87. Ibid., 204.

88. Ibid. On the traumatic aspects of the king's execution and its effects on memory, see Jeanne De Groote, *La mémoire de la mort de Louis XVI au XIXe siècle* (D. E. A. thesis, Université de Paris IV—Sorbonne, 2005).

89. See Kant's "Analytic of the Sublime" in *The Critique of Judgement*, 90–203, especially the following: "Thus, too, the delight in the sublime in nature is only *negative* (whereas that in the beautiful is *positive*): that is to say that it is a feeling of the imagination by its own act depriving itself of its freedom by receiving a final determination in accordance with a law other than that of its empirical employment. In this way it gains an extension and a might greater than that which it sacrifices. But the ground of this is concealed from it, and in its place it *feels* the sacrifice or deprivation, as well as its cause, to which it is subjected. The *astonishment* mounting almost to terror, the awe and thrill of devout feeling that takes hold of one when gazing upon the prospect of mountains ascending to heaven, deep ravines and torrents raging there, deep-shadowed solitudes that invite to brooding melancholy, and the like—all this, when we are assured of our own safety, is not actual fear. Rather is it an attempt to gain access to it through imagination" (121). The "law other than that of empirical employment" had previously been identified as that of reason itself (see 102, 104, 106). For a detailed analysis of these passages, see Strauss, *Subjects of Terror*, 9–12.

90. See, for instance, the analysis of the guillotine and its victims' remains in the historian Jules Michelet's 1853 "Cimetières de la Terreur [*Cemeteries of the Terror*]": "the terror did not increase. Sixty heads, forty, or twenty, the effect was the same. But horror came. I am touching here on a sad topic. Having reached the highest point of the Terror, what I find is like the peak of a great mountain, where there is nothing but extreme aridity, a desert where all life ceases. . . . Pity had disappeared or fallen silent; horror spoke, along with disgust, and the anxiousness of a great city that feared an epidemic. The living took fright. What they did not dare say in the name of humanity, they said in the name of hygiene and salubrity" (in *Histoire de la révolution*, 2:922–3). Terror is a political force that rises above the bodily (the difference between thirty and forty corpses is inconsequential to its purposes) and is best figured by the sort of descriptions associated with the sublime (e.g. the summits of great mountains or vast and deserted spaces). Horror, on the other hand, begins in the aftermath of terror, when its leftovers, the physical remains of its victims, start to inspire disgust and concerns about the diseases that might attach themselves to the living.

91. Hugo, *Les Misérables*, 1071 (trans. modified).

92. Ibid., 1057 (trans. modified). On the political and social significance of sewers in Paris, see Reid. "The sewer, antithesis of the sublime," according to Reid, "became also the seat of sublimation" (4). On Hugo's *Les Misérables*, which Reid interprets in relation to Mary Douglas's notions of "purity and danger," see 20–23.

93. Hugo, *Les Misérables*, 1065 (trans. modified).

94. See ibid., 1057–58 (trans. modified): "the history of men is reflected in the history of cloacae. The Gemoniæ told the story of Rome. The Parisan sewer was an awesome old thing. It was a tomb and it was an asylum. Crime, intelligence, social protest, freedom of conscience, thought, theft, everything that human laws pursue or have pursued has hidden itself in that pit"; and: "the sewer is the conscience of a city. Everything converges there and confronts everything else. In this livid place there are shadows, but there are no more secrets. Everything has its true form, or at least its definitive form" (ibid., 1058, trans. modified).

95. Ibid., 1063 (trans. modified). For some of the associations between Marat and sewers in the public imagination, see Reid, 19.

96. Hugo, *Les Misérables*, 1083 (trans. modified).

97. Ibid.

98. See Immanuel Kant, *Critique of Pure Reason*, trans. Norman Kemp Smith (1929; New York: St. Martin's Press, 1965), 74–91.

99. *Les Misérables*, 1084 (trans. modified).

100. Ibid., 1085 (trans. modified).

101. Sue, *Mystères*, 355–56. The only English translations I have found omit this and the following quotations.

102. Villemin, who demonstrated the contagious nature of tuberculosis, could have had fantasies such as Sue's in mind when he cautioned against demanding

too much from the microscope: "The microscope promises much for the study of pathological physiology, for there is still much to be done. But we must not ask this instrument to show us specific corpuscles or impossible diagnostics that are not in the order of things" (*Du tubercule*, 4). As both Sue and Villemin attest, the revelations of the microscope seem to have given rise to the belief, among doctors and the educated public, that minute and mysterious animals inhabited the body and its environment and that pathological conditions could be explained by these entities.

103. Sue, *Mystères*, 1212.

104. On Eugène Sue's medical career, see Jean-Louis Bory, *Eugène Sue* (1962; Paris: Mémoire du Livre, 2000), 71–127, and Pierre Vallery-Radot, *Chirurgiens d'autrefois: La famille d'Eugène Süe* (Paris: R.-G. Ricou & Ocia Editeurs, 1944), 138–46.

105. Jean-Joseph Sue, *Recherches physiologiques et expériences sur la vitalité. Lues à l'Institut national de France, le 11 Messidor, an V de la République. Suivies d'une nouvelle édition de son Opinion sur le supplice de la guillotine ou sur la douleur qui survit à la décolation* (Paris: chez l'auteur, an VI [1797]). His *Recherches* were successful enough to have appeared in three editions by 1803. By that same year, his paper on the guillotine had gone through four. The title of Cabanis's own study on the guillotine was, in fact, "Note sur l'opinion de MM. Œlsner et Sœmmering, et du citoyen Sue, touchant le Supplice de la Guillotine." On the relation between the Sue family and the medical profession, see Bory, 24–36, and Vallery-Radot, 19–137 and 153–206.

106. Jean-Joseph Sue, "Opinion," in *Recherches physiologiques*, 75–76.

107. See, for instance, Marx and Engels, *Collected Works*, 4:57: "The mystery of the Critical presentation of the *Mystères de Paris* is the mystery of *speculative*, of *Hegelian construction*."

8. WHAT ABJECTION MEANS

1. Alphonse Esquiros, 4.

2. Céline, *Le pont de Londres* (*Guignol's Band*, II) (Paris: Gallimard, 1964), 406; quoted in Julia Kristeva, *Powers of Horror: An Essay on Abjection*, trans. Leon S. Roudiez (New York: Columbia University Press, 1982), 150 (trans. modified).

3. Hegel, *Phenomenology of Spirit*, 60.

4. Ibid., 65.

5. For a general discussion of eating and related subjects (such as nausea) as structuring metaphors in Hegel's philosophy, see Hamacher.

6. Kojève, 39.

7. Kojève writes that man, according to Hegel, "is nothing without the animal that acts as his support, and outside of the natural World he is pure nothingness. And yet he *separates* himself from that World and *opposes* it" (ibid., 546).

8. Sartre, 603.

9. Kojève, 550.

10. Ibid., 560.

11. See Denis Hollier, "The Pure and the Impure: Literature After Silence," in Denis Hollier and Jeffrey Mehlman eds., *Literary Debate: Texts and Contexts* (New York: The New Press, 1999), 7–12.

12. Blanchot, 322–23 (trans. modified).

13. Ibid., 323.

14. See Kant, *Critique of Judgement*: "War itself, provided it is conducted with order and a sacred respect for the lives of civilians, has something sublime about it, and gives nations that carry it on in such a manner a stamp of mind only the more sublime the more numerous the dangers to which they are exposed and which they are able to meet with fortitude" (112–13).

15. Blanchot, 326–27 (trans. modified).

16. See Jacques Lacan, "The Signification of the Phallus: *Die Bedeutung des Phallus*" in *Ecrits*: "let us examine . . . the effects of that presence [of the signifier]. They are, first of all, a deviation of man's needs by the fact that he speaks, in the sense that as far as his needs are subjected to demand, they return to him alienated. This is not the effect of his actual dependence . . . but rather of the sheer fact of putting into signifying form and of the fact that it is from the place of the Other that his message is emitted. What thus among his needs finds itself alienated constitutes an *Urverdrängung* of not being able, hypothetically, to be placed in words; instead it appears as an offshoot that is present in man as desire (*das Begehren*)" (579, trans. modified).

17. Blanchot, 327 (trans. modified).

18. Ibid, 326.

19. Hegel treated the Crusades as the epitome of the Romantic aesthetic and described them as being "of a spiritual tendency, and yet devoid of a truly spiritual aim," because "Christendom is supposed to have its salvation in the spirit alone, in Christ who, risen, has ascended to the right hand of God and has his living actuality, his abode, in the Spirit, not in his grave [i.e. the Holy Sepulcher] and in the visible immediately present places where once he had his temporal abode" (Hegel, *Aesthetics: Lectures in Fine Arts*, vol. 1, trans. T. M. Knox [Oxford: Oxford University Press, 1975], 588).

20. See Hegel, *Philosophy of Mind*, para 458, 213. On the elaborate *tableau* that Madame Necker arranged for her and her husband's corpses, see Antoine de Baecque, *La gloire et l'effroi: Sept morts sous la Terreur* (Paris: Bernard Grasset, 1997), 215–51.

21. Blanchot, 325 (trans. modified).

22. Ibid., 316–17. Cf. the following quotations, also from Blanchot's "Littérature et le droit à la mort," in which he further elaborates the materiality of language: "when [literature] names something, what it designates is suppressed; but what is suppressed is maintained, and the thing has found (in the being that is a word) more of a refuge than a threat" (329, trans. modified). "Literature is a concern for the reality of things, for their unknown, free, and silent existence; literature is their innocence and their forbidden presence" (330). "In this way [i.e. out of a concern for the reality of things], literature allies with the reality of

language, making of it matter without contour, content without form, a capricious and impersonal force that says nothing, reveals nothing, and is satisfied to announce, by its refusal to say anything, that it comes from the night and will return to the night. In itself, this metamorphosis is not a failure [*manquée*]. It is quite true that the words are transformed. They no longer *signify* shadow and earth, they no longer represent the absence of shadow and earth, which is meaning, the clarity of shadows and the transparency of the earth: their answer is opacity, the rustling of folding wings is their speech; physical weight is present in them in the suffocating density of a syllabic mass that has lost all its meaning" (ibid., 330–31, trans. modified).

23. Cf. Gilles Deleuze, *The Logic of Sense*, trans. Mark Lester with Charles Stivale, ed. Constantin Boundas (New York: Columbia University Press, 1990), 166–67, 183–84, 186–87, 239–41.

24. For an analysis of infantile eroticization of the feel of language in the mouth, see Ivan Fonagy, "Les Bases pulsionnelles de la phonation," *Revue française de psychanalyse* (January, 1970): 101–136 and (July 1971): 543–591.

25. Flaubert, *Sentimental Education*, 303 (trans. modified).

26. Ibid., 302.

27. On the materiality of language in the mouth, see Fonagy.

28. Kristeva, *Powers of Horror*, 149 (trans. modified).

29. Céline, 406; quoted in Kristeva, *Powers of Horror*, 150 (trans. modified).

30. Kojève, 550. Cf. Kojève's description of war in Hegel: "War and the condition-of-being-a-soldier are the objectively-real sacrifice of the personal-I, the danger of death for the particular which is the contemplation (*Anschauen*) of his abstract immediate Negativity; just as war is equally the immediately positive personal-I of the particular . . . such [that in it] each individual, insofar as it is a present particular, creates (*macht*) itself as absolute power (*Macht*), contemplates itself as [being] absolutely free, as universal Negativity [existing] for itself and really against another (*Anderes*). It is in war that this is granted (*gewärht* [*sic*]) to the particular: war is [a] crime [committed] *for the Universal* [= the State]; the goal [of war is] the conservation [mediated by the negation] of everything [= the State] against the enemy, who is preparing to destroy that everything. This alienation (*Entäusserung*) [of the Particular from the Universal] must have precisely that abstract form, and be deprived-of-individuality; death must be received and given coldly; not by means of a commented (*statarische*) combat, in which the particular perceives the adversary and kills him out of immediate hatred; no, death is given and received in-the-void (*leer*),—*impersonally*, out of the smoke and powder" (560). The syntax is tortuous but correct, which in itself reveals, perhaps, a torsion caused by that same force that erupts in Céline's text.

31. Letter to Henri Parisot in Artaud, *Œuvres complètes*, vol. 9 (Paris: Gallimard, 1970), 184–86; quoted in Deleuze, 84 (trans. modified).

32. Blanchot, 327 (trans. modified).

33. Letter to Henri Parisot in Artaud, 9:84–6, quoted in Deleuze, 84 (trans. modified).

34. Blanchot, 327 (trans. modified).
35. See Strauss, *Subjects of Terror*, 23–73.
36. Deleuze, 24 (trans. modified).
37. Ibid., 23 (trans. modified).
38. Ibid., 166 (trans. modified). Cf. ibid., 181–83.
39. Ibid., 187 (trans. modified).
40. "Sur les principes de morale politique qui doivent guider la Convention Nationale dans l'administration intérieure de la République, Séance du 17 pluviôse an II [February 5, 1794]" in *Œuvres de Maximilien Robespierre*, vol. 10, ed. Marc Boulouiseau and Albert Soboul (Paris: Presses Universitaires de France, 1967), 354.
41. On the abstraction of the individual in the ideology of the Terror, see "The Reign of Terror against the Anarchy of Horror" in chapter 7.
42. On the invisibility of the guillotine, see Arasse, 35.
43. Hegel, *Phenomenology*, 357.
44. Kojève, 558.
45. Ibid., 550.
46. See Strauss, *Subjects of Terror*, 1–73.
47. Kristeva, *Powers of Horror*, 3–4 (trans. modified).
48. The medieval imagination was probably particularly influenced by this metaphor, which constantly confronted it in the production of texts: the latter were written on skin taken from slaughtered animals and then, if the document lost its value, were scraped off again with pumice stone to make way for another work. The cadaverous skin was what preceded and succeeded the words written on it.
49. Although it varies according to different cultures and periods, the *trait*, or feature, according to Hubert Damisch, is intrinsically related to that most simple of gestures that gives form, like the "abstract line" Redon describes in chapter 6 above. See Damisch, *Traité du trait* (Paris: Edition de la Réunion des Musées Nationaux, 1995), 59: "The *trait* [is] the first and constitutive element of drawing, insofar as the latter is understood to be the 'graphic representation of forms'? The expression could be applied to an entire aspect of painting as it is understood by the literary painters of China (which is, precisely, its 'representative' aspect). If one allows for the fact that the words 'form,' 'representation,' and 'graphism' do not have the same meaning, the same usage, the same resonance here as they do there (supposing that they are even admissible there)."
50. On the belief that certain parts of the body continue to grow autonomously after death, see Ariès, 356, 404.
51. Géraud, 66.
52. Kristeva, *Powers of Horror*, 4 (trans. modified).
53. On the term "fecal stick," see Freud, "On Transformations of Instinct," 131.
54. On babies as equivalent to feces, see "The Sexual Theories of Children" in *The Standard Edition*, 9:219–20, and "On Transformations of Instinct," 128–33.

55. On the rise of hygienic programs in France, Western Europe, and the United States, see Vigarello, 93–231; Corbin, *The Foul and the Fragrant*; and Suellen Hoy, *Chasing Dirt: The American Pursuit of Cleanliness* (Oxford: Oxford University Press, 1995).

56. Kristeva, *Powers of Horror*, 4 (trans. modified).

57. See section 35 of Martin Heidegger, *Being and Time*, trans. John Macquarrie and Edward Robinson (New York: Harper & Row, 1962), 211–14.

58. See Flaubert, "Dictionnaire des idées reçues" in *Œuvres*, 2:999–1023.

59. Hegel, *Phenomenology of Spirit*, 16.

60. Michel Foucault, *The Order of Things: An Archaeology of the Human Sciences* (New York: Random House, 1970), 160.

Abensour, Miguel. *Le procès des maîtres rêveurs; suivi de Pierre Leroux et l'utopie*. Arles: Sulliver, 2000.

Abraham, Karl. *Selected Papers of Karl Abraham M.D.* Translated by Douglas Bryan and Alix Strachey. London: Hogarth Press, 1949.

Ackerknecht, Erwin H. "Hygiene in France, 1815–1848." *Bulletin of the History of Medicine* 22 (March–April 1948): 117–55.

———. *Medicine at the Paris Hospital, 1794–1848*. Baltimore: Johns Hopkins Press, 1967.

Agulhon, Maurice. *The Republican Experiment, 1848–1852*. Translated by Janet Lloyd. Cambridge: Cambridge University Press, 1983.

Albert the Great. *Man and the Beasts: de Animalibus (Books 22–26)*. Translated by James J. Scanlan. Binghamton: MRTS, 1987.

Andrieux. "Fable. Les passagers et le pilote." *Gazette nationale ou le moniteur universel*, no. 134 (February 3, 1796): 533.

Arasse, Daniel. *The Guillotine and the Terror*. Translated by Christopher Miller. London: Allen Lane, 1989.

Arcet, Jean-Pierre-Joseph d'. *Latrines modèles, construites sous un colombier, ventilées au moyen de la chaleur des pigeons, et servant à la préparation de l'engrais*. Paris: L. Mathias, 1843.

Ariès, Philippe. *The Hour of Our Death*. Translated by Helen Weaver. New York: Knopf, 1981.

"Arrest de la cour de parlement extrait des registres du parlement du 21 Mai 1765." Bibliothèque Nationale de France. Fonds Joly de Fleury, 1207, fos. 55–50.

Artaud, Antonin. *Œuvres complètes*. 26 vols. Paris: Gallimard, 1970.

Audidière, Sophie, et al., eds. *Matérialistes français du XVIIIe siècle: La Mettrie, Helvétius, d'Holbach*. Paris: Presses Universitaires de France, 2006.

Aulagnier, Piera. *La violence de l'interprétation: Du pictogramme à l'énoncé*. Paris: Presses Universitaires de France, 1974.

Babon, Hippolyte. "Lettres satiriques et critiques." *La revue nouvelle* (February 1, 1847).

Bachelard, Gaston. *The Formation of the Scientific Mind: A Contribution to a Psychoanalysis of Objective Knowledge*. Translated by Mary McAllester Jones. Manchester: Clinamen, 2002.

———. *La terre et les rêveries du repos: Essai sur les images de l'intimité*. Paris: José Corti, 1948.

Baecque, Antoine de. *La gloire et l'effroi: Sept morts sous la Terreur*. Paris: Bernard Grasset, 1997.

Balzac, Honoré de. *Cousin Bette: Part One of Poor Relations*. Translated by Marion Ayton Crawford. New York: Penguin Books, 1965.

———. *La cousine Bette*. Edited by André Lorant. Paris: GF Flammarion, 1977.

———. *History of the Thirteen*. Translated by Herbert J. Hunt. New York: Penguin, 1974.

———. *Splendors and Miseries of Courtesans*. 2 vols. London: Caxton, 1895.

Banau, Jean-Baptiste and François Turben. *Mémoire sur les épidémies du Languedoc, adressé aux états de cette province*. Paris: Banau, 1786.

Barbey, Auguste. "Odilon Redon." *Mémorial artistique* (April 7, 1894).

Barrera, Albino. *God and the Evil of Scarcity: Moral Foundations of Economic Agency*. Notre Dame, Ind.: University of Notre Dame Press, 2005.

Barthélemy, Marquis de. "Rapport fait à la Chambre par M. le marquis de Barthélemy, au nom d'une commission spéciale chargée de l'examen du projet de loi sur les aliénés." In Ministère de l'Intérieur et des Cultes. *Législation sur les aliénés et les enfants assistés*, vol. 2, 315–50. Paris: Librairie Administrative de Berger-Levrault et Cie., 1881.

Beauregard, Gérard. "Notes d'art: Exposition de M. Odilon Redon." *La Patrie* (April 2, 1894).

Belgrand, Eugène. *Préfecture du département de la Seine. Direction des eaux et égouts. Rapport du directeur sur les emplacements proposés pour de nouveaux cimetières*. Paris: Imprimérie centrale des chemins de fer, A. Chaix et Co., 1876.

Bénichou, Paul. *Le temps des prophètes*. Paris: Gallimard, 1977.

Benjamin, Walter. *Illuminations*. Translated by Harry Zohn. Edited by Hannah Arendt. New York: Schocken, 1969.

Bennington, Geoffrey. "Demanding History." In *Post-structuralism and the Question of History*, edited by Derek Attridge, Geoffroy Bennington, and Robert Young, 15–29. Cambridge: Cambridge University Press, 1987.

Béraud, F.-F.-A. *Les filles publiques de Paris et la police qui les régit*. 2 vols. Paris and Leipzig: Desforges et Cie., 1839.

Bernard, Claude. *Leçons sur les phénomènes de la vie communs aux animaux et aux végétaux*. 1878. Preface Georges Canguilhem. Paris: J. Vrin, 1966.

Bernardin de Saint-Pierre, Henri. *Etudes de la nature*. Paris: Deterville, 1804.

Bernheimer, Charles. *Figures of Ill Repute: Representing Prostitution in Nineteenth-Century France.* Cambridge, Mass.: Harvard University Press, 1989.

Bernstein, Jay. *The Philosophy of the Novel: Lukács, Marxism and the Dialectics of Form.* Brighton: The Harvester Press, 1984.

Bertherand, Emile-Louis. *Mémoire sur la vidange des latrines et des urinoirs publics au point de vue hygiénique, agricole et commercial.* Lille: Lefebvre-Ducrocq, 1858.

Bertholon, Pierre. *De la salubrité de l'air des villes et en particulier des moyens de la procurer.* Montpellier: J. Martel aîné, 1786.

Bibliothèque Nationale de France. Fonds Joly de Fleury, 1207.

Bichat, Xavier. *Anatomie générale.* 3 vols. Paris: Brosson, Gabon, et Cie., 1801.

———. *Physiological Researches on Life and Death.* In *Significant Contributions to the History of Psychology 1750–1920,* vol. 2, edited by Daniel N. Robinson. Translated by F. Gold, i–334. Washington, D.C.: University Publications of America, 1978.

———. *Recherches physiologiques sur la vie et la mort (première partie) et autres textes.* 1800. Edited by André Pichot. Paris: GF-Flammarion, 1994.

Blanchot, Maurice. *The Work of Fire.* Translated by Charlotte Mandell. Stanford: Stanford University Press, 1995.

Bonar, James. *Malthus and His Work.* 1885; London: Frank Cass, 1966.

Bonfils, Jean-Léon. *Essai sur la jurisprudence médicale relative aux aliénés: Thèse Présentée et soutenue à la Faculté de Médecine de Paris, le 17 août 1826, pour obtenir le grade de Docteur en médecine.* Paris: Didot le jeune, 1826.

Borsa, S., and C.-R. Michel. *La vie quotidienne des hôpitaux en France au XIXe siècle.* Paris: Hachette, 1985.

Bory, Jean-Louis. *Eugène Sue.* 1962. Paris: Mémoire du Livre, 2000.

Bouchut, Eugène. *Traité des signes de la mort et des moyens de prévenir les enterrements prématurés.* Paris: J.-B. Baillière, 1849.

Bouillier, Francisque. *Du principe vital et de l'âme pensante ou examen des diverses doctrines médicales et psychologiques sur les rapports de l'âme et de la vie.* Paris: Baillière et fils, 1862.

Boullée, Etienne-Louis. *L'architecte visionnaire et néoclassique.* Edited by J.-M. Pérouse de Montclos. Paris: Hermann, 1993.

Bourdieu, Pierre. *The Rules of Art: Genesis and Structure of the Literary Field.* Translated by Susan Emanuel. Stanford: Stanford University Press, 1995.

Boussel, Patrice. *Balzac et la médecine de son temps.* Exhibition Catalogue. Paris: Ville de Paris, Maison de Balzac, 1976.

Braunstein, Jean-François. *Broussais et le matérialisme: Médecine et philosophie au XIXe siècle.* Paris: Klincksieck, 1986.

Brierre de Boisment, Alexandre-Jacques-François. "Bénédicte-Auguste Morel, *Etudes cliniques.*" In *Annales médico-psychologiques.* 2nd series, vol. 4, 621 (1852).

———. "Remarques médico-légales sur la perversion de l'instinct génésique." *Gazette médicale de Paris* 29 (July 21, 1849): 555–564.

Brouardel, Paul. *La responsabilité médicale: secret médical, déclarations de naissance, inhumations, expertises médico-légales*. Paris: J.-B,. Baillière et Fils, 1898.

Broussais, François. *De l'irritation et de la folie*. 1839; Paris: Fayard, 1986.

Buisson, Mathieu-François-Régis. "Additions aux recherches sur la vie et la mort. De la division la plus naturelle des phénomènes physiques." In *Encyclopédie des sciences médicales*, edited by Alibert et al., Division 1, vol. 4, 121–214. 1802; Paris: Bureau de l'Encyclopédie, 1835.

Bynum, William F. "Médecine et société." In *Du romantisme à la science moderne*, vol. 3 of *Histoire de la pensée médicale en occident*, edited by Mirko D. Grmek, 295–318. Paris: Seuil, 1999.

———. *Science and the Practice of Medicine in the Nineteenth Century*. Cambridge: Cambridge University Press, 1994.

Cabanis, Pierre-Jean-Georges. *Du degré de certitude de la médecine*. 1798. Edited by Jean-Marc Drouin. Paris: Champion-Slatkine, 1989.

———. *Note sur le supplice de la guillotine*. Périgueux: Fanlac, 2002. Reprint of "Note sur l'opinion de MM. Œlsner et Sœmmering, et du citoyen Sue, touchant le Supplice de la Guillotine." 1795.

———. *On the Relations Between the Physical and Moral Aspects of Man*. Vol. 1. Edited by George Mora. Translated by Margaret Duggan Saidi. Baltimore: Johns Hopkins University Press, 1981.

Cadet, Louis-Auguste. *Hygiène, exhumation, crémation ou incinération des corps*. Paris: Baillière, 1877.

Cadet-De-Vaux, Antoine-Alexis. *Mémoire historique et physique sur le cimetière des innocents par M. Cadet de Vaux, Inspecteur Général des Objets de Salubrité, de plusieurs Académies, Censur Royal, &c.&c.; lu à l'Académie Royale des Sciences en 1781. Extrait du Journal de physique 1783*. N.p.: n.p., n.d.

———. *Mémoire sur le méphitisme des puits, par M. Cadet de Vaux, &c. &c. lu à l'Académie royale des sciences, le 25 janvier 1783. Extrait du Journal de physique mars 1783*. N.p.: n.p., n.d.

Cadet-De-Vaux, Antoine-Alexis, Laborie, and Antoine-Augustin Parmentier. *Observations sur les fosses d'aisances et moyens de prévenir les inconvéniens de leur vuidange*. Paris: P.-D. Pierres, 1778.

Canguilhem, Georges. *Ecrits sur la médecine*. Paris: Seuil, 2002.

———. *A Vital Raionalist: Selected Writings from Georges Canguilhem*. Edited by François Delaporte. Translated by Arthur Goldhammer. New York: Zone, 1994.

Carol, Anne. *Les médecins et la mort XIXe–XXe siècle*. Paris: Aubier, 2004.

Carrière, Edouard. "De l'autorité en médecine." *L'union médicale: Journal des intérêts scientifiques et pratiques, moraux et professionels du corps médical* 3, no. 97 (August 14, 1849): 385–86.

———. "De l'autorité en médecine." *L'union médicale: Journal des intérêts scientifiques et pratiques, moraux et professionels du corps médical* 3, no. 111 (September 18, 1849): 441–43.

Carvais, Robert. "La maladie, la loi, et les mœurs." In *Pasteur et la révolution pastorienne*, edited by Claire Salomon-Bayet, 279–330. Paris: Payot, 1986.

Cassirer, Ernst. *The Philosophy of the Enlightenment.* Princeton: Princeton University Press, 1951.

Castel, Robert. *The Regulation of Madness: The Origins of Incarceration in France.* Translated by W. D. Halls. Berkeley: University of California Press, 1988.

Castelnau, Henri de. "Pathologie mentale et médecine légale. Exemple remarquable de monomanie destructive et érotique ayant pour objet la profanation de cadavres humains." *La lancette française: Gazette des hôpitaux civils et militaires.* 3rd series, vol. 1, no. 82 (July 14, 1849): 327–28.

Castle, Terry. *The Female Thermometer: Eighteenth-Century Culture and the Invention of the Uncanny.* Oxford: Oxford University Press, 1995.

Cauchy, Augustin-Louis. *Considérations sur les ordres religieux adressées aux amis des sciences.* Paris: Poussièlgue-Rusand, 1844.

Céline, Louis-Ferdinand. *Le pont de Londres (Guignol's Band, vol. 2).* Paris: Gallimard, 1964.

Certeau, Michel de. *The Writing of History.* Translated by Tom Conley. New York: Columbia University Press, 1988.

Chaban-Delmas, Jacques, ed. *Odilon Redon: 1840–1916.* Exhibition catalogue. Bordeaux: Galérie des Beaux-Arts, 1985.

Chaouat, Bruno. *"Je meurs par morceaux": Chateaubriand.* Villeneuve-d'Ascq: Presses Universitaires du Septentrion, 1999.

Chevalier, Louis. "Paris." In *Le choléra: La première épidémie du XIXe siècle*, edited by Louis Chevalier, 1–46. La Roche-sur-Yon: Imprimerie Centrale de l'Ouest, 1958.

Choderlos de Laclos, Pierre-Ambroise-François. *Les liaisons dangereuses.* Translated by Douglas Parmée. Oxford: Oxford University Press, 1995.

Clark, T .J. *The Painting of Modern Life: Paris in the Art of Manet and His Followers.* New York: Alfred A. Knopf, 1985.

Clayson, Hollis. *Painted Love: Prostitution in French Art of the Impressionist Era.* New Haven: Yale University Press, 1991.

Cloquet, Hippolite. *Osphrésiologie ou traité des odeurs, du sens et des organes de l'olfaction; Avec l'histoire détaillée des maladies du nez et des fosses nasales, et des opérations qui leur conviennent.* Paris: Méquignon-Marvis, 1821.

Coleman, William. *Biology in the Nineteenth Century: Problems of Form, Function, and Transformation.* Cambridge: Cambridge University Press, 1971.

———. *Death is a Social Disease: Public Health and Political Economy in Early Industrial France.* Madison: University of Wisconsin Press, 1982.

Colin, Marcel. "L'anthropologie et la mort." In Christiane Vitani. *Législation de la mort: Travail de l'association lyonnaise de médecine légale*, vii–xv. Paris: Masson & Cie., 1962.

Comte, Auguste. *Système de politique positive ou traité de sociologie instituant la religion de l'humanité*. 4 vols. 1851–1854. Paris: G. Crès, 1912.

Condillac, Etienne de. *Condillac's Treatise on the Sensations*. Translated by Geraldine Carr. Los Angeles: University of Southern California, School of Philosophy, 1930.

Corbin, Alain. *The Foul and the Fragrant: Odor and the French Social Imagination*. Translated by Miriam L. Kochan, Roy Porter, and Christopher Prendergast. Cambridge, Mass.: Harvard University Press, 1986.

———. "Présentation." In Alexandre Parent-Duchâtelet. *La prostitution à Paris au XIXe siècle*. Edited by Alain Corbin, 7–55. Paris: Seuil, 1981.

———. *Women for Hire: Prostitution and Sexuality in France after 1850*. Translated by Alan Sheridan. Cambridge, Mass.: Harvard University Press, 1990.

Coste, Urbain. "La monomanie." *Journal universel de sciences médicales* 43 (July 1826): 53.

Crémieux, Albert. *La révolution de février: Etude critique sur les journées des 21, 22, 23 et 24 février 1848*. Paris: Edouard Cornély, 1912.

Cruchet, René. *La médecine dans la littérature française*. Bordeaux: Delmas, 1939.

Dagognet, François. *Méthodes et doctrine dans l'œuvre de Pasteur*. Paris: Presses Universitaires de France, 1967.

———. *Pasteur sans la légende*. Paris: Géraldine Billon, 1994.

Dalboussière, Charles. "De la responsabilité médicale. Affaire Thouret-Noroy." *Annales d'hygiène publique et de médecine légale* 12, no. 2 (October 1834): 406–456.

Damisch, Hubert. *Traité du trait*. Paris: Editions de la Réunion des Musées Nationaux, 1995.

Dansel, Michel. *Le cas du sergent Bertrand: Un nécrophile conséquent*. Paris: Bibliothèque de l'homme, 1999.

Darwin, Charles. *The Power of Movement in Plants*. Vol. 27 of *The Works of Charles Darwin*. Edited by Paul H. Barrett and R. B. Freeman. London: William Pickering, 1989.

Daston, Lorainne, and Fernando Vidal. "Introduction: Doing What Comes Naturally." In *The Moral Authority of Nature*, edited by Lorraine Daston and Fernando Vidalds, 1–20. Chicago: University of Chicago Press, 2004.

Debreyne, Pierre-Jean-Corneille. *Etude de la mort ou Initiation du prêtre à la connaissance pratique des maladies graves et mortelles et de tout ce qui, sous ce rapport, peut se rattacher à l'exercice difficile du saint ministère*. 1845. Paris: M. V. Poussielgue-Ronsard, 1864.

———. *La théologie morale et les sciences médicales*. 1842. Edited by A. Ferrand. Paris: Poussielgue Frères, 1884. Reprint of *Essai sur la théologie morale, considérée dans ses rapports avec la physiologie et la médecine, ouvrage spécialement destiné au clergé*. 1842.

De Groote, Jeanne. *La mémoire de la mort de Louis XVI au XIXe siècle*. D. E. A. thesis. Université de Paris IV–Sorbonne, 2005.

Delamare, Jean, and Thérèse Delamare-Riche. *Le grand renfermement: Histoire de l'hospice de Bicêtre 1657–1974*. Paris: Maloine, 1990.

Delaporte, François. *Disease and Civilization: The Cholera in Paris, 1832*. Translated by Arthur Goldhammer. Cambridge, Mass.: MIT Press, 1986.

———. *Figures de la médecine*. Preface Emmanuel Fournier. Paris: Cerf, 2009.

Deleuze, Gilles. *The Logic of Sense*. Trans. Mark Lester with Charles Stivale. Edited by Constantin Boundas. New York: Columbia University Press, 1990.

De Man, Paul. *The Resistance to Theory*. Minneapolis: University of Minnesota Press, 1986.

———. *Allegories of Reading: Figural Language in Rousseau, Nietzsche, Rilke, and Proust*. New Haven and London: Yale University Press, 1979.

Derrida, Jacques. *The Gift of Death: Second Edition & Literature in Secret*. Translated by David Wills. Chicago: University of Chicago Press, 2008.

———. *Glas*. Translated by John P. Leavey, Jr. and Richard Rand. Lincoln, Nebr.: University of Nebraska Press, 1986.

———. *Margins of Philosophy*. Trans. Alan Bass. Chicago: University of Chicago Press, 1982.

Desrosières, Pierre. "A propos d'un cas de nécrophilie: Place du corps mort dans les perversions: Nécrophilie, nécrosadisme et vampirisme." Doctoral thesis in medicine. Université de Paris, Val de Marne, Faculté de Médecine de Créteil, 1974, no. 37.

Destutt de Tracy, Antoine-Louis-Claude. *Eléments d'idéologie*. 3 vols. Brussels: n.p., 1826.

Devergie, Alphonse. *Notions générales sur la morgue de Paris: Sa description, son système hygiénique; de l'autopsie judiciaire comparée à l'autopsie pathologique*. Paris: F. Malteste, 1877.

Dhombres, Nicole, and Jean Dhombres. *Naissance d'un nouveau pouvoir: sciences et savants en France (1793–1824)*. Paris: Payot, 1989.

Diderot, Denis, et al., eds. *Encyclopédie ou dictionnaire raisonné des sciences et des métiers*. 28 vols. Neufchastel: Samuel Faulche & Co., 1765.

Dinet-Lecomte, Marie-Claude. *Les sœurs hospitalières en France aux XVIIe et XVIIIe siècles: La charité en action*. Paris: Honoré Champion, 2005.

Dobo, Nicolas, and André Role. *Bichat: La vie fulgurante d'un génie*. Paris: Perrin, 1989.

Dondey, Théophile (pseudonym Philothée O'Neddy). *Feu et flamme*. 1833. Edited by Marcel Hervier. Reprint, Paris: Editions des Presses Françaises, 1926.

Dorra, Henri, ed. *Symbolist Art Theories: A Critical Anthology*. Berkeley: University of California Press, 1994.

Douglas, Mary. *Purity and Danger: An Analysis of the Concepts of Pollution and Taboo.* 1966. London: Routledge, 1996.

Downing, Lisa. *Desiring the Dead: Necrophilia and Nineteenth-Century French Literature.* Oxford: Legenda, 2003.

Druick, Douglas W., and Peter Kort Zegers. "In the Public Eye." In *Odilon Redon: Prince of Dreams, 1840–1916,* edited by Douglas W. Druick, 137–45. Chicago: The Art Institute of Chicago & Harry N. Abrams, 1994.

Du Camp, Maxime. *Souvenirs de l'année 1848: La révolution de février, le 15 mai, l'insurrection de juin.* Paris: Hachette, 1876.

———. *Souvenirs littéraires, Tome I: 1822–1850.* Paris: L'Harmattan, 1993.

Ducreux, Robert. *Le médecin radoteur ou les pots pourris et autres textes.* Edited by Rodolphe Trouilleux and Jean-Michel Roy. Paris: Honoré Champion, 1999.

Du Roselle, Hippolyte. *Les eaux, les égouts et les fosses d'aisances dans leurs rapports avec les épidémies.* Amiens: T. Jeunet, 1867.

Du Tennetar, Michel. *Mémoire sur l'état de l'atmosphère à Metz et ses effets sur les habitans de cette ville, ou réflexions sur les dangers d'une atmosphère habituellement froide et humide, et les moyens de les prévenir.* Nancy: C.-S. Lamort, 1778.

Duveau, Georges. *1848: The Making of a Revolution.* Translated by Anne Carter. New York: Random House, 1967.

Eigeldinger, Marc. *La philosophie de l'art chez Balzac.* 1957; Geneva: Slatkine Reprints, 1998.

Eisenman, Stephen F. *The Temptation of Saint Redon: Biography, Ideology, and Style in* the Noirs *of Odilon Redon.* Chicago: University of Chicago Press, 1992.

Enriquez, Eugène. *De la horde à l'état: Essai de psychanalyse du lien social.* Paris: Gallimard, 1983.

Epaulard, Alexis. *Vampirisme, nécrosadisme, nécrophagie.* Lyon: A. Storck, 1901.

Esquiros, Alphonse. *Les vierges folles.* Paris: Auguste Le Galloir, 1840.

Etlin, Richard A. *The Architecture of Death: The Transformation of the Cemetery in Eighteenth-Century Paris.* Cambridge, Mass.: MIT Press, 1984.

Factums of the Bibliothèque Nationale de France: 8 Fm 3159, 8 Fm 3160, and 8 Fm 3161.

"Faits divers." *Le Courrier français.* March 23, 1849.

Farge, Arlette. *Le goût de l'archive.* Paris: Seuil, 1997.

———. "Signe de vie, risque de mort. Essai sur le sang et la ville au XVIIIe siècle." *Urbi* no. 2 (December, 1979): xv–xxii.

Faure, Olivier. *Les Français et leur médecine au XIXe siècle.* Paris: Belin, 1993.

———. *Genèse de l'hôpital moderne: les hospices civils de Lyon de 1802 à 1845.* Lyon: Presses Universitaires de Lyon [1981].

———. *Histoire sociale de la médecine.* Paris: Anthropos-Economica, 1994.

Fauve-Chamoux, Antoinette, ed. *Malthus hier et aujourd'hui: Congrès international de démographie historique CNRS, mai 1980.* Paris: CNRS, 1984.

Favre, Robert. *La mort dans la littérature et la pensée françaises au siècle des lumières.* Lyon: Presses Universitaires de Lyon [1978].

Fehér, Ferenc. *The Frozen Revolution: An Essay on Jacobinism.* Cambridge: Cambridge University Press, 1987.

———. "Justice révolutionnaire." In Michael Walzer. *Régicide et révolution: Le Procès de Louis XVI.* Translated by J. Debouzy, 351–80. Paris: Payot, 1989.

Fernand, Jacques. *Les cimetières: Supprimer la fosse commune et les fosses temporaires. Pétition addressée à l'assemblée nationale au conseil de Paris et aux autres conseils municipaux pour supprimer les fosses temporaires et la fosse commune, et donner gratis aux pauvres le repos et le terrain à perpétuité, les riches paieront plus chers.* Paris: C. Vanier, 1874.

Fiaux, Louis. *La femme, le mariage et le divorce: Etude de physiologie et de sociologie.* Paris: Germer Baillière et Cie., 1880.

Figura, Starr. "Redon and the Lithographed Portfolio." In *Beyond the Visible: The Art of Odilon Redon,* edited by Jodi Hauptman, 76–95. New York: The Museum of Modern Art, 2005.

Flaubert, Gustave. *Correspondance.* 4 vols. Edited by Jean Bruneau. Paris: Gallimard (Pléiade), 1973.

———. *Œuvres.* 2 vols. Edited by A. Thibaudet and R. Dumesnil. Paris: Gallimard (Pléiade), 1952.

———. *Sentimental Eduction.* Translated by Robert Baldick. New York: Penguin, 2004.

———. *La tentation de Saint Antoine.* Paris: Ambroise Vollard, 1938.

Fodéré, François-Emmanuel. *Les lois éclairées par les sciences physiques, ou traité de médecine légale et d'hygiène publique.* 3 vols. Paris: Croullebois, 1798.

Fonagy, Ivan. "Les Bases pulsionnelles de la phonation." *Revue française de psychanalyse* (January, 1970): 101–36 and (July 1971): 543–91.

Foucault, Michel. *Abnormal: Lectures at the Collège de France.* Edited by Valerio Marchetti and Antonella Salomoni. Translated by Graham Burchell. New York: Picador, 2003.

———. *The Birth of the Clinic: An Archaeology of Medical Perception.* Translated by A. M. Sheridan Smith. New York: Random House 1973.

———. *Dits et écrits: 1954–1988.* 4 vols. Edited by Daniel Defert, François Ewald, and Jacques Lagrange. Paris: Gallimard, 1994.

———. *Histoire de la folie à l'âge classique.* Paris: Gallimard, 1972.

———. *The History of Sexuality: Volume I: An Introduction.* Translated by Robert Hurley. 1978; New York: Random House, 1990.

———. *Madness and Civilization: A History of Insanity in the Age of Reason.* Translated by Richard Howard. 1965; New York: Random House, 1973.

———. *Naissance de la bio-politique: cours au Collège de France (1978–1979).* Edited by François Ewald, Alessandro Fontana, and Michel Senellart. Paris: Gallimard, 2004.

———. *The Order of Things: An Archaeology of the Human Sciences.* New York: Random House, 1970.

Freud, Sigmund. *Beyond the Pleasure Principle.* In *The Standard Edition of the Complete Psychological Works of Sigmund Freud.* Vol. 18. Edited and translated by James Strachey, 1–64. London: Hogarth Press, 1955.

———. *From the History of an Infantile Neurosis.* In *The Standard Edition of the Complete Psychological Works of Sigmund Freud.* Vol. 17. Edited and translated by James Strachey. 1–122. London: Hogarth Press, 1955.

———. "On Transformations of Instinct as Exemplified in Anal Erotism." In *The Standard Edition of the Complete Psychological Works of Sigmund Freud.* Vol. 17. Edited and translated by James Strachey, 125–133. London: Hogarth Press, 1955.

———. "The Sexual Theories of Children." In *The Standard Edition of the Complete Psychological Works of Sigmund Freud.* Vol. 9. Edited and translated by James Strachey, 205–26. London: Hogarth Press, 1955.

Gallagher, Catherine. *The Body Economic: Life, Death, and Sensation in Political Economy and the Victorian Novel.* Princeton: Princeton University Press, 2006.

Gannal, Félix. *Les cimetières depuis la fondation de la monarchie française jusqu'à nos jours. Histoire et législation.* Paris: Muzard et fils, 1884.

———. *Moyens de distinguer la mort réelle de la mort apparente.* Paris: Jules-Juteau et Fils, 1868.

Garnier-Pagès, Louis-Antoine. *Histoire de la révolution de 1848.* 2 vols. Paris: Degorce-Cadot, 1868.

Gauchet, Marcel and Gladys Swain. *Madness and Democracy: The Modern Psychiatric Universe.* Translated by Catherine Porter. Princeton: Princeton University Press, 1999.

Gautier, Théophile. *Romans, contes et nouvelles.* 2 vols. Edited by Pierre Laubriet et al. Paris: Gallimard (Pléiade), 2002.

Géraud, Mathieu. *Essai sur la suppression des fosses d'aisances et de toute espèce de voirie, sur la manière de convertir en combustibles les substances qu'on y renferme.* Amsterdam: n.p., 1786.

Gervais, Robert. "Le microbe et la responsabilité médicale." In *Pasteur et la révolution pastorienne,* edited by Claire Salomon-Bayet, 217–75. Paris: Payot, 1986.

Gilbert, Geoffrey. *Malthus: Critical Responses.* 4 vols. New York: Routledge, 1998.

Gilbert, Nicolas-Pierre. *Quelques réflexions sur la médecine légale et son état actuel en France.* Paris: Villier, 1800.

Goldstein, Jan. *Console and Classify: The French Psychiatric Profession in the Nineteenth Century.* Cambridge: Cambridge University Press, 1987.

Gordon, Bruce and Peter Marshall. "Introduction: Placing the Dead in Late Medieval and Early Modern Europe." In *The Place of the Dead: Death and Remembrance in Late Medieval and Early Modern Europe,* edited by Bruce Gordon and Peter Marshall, 1–16. Cambridge: Cambridge University Press, 2000.

Grenville, G.A.S. *Europe Reshaped: 1848–1878*. Oxford: Blackwell, 2000.

Guillaume, Pierre. *Médecins, église et foi depuis deux siècles*. Paris: Aubier, 1990.

Guyot, Yves. *La prostitution*. Paris: G. Charpentier, 1882.

Haeckel, Ernst. *Generelle Morphologie der Organismen: allgemeine Grundzüge der organischen Formen-Wissenschaft: mechanisch begründet durch die von Charles Darwin reformirte Descendenz-Theorie*. 2 vols. Berlin: G. Reimer, 1866.

———. *Kunstformen der Natur*. 2 vols. Leipzig and Vienna: Bibliographisches Institut, 1899–1904.

———. *The Wonders of Life: A Popular Study of Biological Philosophy*. Translated by Joseph McCabe. New York: Harper & Row, 1904.

Haguenot, H. *Mémoires sur les dangers des inhumations*. N.p.: n.p., 1744.

Hales, Stephen. *A Treatise on Ventilators: Wherein an Account Is Given of the Happy Effects of the Several Trials That Have Been Made of Them*. London: Richard Manby, 1758.

———. *Vegetable Staticks: or, an Account of Some Statical Experiments on the Sap in Vegetables: Being an Essay Towards a Natural History of Vegetation*. London: W. & J. Innys, 1727.

Hamacher, Werner. *Pleroma: Reading in Hegel*. Translated by Nicholas Walker and Simon Jarvis. Stanford, Calif.: Stanford University Press, 1998.

Hannaway, Caroline and Owen Hannaway. "La fermeture du cimetière des innocents." In *XVIIIe siècle*. 1977. 181–92.

Harris, Ruth. *Murders and Madness: Medicine, Law, and Society in the* Fin de Siècle. Oxford: Clarendon Press, 1989.

Harsin, Jill. *Policing Prostitution in Nineteenth-Century Paris*. Princeton: Princeton University Press, 1985.

Hegel, Georg Wilhelm Friedrich. *Aesthetics: Lectures in Fine Arts*. 2 vols. Translated by T. M. Knox. Oxford: Oxford University Press, 1975.

———. *Hegel's Philosophy of Mind: Part Three of the Encyclopaedia of the Philosophical Sciences*. Translated by William Wallace. Oxford: Clarendon Press, 1971.

———. *Phenomenology of Spirit*. Translated by A. V. Miller. Oxford: Oxford University Press, 1981.

Heidegger, Martin. *Being and Time*. Translated by John Macquarrie and Edward Robinson. New York: Harper & Row, 1962.

Hennequin, Emile. "Beaux-arts: Odilon Redon." *Revue littéraire et artistique*, 5 (March 4, 1882): 136–38.

Henry, Christophe. " 'De la fumée surgit la lumière.' Sources théoriques et fonctions poétiques du clair-obscur boulléen." In *Claude Nicolas Ledoux et le livre d'architecture en français. Etienne Louis Boullée l'utopie et la poésie de l'art*, edited by Daniel Rabreau and Dominique Massounie, 278–99. Paris: Editions du patrimoine, 2006.

Hoffhaus, Charles E. "A Homogeneous Theory of the Origin of Vertebrates." *Journal of Paleontology* 37, no. 2 (March 1963): 458–71.

Hollier, Denis. "The Pure and the Impure: Literature After Silence." In *Literary Debate: Texts and Contexts*, edited by Denis Hollier and Jeffrey Mehlman, 3–26. New York: The New Press, 1999.

Horne, Jacques de. *Mémoire sur quelques objets qui intéressent plus particulièrement la salubrité de la ville de Paris*. Paris: J.-C. Dessaint, 1788.

Hoy, Suellen. *Chasing Dirt: The American Pursuit of Cleanliness*. Oxford: Oxford University Press, 1995.

Huard, Pierre. "L'enseignement médico-chirurgical." In *Enseignement et diffusion des sciences en France au XVIIIe siècle*, edited by René Taton, 169–236. Paris: Hermann, 1964.

Huet, Marie-Hélène. "Chateaubriand and the Politics of (Im)mortality." *Diacritics* 30, no. 3 (Fall 2000): 28–39.

———. *Mourning Glory: The Will of the French Revolution*. Philadelphia: University of Pennsylvania Press, 1997.

Hugo, Victor. *Les Misérables*. Translated by Charles E. Wilbour. New York: Modern Library, n.d.

———. *Théâtre complet*. Edited by J.-J Thierry and Josette Mélèze. Paris: Gallimard (Pléiade), 1963.

Huneman, Philippe. *Bichat, la vie et la mort*. Paris: Presses Universitaires de France, 1998.

Huysmans, Joris-Karl. *Against Nature (A rebours)*. Translated by Robert Baldick. New York: Penguin, 2003.

———. *L'art moderne*. Vol. 6 of *Œuvres complètes françaises*. Paris: G. Crès, 1929.

———. *Becalmed*. Translated by Terry Hale. London: Atlas, 1992.

"Intérieur." *Le constitutionnel*. March 19, 1849.

Jacyna, L. S. "Romantic Thought and the Origins of Cell Theory." In *Romanticism and the Sciences*, edited by Andrew Cunningham and Nicholas Jardine, 161–68. Cambridge: Cambridge University Press, 1990.

Jameson, Fredric R. "*La cousine Bette* and Allegorical Realism." *PMLA* 86 (1971): 241–54.

Jeorger, Muriel. "La structure hospitalière en France sous l'Ancien Régime." *Annales économies sociétés civilisations* 32, no. 5 (September/October 1977): 1025–1051.

"Les Jeunes France." *Le Figaro*. August 30, 1831.

Jones, Colin. *The Charitable Imperative: Hospitals and Nursing in Ancien Régime and Revolutionary France*. New York: Routledge, 1989.

Jones, Ernest. *Papers on Psycho-analysis*. New York: William Wood & Co., 1923.

Jorland, Gérard. *Une société à soigner: Hygiène et salubrité publiques en France au XIXe siècle*. Paris: Gallimard, 2010.

Jourdan, A. "Mélanges." *Gazette nationale ou le moniteur universel* no. 288 (July 6, 1796): 1130.

Kaës, René. "Quatre études sur la fantasmatique de la formation et le désir de former." In *Fantasme et formation*, edited by René Kaës, et al., 1–75. 1979; Paris: Dunod, 2001.

Kant, Immanuel. *The Conflict of the Faculties: Der Streit der Fakultäten*. Translated by Mary J. Gregor. New York: Abaris Books, 1979.

———. *The Critique of Judgement*. Translated by James Creed Meredith. Oxford: Oxford University Press, 1952.

———. *Critique of Pure Reason*. Translated by Norman Kemp Smith. 1929; New York: St. Martin's Press, 1965.

Kaufmann, Emil. *Three Revolutionary Architects, Boullée, Ledoux, and Lequeu*. In *Transactions of the American Philosophical Society*. New series, vol. 42 (1952). 429–564.

Keel, Omar. "L'essor de l'anatomie pathologique et de la clinique en Europe de 1750 à 1800: Nouveau bilan." In *La Médecine des lumières: Tout autour de Tissot*, edited by Vincent Barras and Micheline Louis-Courvoisier, 69–92. Geneva: Georg, 2001.

Kelly, Dorothy. *Fictional Genders: Role & Representation in Nineteenth-Century French Narrative*. Lincoln: University of Nebraska Press, 1989.

Kératry, Auguste-Hilarion de. *De l'âme humaine et de la vie future (Extrait de la Revue contemporaine, liv. du 15 décembre)*. Paris: La Revue contemporaine, 1852.

———. *Les derniers des Beaumanoir, ou la tour d'Helvin*. 4 vols. Paris: Bossange frères, 1825.

———. *Examen philosophique des considérations sur le sentiment du sublime et du beau, dans le rapport des caractères, des tempéraments, des sexes, des climats, et des religions, d'Emmanuel Kant*. Paris: Bossange frères, 1823.

———. *Inductions morales et physiologiques*. Paris: C. Gosselin, 1841.

Knight, Diana. "Reading as an Old Maid: *La cousine Bette* and Compulsory Heterosexuality." *Quinquereme* 12, no. 1 (1989): 67–79.

Koch, Robert. *Die Aetiologie der Milzbrandkrankheit, begrundet auf die Entwicklungsgeschichte des* Bacillus Anthracis. In *Beiträge zur Biologie der Pflanzen*, edited by Ferdinand Cohn. Vol. 2, no. 2, 277–310. Breslau: J. U. Kerns, 1876.

Kojève, Alexandre. *Introduction à la lecture de Hegel: Leçons sur la* Phénomenologie de l'Esprit *professées de 1933 à 1939 à l'Ecole des Hautes Etudes*. Edited by Raymond Queneau. Paris: Gallimard, 1947.

Kristeva, Julia. *Powers of Horror: An Essay on Abjection*. Translated by Leon S. Roudiez. New York: Columbia University Press, 1982.

Kselman, Thomas. *Death and the Afterlife in Modern France*. Princeton: Princeton University Press, 1993.

Kudlick, Catherine J. *Cholera in Post-Revolutionary Paris: A Cultural History*. Berkeley: University of California Press, 1996.

Lacan, Jacques. *Ecrits: The First Complete Translation in English*. Translated by Bruce Fink et al. New York: W. W. Norton, 2002.

————. *On Feminine Sexuality: The Limits of Love and Knowledge: Book XX: Encore 1972–1973*. Translated by Bruce Fink. New York: W. W. Norton, 1998.

————. "Radiophonie." In *Scilicet* 2/3 (1970): 55–99.

————. "Pour une Logique du fantasme." In *Scilicet* 2/3 (1970): 223–73.

————. *The Seminar of Jacques Lacan Book VII: The Ethics of Psychoanalysis*. Edited by Jacques-Alain Miller. Translated by Dennis Porter. New York: W. W. Norton, 1992.

Lachaise, Claude. *Topographie médicale de Paris ou examen général des causes qui peuvent avoir une influence marquée sur la santé des habitans de cette ville, le caractère de leurs maladies, et le choix des précautions hygiéniques qui leur sont applicables*. Paris: J.-B. Baillière, 1822.

Laingui, André and Jean Illes. "La responsabilité du médecin dans l'ancien droit." In *Etudes de droit et d'économie de la santé*, edited by Didier Truchet, 1–15. Paris: Economica, 1982.

Laissus, Yves. "Le jardin du roi." In *Enseignement et diffusion des sciences en France au XVIIIe siècle*, edited by René Taton, 287–341. Paris: Hermann, 1964.

Lamartine, Alphonse de. *Histoire de la révolution de 1848*. 2 vols. Paris: Perrotin, 1849.

Langer, William L. *Political and Social Upheaval: 1832–1852*. New York: Harper & Row, 1969.

Laplanche, Jean, and J.-B. Pontalis. *Fantasme originaire fantasme des origines origines du fantasme*. 1964. Paris: Hachette, 1985.

Larson, Barbara. *The Dark Side of Nature: Science, Society, and the Fantastic in the Work of Odilon Redon*. University Park, Penn.: Pennsylvania State University Press, 2005.

Latour, Amédée. "De l'autorité en médecine." *L'union médicale. Journal des intérêts scientifiques et pratiques, moraux et professionnels du corps médical* 3, no. 98 (August 16 and 18, 1849): 389–90.

————. "De l'autorité en médecine." *L'union médicale. Journal des intérêts scientifiques et pratiques, moraux et professionnels du corps médical* 3, no. 112 (September 20, 1849): 444–46.

————. "Note du rédacteur en chef." *L'union médicale. Journal des intérêts scientifiques et pratiques, moraux et professionnels du corps medical*, 3, no. 97 (August 14, 1849): 387.

Latour, Bruno. *The Pasteurization of France*. Translated by Alan Sheridan and John Law. Cambridge, Mass.: Harvard University Press, 1988.

Laubriet, Pierre. *L'intelligence de l'art chez Balzac*. 1961. Paris: Slatkine Reprints, 1980.

Lécuyer, Bernard Pierre. "L'hygiène en France avant Pasteur 1750–1850." In *Pasteur et la révolution pastorienne*, edited Claire Salomon-Bayet, 65–142. Paris: Payot, 1986.

———. "Pierre Leroux pourfendeur de Malthus inspirateur de Lacordaire dans *Malthus et les économistes, ou y aura-t-il toujours des pauvres?*" In *Malthus hier et aujourd'hui: Congrès international de démographie historique CNRS, mai 1980*, edited by Antoinette Fauve-Chamoux, 349–55. Paris: CNRS, 1984.

Ledoux, Claude-Nicolas. *L'architecture considéré sous le rapport de l'art, des moeurs et de la léglislation*. Paris: chez l'auteur, 1804.

Legallois, César-Julien-Jean. "Expériences sur le principe de la vie, notamment sur celui des mouvements du cœur, et sur le siége de ce principe." In *Encyclopédie des sciences médicales*, edited by Alibert et al., 215–327. Division 1, vol. 4. Paris: Bureau de l'Encyclopédie, 1835.

Légouvé. "La sépulture." *Gazette nationale ou le moniteur universel*, no. 42 (November 2, 1796): 166.

Legrand du Saulle, Henri. *La folie devant les tribunaux*. Paris: F. Savy, 1864.

Lenormand, Léonce. *Des inhumations précipités*. Mâcon: D. Ceville, 1843.

Léonard, Jacques. "Femmes, religion et médecine: les religieuses qui soignent." In *Annales économies sociétés civilisations* 32, no. 5 (September/October 1977): 887–907.

———. *La France médicale: médecins et malades au XIXe siècle*. Paris: Gallimard, 1978.

———. *La médecine entre les savoirs et les pouvoirs: Histoire intellectuelle et politique de la médecine française au XIXe siècle*. Paris: Aubier Montaigne, 1981.

Léonard, Jacques, Roger Darquenne, and Louis Bergeron. "Médecins et notables sous le consulat et l'empire." *Annales économies sociétés civilisations* 32, no. 5 (September/October 1977): 887–907.

Leroux, Jules. "Préface." In Pierre-Henri Leroux. *Malthus et les économistes, ou y aura-t-il toiujours des pauvres*. Vol. 1. Paris: Librairie de la Bibliothèque nationale, 1897.

Leroux, Pierre-Henri. *Aux états de Jersey, sur un moyen de quintupler, pour ne pas dire plus, la production agricole du pays, par Pierre Leroux*. London: Universal Library, 1853.

———. *Malthus et les économistes, ou y aura-t-il toiujours des pauvres*. 2 vols. Paris: Librairie de la Bibliothèque nationale, 1897.

Levie, Françoise. *Etienne-Gaspard Robertson: La vie d'un fantasmagore*. Paris: Editions du Préambule, 1990.

Levinas, Emmanuel. *Totality and Infinity: An Essay on Exteriority*. Translated by Alphonso Lingis. Pittsburgh: Duquesne University Press, 1969.

Le Yaouanc, Moïse. *Nosographie de l'humanité balzacienne*. Paris: Librairie Maloine, 1959.

Lombroso, Cesare. *L'homme criminel, criminel-né, fou moral, épileptique: Etude anthropologique et médico-légale*. 2 vols. Translated by M. Bournet. Paris: F. Alcan, 1887.

Lorant, André. "Introduction." In Honoré de Balzac. *La cousine Bette*. Edited by André Lorant. Paris: GF Flammarion, 1977.

Loraux, Nicole. *The Invention of Athens: The Funeral Oration in the Classical City*. Trans. Alan Sheridan. Cambridge, Mass.: Harvard University Press, 1986.

Lorrain, Jean. "Un étrange jongleur." *L'écho de Paris*. April 10, 1894.

Louis, Antoine. *Lettres sur la certitude des signes de la mort, où l'on rassure les citoyens de la crainte d'être enterrés vivans avec des observations et des expériences sur les noyés*. Paris: M. Lambert, 1752.

Lucey, Michael. *The Misfit of the Family: Balzac and the Social Forms of Sexuality*. Durham: Duke University Press, 2003.

Lucy, Marth. "The Evolutionary Body." PhD Diss. New York University, 2004.

Lukács, Georg. *Studies in European Realism: A Sociological Survey of the Writings of Balzac, Stendhal, Zola, Tolstoy, Gorki, and Others*. Translated by Edith Bone. 1950; London: Merlin Press, 1978.

Lunier, Ludger. "Examen médico-légal d'un cas de monomanie instinctif. Affaire du sergent Bertrand." *Annales médico-psychologiques* 1 (1849): 351–79.

Malthus, Thomas Robert. *An Essay on the Principle of Population, as it Affects the Future Improvement of Society with Remarks on the Speculations of Mr. Godwin, M. Condorcet, and Other Writers*. London: J. Johnson, 1798.

Manning, Stephen. "'I Sing of a Myden.'" *PMLA* 75 (1960): 8–12.

Marchant, F.-M. *Le conducteur de l'étranger à Paris*. Paris: Moronval, 1811.

Marder, Elissa. *Dead Time: Temporal Disorders in the Wake of Modernity (Baudelaire and Flaubert)*. Stanford, Calif.: Stanford University Press, 2001.

Maret, Jean-Philibert. *Mémoire sur l'usage où l'on est d'enterrer les morts dans les églises et dans l'enceinte des villes*. Dijon: Cause, 1773.

Martin, Didier, and Sylviane Martin. "Parcours sanitaire du code civil." In *Etudes de droit et d'économie de la santé*, edited by Didier Truchet, 17–25. Paris: Economica, 1982.

Marx, Karl and Frederick Engels. *Collected Works*. 47 vols. Edited by James S. Allen et al. New York: International Publishers, 1975–1995.

Matlock, Jann. "Ghostly Politics." *Diacritics* 30, no. 3 (Fall 2000): 53–71.

———. "The Invisible Woman and Her Secrets Unveiled." *Yale Journal of Criticism* 9, no. 2 (1996): 175–221.

———. "Reading Invisibility." In *Field Work: Sites in Literary and Cultural Studies*, edited by Marjorie Garber, Paul B. Franklin, and Rebecca L. Walkowitz, 183–95. New York: Routledge, 1996.

———. *Scenes of Seduction: Prostitution, Hysteria, and Reading Difference in Nineteenth-Century France*. New York: Columbia University Press, 1994.

———. "Voir aux limites du corps: Fantasmagories et femmes invisibles dans les spectacles de Robertson." In *Lanternes magiques, tableaux transparents*, edited by Ségolène Le Men et al., 85–99. Paris: Réunion des Musées nationaux, 1995.

Maulitz, Russel C. *Morbid Appearances: The Anatomy of Pathology in the Early Nineteenth Century*. Cambridge: Cambridge University Press, 1987.

Maza, Sara C. *The Myth of the French Bourgeoisie: An Essay on the Social Imaginary 1750–1850.* Cambridge, Mass.: Harvard University Press, 2003.

Mellerio, André. "Les artistes à l'atelier: Odilon Redon." *L'art dans les deux mondes.* July 4, 1891.

———. *Odilon Redon, peintre, dessinateur et graveur.* Paris: H. Floury, 1923.

———. *Odilon Redon.* 1913. Reprint, New York: Da Capo Press, 1968.

———. "Odilon Redon." In *Exposition Odilon Redon.* Exhibition catalogue. Galeries Durand-Ruel, Paris, 1894.

"Mémoire des curés de Paris à l'occasion des arrêts du 12 mars 1763, 21 mai, 23 septembre 1765 sur le déplacement des cimetières." Bibliothèque Nationale de France. Fonds Joly de Fleury, 1207, fol. 18.

Mercier, Louis-Sébastien. *Tableau de Paris.* 12 vols. Amsterdam [i.e. in France]: n.p., 1783–88.

Michéa, Claude-François. "Des déviations maladives de l'appétit vénérien." *L'union médicale* 3, no. 85 (July 17, 1849): 338a–339c.

Michelet, Jules. *Histoire de la révolution.* 2 vols. Edited by Gérard Walter. Paris: Gallimard (Pléiade), 1952.

———. *Œuvres complètes.* 16 vols. Edited by Paul Viallaneix. Paris: Flammarion, 1974.

Milanesi, Claudio. *Mort apparente, mort imparfaite: Médecine et mentalités au XVIIIe siècle.* Paris: Payot, 1991.

Miller, D. A. *The Novel and the Police.* Berkeley: University of California Press, 1988.

Milner, Max. *La fantasmagorie: Essai sur l'optique fantastique.* Paris: Presses Universitaires de France, 1982.

Ministère de l'Intérieur et des Cultes. *Législation concernant les aliénés et les enfants assistés.* 3 vols. Paris: Berger-Levrault, 1880.

Mirbeau, Octave. *Torture Garden.* Translated by Michael Richardson. Sawtry: Dedalus, 1995.

Mireur, Hippolyte. *La prostitution à Marseille: Histoire, administration et police, hygiène.* Paris: E. Dentu, 1882.

———. *La syphilis et la prostitution dans leurs rapports avec l'hygiène, la morale et la loi.* Paris: Masson, 1888.

M. L. N**. *L'hygiène, ou l'art de conserver la santé.* Chatillon-sur-Seine: C. Cornillac, 1840.

Mora, George. "Cabanis, Neurology and Psychiatry." In Pierre-Jean-George Cabanis. *On the Relations Between the Physical and Moral Aspects of Man,* xlv–xc.

Moravia, Sergio. "Cabanis and His Contemporaries." Translated by George Mora. In Pierre-Jean-George Cabanis. *On the Relations Between the Physical and Moral Aspects of Man,* vii–xliv.

Moreau, François-Marc. *Histoire statistique du choléra-morbus dans le quartier du faubourg Saint-Denis (5e arrondissement), pendant les mois d'avril, mai, juin, juillet, août et septembre.* Paris: Chez l'auteur, 1833.

Morel, Bénédicte-Auguste. "Considérations médico-légales sur un imbécile érotique convaincu de profanation de cadavres, par le docteur Morel, médecin en chef de l'asile de Saint-Yon. A M. le docteur Bédor, médecin de l'hospice civil à Troyes, membre correspondant de l'Académie impériale de médecine, médecin du dépôt provisoire d'aliénés de l'Hôtel-Dieu de Troyes, etc. Première lettre." *Gazette hébdomadaire de médecine: Bulletin de l'enseignement médical* 4, no. 8 (February 20, 1857): 123–25.

———. "Considérations médico-légales . . . Deuxième lettre." *Gazette hébdomadaire de médecine et de chirurgie: Bulletin de l'enseignement médical* 4, no. 11 (March 13, 1857): 185–87.

———. "Considérations médico-légales . . . Troisième lettre (*Deuxième partie*)." *Gazette hébdomadaire de médecine: Bulletin de l'enseignement medical*, 4, no. 8 (February 20, 1857): 197–200.

———. *Traité des maladies mentales*. Paris: Victor Masson, 1860.

Mutigny, Jean de. *Victor Hugo et le spiritisme*. Paris: Fernand Nathan, 1981.

Nasio, J.-D. *Le fantasme: Le plaisir de lire Lacan*. Paris: Payot, 1992.

Navet, Georges. *Pierre Leroux, politique, socialisme et philosophie*. Paris: Publications de la Société P.-J. Proudhon, 1994.

Pajot, Dr. [Charles?]. "A Monsieur le rédacteur en chef." *Gazette hébdomadaire de médecine* 4, no. 8 (February 20, 1857): 200.

Parent-Duchâtelet, Alexandre-Jean-Baptiste. *De la prostitution dans la ville de Paris considérée sous le rapport de l'hygiène publique, de la morale et de l'administration*. 2 vols. 1836. Paris: J.-B. Baillière, 1837.

———. *La prostitution à Paris au XIXe siècle*. Edited by Alain Corbin. Paris: Seuil, 1981.

Pasteur, Louis. *Correspondance de Pasteur 1840–1895*. Edited by Pasteur Vallery-Radot. 4 vols. Paris: Flammarion, 1951.

Pellieux, Augustin. "Observations sur les gaz méphitiques des caveaux mortuaires des cimetières de Paris." *Annales d'hygiène publique* 41 (January 1849): 127–40.

Peillon, Vincent. *Pierre Leroux et le socialisme républicain*. Latresne: Le Bord de l'eau, 2003.

Pérouse de Montclos, Jean-Marie. *Etienne-Louis Boullée*. Paris: Flammarion, 1994.

Petrucci, Armando. *Writing the Dead: Death and Writing Strategies in the Western Tradition*. Translated by Michael Sullivan. Stanford, Calif.: Stanford University Press, 1998.

Piattoli, Scipione. *Essai sur les lieux et les dangers des sépultures*. Translated by Félix Vicq d'Azyr. Paris: P. Fr. Didot, Libraire de la Société Royale de Médecine, 1778.

Pichot, André. "Présentation." In *Recherches physiologiques sur la vie et la mort (première partie) et autres texts* by Xavier Bichat, edited by André Pichot, 7–52. Paris: GF-Flammarion, 1994.

Piis, le citoyen. "La pâque naturelle: hymne à l'usage des philosophes." *Gazette nationale ou le moniteur universel*, no. 190 (March 30, 1796): 757–58.

Pike, David L. "Medical Mapping: the Thames, the Body and Our Mutual Friend." In *Filth: Dirt, Disgust, and Modern Life*, edited by William A. Cohen and Ryan Johnson, 51–77. Minneapolis: University of Minnesota Press, 2005.

Pinard, M. *Le cimetière du sud (Montparnasse)*. Paris: Retaux Frères, 1866.

Pinel, Philippe. "Résultats d'observations pour servir de base aux rapports juridiques dans les cas d'aliénation mentale." In *Mémoires de la Société médicale d'émulation de Paris*. Vol. 8. N.p.: n.p., 1817.

Plato. *Collected Dialogues Including the Letters*. Edited by Edith Hamilton and Huntington Cairns. Princeton: Princeton University Press, 1963.

Poe, Edgar Allan. *Poetry and Tales*. Edited by Patrik F. Quinn. New York: Library of America, 1984.

Pontmartin, A. de. "Semaines littéraires." *La gazette de France*, June 11, 1865.

Porée, Charles Gabriel. *Lettres sur la sépulture dans les églises. A Monsieur de C . . . . . .* Caen: Jean-Claude Pyron, 1745.

Proust, Marcel. *Jean Santeuil*. Edited by Pierre Clarac and Yves Sandre. Paris: Gallimard (Pléiade), 1971.

Pyle, Andrew, ed. *Population: Contemporary Responses to Thomas Malthus*. Bristol: Thoemmes Press, 1994.

Rabreau, Daniel. *Claude-Nicolas Ledoux (1736–1806). L'architecture et les fastes du temps*. Paris: Centre Ledoux, Université de Paris-I Panthéon-Sorbonne, 2000.

Raimond, Jean. "Feuilleton." *L'union médicale: Journal des intérêts scientifiques et pratiques, moraux et professionnels du corps medical*, 3, no. 92 (August 2, 1849): 365–66.

Ramsey, Mathew. "Le médecin, le peuple, l'état: la question du monopole professionnel." In *La médecine des lumières: Tout autour de Tissot*, edited by Vincent Barras and Micheline Louis-Courvoisier, 27–40. Geneva: Georg, 2001.

———. "The Popularization of Medicine in France, 1650–1900." In *The Popularization of Medicine 1650–1850*, edited by Roy Porter, 97–133. London: Routeledge, 1992.

———. "Property Rights and the Right to health: The Regulation of Secret Remedies in France, 1789–1815." In *Medical Fringe & Medical Orthodoxy 1750–1850*, edited by W. F. Bynum and Roy Porter, 79–105. London: Croom Helm, 1987.

Redon, Odilon. *A soi-même: journal 1867–1915: Notes sur la vie, l'air et les artistes*. Paris: José Corti, 1961.

———. *A Edgar Poe*. Paris: G. Fischbacher, 1882.

Regnault, Elias. *Du degré de compétence des médecins dans les questions judiciaires relatives aux aliénations mentales, et des théories physiologiques sur la monomanie*. Paris: R. Warée fils ainé, 1828.

Reid, Donald. *Paris Sewers and Sewermen: Realities and Representations*. Cambridge, Mass.: Harvard University Press, 1991.

Richardson, Ruth. *Death, Dissection and the Destitute*. Chicago: University of Chicago Press, 2000.

Rivail, Hippolyte (pseud. Allan Kardec). *Le livre des esprits*. 1857. Paris: Didier et Cie., 1867.

Robertson, Etienne-Gaspard. *Mémoires récréatifs, scientifiques et anecdotiques d'un physicien-aéronaute. I. La fantasmagorie. 1831–1833*. Langres: Café, Clima, 1985.

Robespierre, Maximilien. *Œuvres de Maximilien Robespierre*. 10 vols. Edited by Marc Bouloiseau and Albert Soboul. Paris: Presses Universitaires de France, 1967.

———. *Pour le bonheur et pour la liberté: Discours*. Edited by Yannick Bosc, Florence Gauthier, and Sophie Wahnich. Paris: La Fabrique, 2000.

Robiano de Borsbeek, Louis François de Paule-Marie-Joseph de. *De la violation des cimetières*. Louvain: Vanlinthout et Vandenzanden, 1824.

Rodenbach, Georges. *Bruges-la-morte*. Translated by Philip Mosley. Scranton, Penn.: University of Scranton Press, 2007.

Romanes, George J. *Animal Intelligence*. London: Kegan Paul, Trench, & Co., 1882.

Ronesse, Jacques-Hippolyte. *Vues sur la propreté de Paris*. N.p.: n.p., 1782.

Rosario, Vernon A. *The Erotic Imagination: French Histories of Perversity*. Oxford: Oxford University Press, 1997.

Rose, Gillian. *Mourning Becomes the Law: Philosophy and Representation*. Cambridge: Cambridge University Press, 1996.

Rousseau, Jean-Jacques. *Discourse on the Origins of Inequality*. In *Discourse on the Origins of Inequality (Second Discourse), Polemics, and Political Economy*. In *The Collected Writings of Rousseau*. Vol. 3. Edited by Roger D. Masters and Christopher Kelly. Translated by Judith R. Bush et al. Hanover, New Hampshire: University Press of New England, 1992.

———. *Social Contract, Discourse on the Virtue Most Necessary for a Hero, Political Fragments, and Geneva Manuscript*. In *The Collected Writings of Rousseau*. Vol. 4. Edited by Roger D. Masters and Christopher Kelly. Translated by Judith R. Bush, et al. Hanover, New Hampshire: University Press of New England, 1994.

Royer-Collard, Hippolyte-Louis. *Cours d'hygiène professé à la Faculté de médecine*. Paris: Lacrampe, 1846.

S. . . . , Dr. "Hôpital militaire du Val-de-Grâce. Service de M. Baudens. Coup de feu compliqué chez un sous-officier du 74e de ligne, soupçonné d'être l'auteur de la profanation commise au cimetière Mont-Parnasse." *La lancette française: Gazette des hôpitaux civils et militaires*. 3rd series, vol. 1, no. 36 (March 27, 1849): 144.

Saint-Just, Louis-Antoine-Léon. *Discours et rapports*. Edited by Albert Soboul. Paris: Editions Sociales, 1957.

Salomon-Bayet, Claire, ed. *Pasteur et la révolution pastorienne*. Paris: Payot, 1986.

Samuels, Maurice. *The Spectacular Past: Popular History and the Novel in Nineteenth-Century France*. Ithaca: Cornell University Press, 2004.

Sandström, Sven. *Le monde imaginaire d'Odilon Redon: Etude iconologique.* Lund: n.p., 1955.

"Le Sergent Bertrand." *Le siècle* 14, no. 181 (July 11, 1849): 4–5.

Sartre, Jean-Paul. *Being and Nothingness: An Essay on Phenomenological Ontology.* Translated by Hazel E. Barnes. New York: Philosophical Library, 1956.

Schotsman, H. D. "Clavaud, sa vie, son œuvre." *Bulletin du Centre de Recherches Scientifiques de Biarritz* 8, no. 4 (May 2, 1881): 335–36

Schwartz, Vanessa R. *Spectacular Realities: Early Mass Culture in* Fin-de-Siècle *Paris.* Berkeley: University of California Press, 1998.

Scotti, Angelo Antonio. *Le médecin chrétien, ou Médecine et religion.* Translated by Bernardin Gassiat. Paris: V. Palmé, 1881.

Seignobos, Charles. *Histoire de la France contemporaine depuis la révolution jusqu'à la paix de 1919.* Vol. 6. Edited by Ernest Lavisse. Paris: Hachette, 1921.

Shapin, Steven. *Never Pure: Historical Studies of Science as if It Was Produced by People with Bodies, Situated in Time, Space, Culture, and Society, and Struggling for Credibility and Authority.* Baltimore: Johns Hopkins University Press, 2010.

Sigmann, Jean. *1848: The Romantic and Democratic Revolutions in Europe.* Translated by Lovette F. Edwards. New York: Harper & Row, 1973.

Sournia, Jean-Charles. *La médecine révolutionnaire 1789–1799.* Paris: Payot, 1989.

Stallybrass, Peter, and Allon White. *The Politics and Poetics of Transgression.* Ithaca, N.Y.: Cornell University Press, 1986.

Starkie, Enid. *Petrus Borel the Lycanthrope: His Life and Times.* London: Faber and Faber, 1954.

Stearns, Peter N. *1848: The Revolutionary Tide in Europe.* New York: W. W. Norton, 1974.

Strauss, Jonathan. "After Death." *Diacritics* 30, no. 3 (Fall 2000): 90–104.

———. "Antigone et l'état cadavérique." In *Lire, écrire la honte,* edited by Bruno Chaouat, 185–206. Lyon: Presses Universitaires de Lyon, 2007.

———. "Political Force and the Grounds of Identity From Rousseau to Flaubert." *MLN* 117, no. 4 (September 2002): 808–35.

———. "Preface." *Diacritics* 30, no. 3 (Fall 2000): 3–11.

———. *Subjects of Terror: Nerval, Hegel, and the Modern Self.* Stanford, Calif.: Stanford University Press, 1998.

Sue, Eugène. *Les Mystères de Paris.* Edited by Francis Lacassin. Paris: Robert Laffont (Bouquins), 1989.

Sue, Jean Joseph. *Recherches physiologiques et expériences sur la vitalité. Lues à l'Institut national de France, le 11 messidor, an V de la république. Suivies d'une nouvelle édition de son Opinion sur le supplice de la guillotine ou sur la douleur qui survit à la décolation.* Paris: chez l'auteur, an VI (1797).

Swenson, James. *On Jean-Jacques Rousseau Considered as One of the First Authors of the Revolution.* Stanford, Calif.: Stanford University Press, 2000.

Swift, David L. "Priestley and Lavoisier: Oxygen and Carbon Dioxide." In *A History of Breathing Physiology*, edited by Donald F. Proctor, 223–38. New York: M. Dekker, 1995.

Sydenham, Thomas. *The Works of Thomas Sydenham, M.D.* Vol. 1. Translated by R. G. Latham. London: Sydenham Society, 1848.

Taine, Hippolyte. *Essais de critique et d'histoire.* Paris: Hachette, 1858.

Tardieu, Ambroise. *Etude médico-légale sur les attentats aux mœurs.* Paris: J.-B. Baillière et Fils, 1878.

———. "Traité des signes de la mort d'Eugène Bouchut." *Annales d'hygiène publique et de médecine légale* 41 (January 1849): 474.

———. *Voiries et cimetières: Thèse présentée au concours pour la chaire d'hygiène à la faculté de médecine de Paris, et soutenue le 1er mars 1852.* Paris: J.-B. Baillière, 1852.

Thierry de Faletans, Hippolyte de. *Fables et contes: Essais.* Paris: Lemercier et Cie., 1871.

Thoré, Théophile. *Le salon de 1847 précédé d'une lettre à Firmin Barrion.* Paris: Alliance des Arts, 1847.

Thouret, Jacques-Guillaume. *Rapport sur les exhumations du cimetière et de l'église des Saints-Innocents; Lu dans la séance de la Société Royale de Médecine, tenue au Louvre le 3 mars 1789.* Paris: Ph.-Denys Pierres, 1789.

Tillie, Jules. *Manuel de médecine à l'usage du clergé paroissial, suivi des soins à donner dans les cas urgents.* Saint-Omer: H. d'Homont, 1891.

Tocqueville, Alexis de. *Œuvres.* 3 vols. Edited by François Furet and Françoise Mélonio. Paris: Gallimard (Pléiade), 2004.

Trélat, Emile. "Rapport de M. Emile Trélat sur l'évacuation des vidanges par la voie publique." In *De l'évacuation des vidanges dans la ville de Paris*, edited by Emile Trélat, A. Hudelo, and Henri Gueneau de Mussy, 17–126. Paris: G. Masson, 1882.

Trouilleux, Rodolphe, and Jean-Michel Roy. "Préface." In *Le médecin radoteur ou les pots pourris et autres textes* by Robert Ducreux, edited by Rodolphe Trouilleux et Jean-Michel Roy, 13–69. Paris: Honoré Champion, 1999.

Truchet, Didier. "L'autorité juridique des principes d'exercice de la médecine." In *Etudes de droit et d'économie de la santé*, edited by Didier Truchet, 43–54. Paris: Economica, 1982.

Usk, Thomas. *The Testament of Love.* Edited by R. Allen Shoaf. Kalamazoo, Michigan: Medieval Institute Publications, 1998.

Valabrega, Jean-Paul. *Phantasme, mythe, corps et sens: Une théorie psychanalytique de la connaissance.* 1980. Reprint, Paris: Payot, 1992.

Vallery-Radot, Pierre. *Chirurgiens d'autrefois: la famille d'Eugène Süe.* Paris: R.-G. Ricou & Ocia Editeurs, 1944.

Van Zuylen, Marina. *Monomania: The Flight from Everyday Life in Literature and Art.* Ithaca, N.Y.: Cornell University Press, 2005.

Works Cited 381

———. "The Secret Life of Monsters." In *Beyond the Visible: The Art of Odilon Redon*, edited by Jodi Hauptman, 57–73. New York: Museum of Modern Art, New York, 2005.

Verdier, Jean. *La jurisprudence de la médecine en France, ou traité historique et juridique des établissements, reglemens, police, devoirs, fonctions, honneurs, droits & privileges des trois corps de médecine; avec les devoirs, fonctions & autorité des juges à leur égard.* 2 vols. Paris: Malassis le jeune, 1762.

Vicq d'Azyr, Félix. "Discours préliminaire." In Scipione Piattoli. *Essai sur les lieux et les dangers des sépultures.* Translated by Félix Vicq-d'Azyr, i–cxlvii. Paris: P. Fr. Didot, Libraire de la Société Royale de Médecine, 1778.

Vicq d'Azyr, Félix, and Jacques-Louis Moreau (de la Sarthe). *Médecine.* 13 vols. Paris: Panckoucke, 1787–1830.

Vidler, Anthony. *Claude-Nicolas Ledoux: Architectural Reform at the End of the Ancien Régime.* Cambridge, Mass.: MIT University Press, 1990.

Vigarello, Georges. *Concepts of Cleanliness: Changing Attitudes in France since the Middle Ages.* Translated by Jean Birrell. Cambridge: Cambridge University Press, 1988.

Vigier, Philippe. *La vie quotidienne en province et à Paris pendant les journées de 1848: 1847–1851.* Paris: Hachette, 1982.

Vila, Anne C. *Enlightenment and Pathology: Sensibility in the Literature and Medicine of Eighteenth-Century France.* Baltimore: Johns Hopkins University Press, 1998.

Villemin, Jean-Antoine. *Du rôle de la lésion organique dans les maladies.* Strasbourg: Vve Berger-Levrault, 1862.

———. *Du tubercule au point de vue de son siége, de son évolution et de sa nature.* Paris: J.-B. Baillière et fils, 1861.

Viola, Jerome. "Redon, Darwin and the Ascent of Man." *Marsyas* 11 (1962–64): 42–57.

Vitani, Christiane. *Législation de la mort: Travail de l'association lyonnaise de médecine légale.* Paris: Masson & Cie., 1962.

Vona, Costantino. "La *Margarita Pretiosa* nella interpretazione di alcuni scrittori ecclesiastici." *Divinitas* 1 (1957): 118–60.

Vovelle, Robert. *La mort et l'Occident de 1300 à nos jours. Précédé de: La mort, état des lieux.* 1983. Reprint, Paris: Gallimard, 2000.

Walzer, Michael. *Régicide et révolution: Le procès de Louis XVI.* Translated by J. Debouzy. Paris: Payot, 1989.

Weber, Caroline. *Terror and Its Discontents: Suspect Words In Revolutionary France.* Minneapolis and London: University of Minnesota Press, 2003.

Weiner, Dora B. *The Citizen-Patient in Revolutionary and Imperial Paris.* Baltimore: Johns Hopkins University Press, 1993.

———. *Comprendre et soigner: Philippe Pinel (1745–1826) La médecine de l'esprit.* Paris: Fayard, 1999.

Weisz, George. *Divide and Conquer: A Comparative History of Medical Specialization.* Oxford: Oxford University Press, 2006.

———. *The Medical Mandarins: The French Academy of Medicine in the Nineteenth and Early Twentieth Centuries.* Oxford: Oxford University Press, 1995.

Winnock, Michel. *La France et les juifs de 1789 à nos jours.* Paris: Seuil, 2004.

Winslow, Jacob Benignus. *Dissertation sur l'incertitude des signes de la mort et l'abus des enterremens et embaumemens précipités.* Translated by Jacques-Jean Bruhier. Paris: C.-F. Simon, fils, 1742.

Zacchia, Paolo. *Quaestiones medico-legales.* Venice: M. D. Horstius, 1637.

Zola, Emile. *Nana.* Translated by George Holden. New York: Penguin, 1972.

———. *Œuvres complètes.* 10 vols. Edited by Henri Mitterand. Paris: Cercle du Livre Précieux, 1968.

———. *Thérèse Raquin.* London: William Heinemann, 1955.

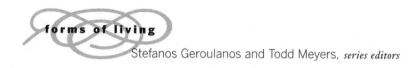

forms of living

Stefanos Geroulanos and Todd Meyers, *series editors*

Georges Canguilhem, *Knowledge of Life*. Translated by Stefanos Geroulanos
  and Daniela Ginsburg, Introduction by Paola Marrati and Todd Meyers
Henri Atlan, *Selected Writings: On Self-Organization, Philosophy, Bioethics, and
  Judaism*. Edited and with an Introduction by Stefanos Geroulanos and
  Todd Meyers
Georges Canguilhem, *Writings on Medicine*. Translated and with an
  Introduction by Stefanos Geroulanos and Todd Meyers
Jonathan Strauss, *Human Remains: Medicine, Death, and Desire in Nineteenth-
  Century Paris*